NAMASTE
HUMANISM IN CHILD NEUROLOGY

DAVID L COULTER MD
ALCY TORRES MD

NAMASTE

HUMANISM IN CHILD NEUROLOGY

Project Manager: Relfa Proano, MD

The authors would like to thank Relfa Proano, MD for her assistance with the Spanish translation and her assistance with the manuscript preparation and Nancy Gardella for various suggestions and grammatical corrections.

First published in this edition 2021

ISBN: 978-1-915147-01-1 (Ebook)
ISBN: 978-1-915147-00-4 (Paperback)

Project Manager: Relfa Proano
Managing Editor: Biju Hameed

NAMASTE

HUMANISM IN CHILD NEUROLOGY

Edited by

David L. Coulter,MD
Harvard University; Boston Children Hospital,
Boston, MA, USA

Alcy R. Torres,MD
Boston University; Boston Medical Center,
Boston, MA, USA

2021

INTERNATIONAL CHILD NEUROLOGY ASSOCIATION

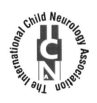

Contents

PART 1
REGIONAL PERSPECTIVE

PART 2
RELIGIOUS PERSPECTIVE ABOUT HUMANISM IN CHILD NEUROLOGY

PART 3
HUMANISM IN CLINICAL PRACTICE

PART 4
GLOBAL HUMANISTIC STORIES IN CHILD NEUROLOGY

DEDICATORY

To our patient, the source of the inspiration and to our families for the selfless support.

LIST OF CONTRIBUTORS

Alcy Torres Catefort, MD
Past President of the Ecuadorian Pediatric Society
Past Ecuadorian Representative of the Latin American
Pediatric Association (ALAPE)
Past President of the VI Course and II Congress of the
Iberoamerican Academy of Pediatric Neurology (AINP) 1994
Professor of Pediatrics, Universidad Central del Ecuador
Carlos Andrade Marin Hospital
Quito, Ecuador

Alcy R. Torres, MD, FAAP
Associate Professor of Pediatrics and Neurology
Assistant Dean of Diversity and Inclusion
Director of the Pediatric Traumatic Injury, International and
Bilingual Programs
Boston University School of Medicine
Boston Medical Center
Boston, MA, USA

Candace Cole-McCrea Ph.D
Professor Emeritus, Great Bay Community College
Portsmouth, NH, USA

Caley Mikesell, BPH
School of Medicine, Universidad San Francisco de Quito
Quito, Ecuador

Charles K. Hammond, MD
Department of Child Health, School of Medicine and
Dentistry
Kwame Nkrumah University of Science and Technology
Kumasi, Ghana

David L. Coulter, MD
Associate Professor of Neurology at Harvard Medical School
Senior Associate at Boston Children's Hospital
Boston Children's Hospital
Boston, MA, USA

Daniel San Juan Orta, MD, MSc, FACNS
President of Mexican Chapter International League Against
Epilepsy
Consultant in the Epilepsy Clinic at the National Institute of
Neurology
and Neurosurgery (NINN),
Associate Professor of the Fellowships of Epilepsy Surgery
and Clinical
Neurophysiology ,Sub-specialty, at NINN
Mexico City, Mexico

Dídac Casas-Alba, MD
Master in Pediatric Neurology
Neuropediatric Department
Hospital Sant Joan de Déu (University of Barcelona)
Barcelona, Spain

Edgard Andrade, MD, MS, FAAP
Pediatric Neurologist and Epileptologist
Institute of Pediatric Neurosciences
Ocala, FL, USA

Efraín Olivas Peña, MD
Physician assigned to the Department of Neurosciences
National Institute of Perinatology
Associate Professor in the subspecialty of Neonatology
National Institute of Perinatology
Autonomous University of Mexico
Mexico City, Mexico

Edward Kija, MD
Department of Pediatrics and Child Health
Muhimbili University of Health and Allied Sciences
Dar Es Salaam, Tanzania

Felipe Roman Larrea
Doctor in Spiritual Theology (2021), Pontifica University of
the Holy Cross
Rome, Italy

Forrest P. Beaulieu, MD
PL-1, Pediatrics/Child Neurology
Children's Hospital of Philadelphia
Philadelphia, PA, USA

Ghada Ahmed Saad Elhawary, MBBch
Pediatrics department, Faculty of Medicine, Ain Shams
University, Cairo, Egypt
Faculty of Medicine, Ain Shams University
Cairo, Egypt

Gladys Guerrero de Torres
Past President of the Committee of Pediatrics Ladies
Quito,Ecuador

Grace Akello, PhD
Medical Anthropologist and Associate Professor
Coordinator of Master of Medical Anthropology Program
Gulu University Faculty of Medicine

P. O. Box 166
Gulu, Uganda

Hari Conjeevaram, MD, MSc, FACP, FACG
Program Director, GI Fellowship Program
Medical Director, Student Run Free Clinic
Professor of Medicine Division of Gastroenterology
and Hepatology
University of Michigan
Ann Arbor, MI, USA

Hector Jose Castaneda, MD
Director Instituto de Neurociencias, El Salvador
Medical Director, Hospital Diagnostico, San Salvador, El
Salvador
Medical Director, Free Sai Clinic
San Salvador, El Salvador

Jaume Campistol MD, PhD
Professor of Pediatrics, Barcelona University
Director of the Master in Pediatric Neurology
Neuropediatric Department
Hospital Sant Joan de Déu (University of Barcelona)
Barcelona, Spain

Jaskaran Singh Lamba
Undergraduate student
Frederick S Pardee School of Global Studies
Boston University
Boston, MA, USA

Javeria Raza Alvi, Dr
Department of Pediatric Neurology
The Children's Hospital & Institute of Child Health
Fellow, Pediatric Neurology
Institute of Child Health, Children Hospital of Lahore
National Delegate, AOCNA

Secretary General, Pakistan Pediatric Association
Lahore, Pakistan

Jo M, Wilmshurst, MB BS, MD
Professor of Paediatric Neurology, Neuroscience Institute,
University of Cape Town
Head of Paediatric Neurology, Red Cross War Memorial
Children's Hospital
Director of the African Paediatric Fellowship Program
President of the International Child Neurology Association
(2018-2022)
Cape Town, South Africa

Joseph R. Deacon III, Ph.D., LP, BCBA-D
Retired, Supervising Psychologist/Director of Research
Pauls Valley State School, Pauls Valley, OK, USA
J. Iverson Riddle Developmental Center
Member of American Association on Intellectual and
Developmental Disabilities
Morganton, NC, USA

Joel Fernando Mendoza Cruz, MD
Pediatrician Neurologist
Head of the Neurology Service of the Morelia Children's
Hospital
Associate Professor of Neurology
Member of the Bioethics Committee of the Morelia Children's
Hospital
Founder of the School for Parents of the Morelia Children's
Hospital
Founding Member of the Mexican Society of Pediatric
Neurology
Founding Member of the Michoacan Neuroscience Society
ICNA member since 1985
Morelia,Mexico

Jorge Vidaurre MD, FACNS, FAES
Director, Pediatric Clinical Neurophysiology Program
Director, EEG laboratory
Associate Professor, Pediatric Neurology
Nationwide Children's Hospital – The Ohio State University
Columbus, OH, USA

Juan David Naranjo, MD
Pontificia Universidad Católica del Ecuador
Quito, Ecuador

J.M.F. Niermeijer, MD, PhD
Pediatric Neurologist
Department of Neurology
ETZ St Elisabeth Twee Steden Hospital
Tilburg, Netherlands

J. W. Gorter, MD
CanChild Centre for Childhood Disability Research, McMaster
University
Hamilton, ON, Canada
NetChild Network for Childhood Disability Research
Utrecht, Netherlands

K P Vinayan, MD, DNB,DM
Professor and Head
Department of Pediatric Neurology
Amrita Institute of Medical Sciences ,Amrita
University Cochin
Conver, Pediatric Neurology sub section, Indian Academy of
Neurology
Member, Commission for Diagnostic Methods, International
League Against Epilepsy (ILAE)
Member, Asian Epilepsy Academy (ASEPA)
Treasurer, Indian Epilepsy Society,Kerala, India

Kshitij Mankad MD, MRCP, FRCR, PG Dip Hospital &
Healthcare Mgmt.

Lean 6 Sigma (Black Belt)
Clinical Lead for Paediatric Neuroradiology & Associate
Professor
Great Ormond Street Hospital, University College London
Hospital
London, England

Leon G. Epstein, MD
Member and Past-Chair, CNS Ethics Committee
Northwestern University Feinberg School of Medicine
Ann & Robert H. Lurie Children's Hospital of Chicago
Chicago, IL, USA

Mae Chee Sansanee Sthirasuta Venerable
Founder of Sathira-Dhammasathan
Founder of Bodhisattva Valley (Sathira-Dhammasathan2),
Phetchaburi, Thailand
Co-Chair of Global Peace Initiative of Women
Bangkok, Thailand

Mandeep Rana, MD
Assistant Professor Pediatrics
Boston University School of Medicine
Boston Medical Center
Boston, MA, USA

Matthew P. Kirschen, MD PhD
Assistant Professor, Departments of Anesthesiology and
Critical Care Medicine
Neurology, and Pediatrics
Associate Director, Pediatric Neurocritical Care
Perelman School of Medicine at the University of
Pennsylvania
Attending Physician, Pediatric Critical Care Medicine
Children's Hospital of Philadelphia
Philadelphia,PA USA

Mario Tomas Rodríguez, MD
Consultant Physician in Child Neurology
Former Head of Pediatrics Service, and Teaching and Research
Hospital General de Agudos de Lanus
Director of Degree of University Specialist in Pediatrics
Children's Medicine Academic discipline Universidad Nacional de Buenos Aires
Full Member of the Argentine Society of Children's Neurology
Buenos Aires, Argentina

Margie A Ream, MD, PhD
Assistant Professor of Pediatrics, Division of Neurology
Nationwide Children's Hospital – The Ohio State University
Director of Nationwide Children's Hospital's Child Neurology Residency
Member of the Editorial board of the Journal of Child Neurology
Columbus, OH, USA

Mariette Debeij, MD
Pediatric neurologist at Kempenhaeghe
Academic Centre for Epileptology University of Maastricht
Heeze, Netherlands

Masanori Takeoka, MD, FAES
Department of Neurology ,Boston Children's Hospital
Harvard Medical School
Boston, MA, USA

Michelle Grunauer, MD, PhD
Professor and Dean, Critical Care, Ethics, Palliative Care
School of Medicine at Universidad San Francisco de Quito
Academic Director and Attending Physician, Critical Care and Palliative Care
Hospital de los Valles, Quito, Ecuador

Professor (by courtesy), Johns Hopkins Carey Business School
Adjunct Clinical Professor, Zucker School of Medicine, Hofstra/Northwell
Quito, Ecuador

Melissa Cowgill / Melissa Hinostroza Saenz, MD/MBBS
Ricardo Palma University
Lima, Peru

Milatz Marjon
Teacher and Ambulatory Educationalist at Educational Center of Expertise De Berkenschutse
A special Ambulatory Educationalist School Guidance service for children with epilepsy
Heeze, Netherlands

Michel N. Fayad, MD
Assistant Professor of Neurology
Harvard Medical School
Staff Neurologist, Boston Children's Hospital
Boston, MA, USA

Nicolas Garofalo Gomez, MD, PhD
Second Degree Specialist in Neurology
Associate Professor ,Neuro Pediatrics Service
Instituto de Neurologia y Neurocirugia de Cuba
Habana, Cuba

Nina A. Fainberg, MD
Fellow Physician, Pediatric Critical Care Medicine
Department of Anesthesiology and Critical Care Medicine
Children's Hospital of Philadelphia
Philadelphia,PA USA

Oscar Ignacio Doldán Pérez, MD
Intensive Care Pediatrician, La Costa Medical Center
Asunción, Paraguay

Ornella Ciccone, (SFMA) MD
Consultant Paediatric Neurologist ,Istituto Serafico, Assisi,
Italy
University Teaching Hospitals - Children's Hospital
Lusaka, Zambia

Phillip L Pearl, MD
President, CNS
Boston Children's Hospital and Harvard Medical School
Boston, MA, USA

Pedro Weisleder, MD, PhD
Professor of Pediatrics
Division of Neurology
Nationwide Children's Hospital – The Ohio State University
Director of Nationwide Children's Hospital's Center for
Pediatric Bioethics
Editor-in-Chief, Seminars in Pediatric Neurology
Columbus,OH,USA

Rabbi Sharon Clevenger
The Rashi School
Dedham, MA,USA

Rekha Mittal, MD
Additional Director (Pediatric Neurology)
Madhukar Rainbow Children's Hospital,
President, Association of Child Neurology (India)
New Delhi, India

Relfa Proano Ponce, MD
BostonMedical Center
BostonUniversity School of Medicine
Boston,MA, USA

Rinat Jonas, MD
Assistant Professor of Pediatrics and Neurology
Director, Child Neurology Residency Program

Director, Pediatric EEG
BostonMedical Center
Boston, MA, USA

Ronnie E. Baticulon, MD
Pediatric Neurosurgeon, Division of Neurosurgery,
Department of Neurosciences
Associate Professor of Anatomy, Philippine General Hospital
University of the Philippines Manila
Manila,Phillipines

Roxana Orbe, MD
Child and Adolescents Psychiatry Resident
Hospital General de Niños Pedro de Elizalde
Buenos Aires, Argentina

Rosana Huerta Albarrán, M.D., MSc
Representative of the Young Epilepsy Section (YES) of
Mexican Chapter International League Against Epilepsy
,Associate Professor of Pediatrics and Sleep Medicine
Coordinator of Research in Pediatrics Unit at General
Hospital of Mexico

Dr. Eduardo Liceaga
Staff Pediatric Neurologist at General Hospital of México Dr.
Eduardo Liceaga and Sleep Medicine Clinic of National
Autonomous University of Mexico
Mexico City, Mexico.

Sarah Hisham Hassan Wagdy, BA
Faculty of Al-Alsun Ain Shams University,
Cairo, Egypt.

Sahar Mohamed Ahmed Hassanein, MD, PhD
Pediatrics Department, Faculty of Medicine, Ain Shams
University Cairo, Egypt
Faculty of Medicine, Ain Shams University
Cairo, Egypt

Simone L. Ardern-Holmes, MBChB, PhD, FRACP
Senior Clinical Lecturer
University of Sydney Faculty of Medicine and Health
Staff Specialist Neurologist, The Children's Hospital at
Westmead
Westmead, NSW Australia

Shen Yan-Wen, MD, PhD
Pediatric Neurologist
Department of Pedeatric
The First Medical Center of PLA General Hospital
Beijing, China

Tipu Sultan,MD.
Department of Pediatric Neurology
The Children's Hospital & Institute of Child Health
Professor of Pediatric Neurology & Institute of Child Health
Children Hospital, Lahore
National Delegate ,AOCNA
Secretary General, Pakistan Pediatric Association
Lahore, Pakistan

Tirso Zúñiga Santamaría, MD., PhD
Neuro-genetic Department, at the National Institute of
Neurology and Neurosurgery (NINN), Mexico City, Mexico

Thasanporn Toemthong, DDS
Rajanukul Institute, Department of Mental Health, Ministry
of Public Health, Thailand
Recipient of a scholarship from Department of Foreign
Affairs and Trade, Australian
Government in Intellectual & Developmental Disabilities to
join 2016 IASSIDD World
Congress in Melbourne
Bangkok, Thailand

Thananchai Tejapañño Sugsai, BA
Phrakru Dhammarata, The Ecclesiastical Honorific Rank

Wat Nyanavesakavan, Teacher
Bachelor of Communication Arts, Bangkok University
Graduate Diploma of Tripitaka Studies,
Mahachulalongkornrajavidyalaya University
Dhamma Scholar, Advanced Level
Pali Scholar, Level 3
Bangkok, Thailand

Varnit Shanker, MD
MBBS, DCH (UK), MRCPCH
ALM Biology degree candidate, HES, Harvard University
Consultant, Department of Neonatal Neurocritical Care,
DACH
Jaipur, India

Vishal Sondhi, MD, DM
Associate Professor ,Department of Pediatrics
Armed Forces Medical College,
Pune, India

Victor Alejandro Gaona, MD
Neuropediatrician
President of the Ibero-American Academy of Pediatric
Neurology
Professor of Physiology, National University of Asuncion
Department of Pediatric Neurology and Neurophysiology
La Costa Medical Center
Asuncion, Paraguay

William D. Graf, MD
Chair, CNS Ethics Committee
Connecticut Children's and the University of Connecticut
Farmington, CT, USA

Wynne Morrison, MD MBE
Associate Professor, Department of Anesthesiology and
Critical Care Medicine
Perelman School of Medicine at the University of

Pennsylvania
Attending Physician, Pediatric Critical Care Medicine and
Palliative Care Medicine
Justin Michael Ingerman Endowed Chair in Palliative Care
Medicine
Children's Hospital of Philadelphia
Philadelphia, PA, USA

Yasmine Elhefnawy, MD
Pediatric Neurologist at Boston Medical Center
Boston University School of Medicine
Boston, MA, USA

Zakir I. Shaikh, MBBS
Resident Physician
Department of Neurology
UMass Medical School
Worcester, MA, USA

Zhao Liu, MD, PhD
Division Head, Pediatric Neurology
Department of Pediatrics
University of Illinois
Peoria, IL, USA

FOREWORD

So often in our busy schedules we, the medical profession, interface with the underlying etiology for a child's state rather than the actual child e.g. "the GBS patient," "the spasms child." Remembering and practicing humanism re-centres an approach to the individual and holistic needs of a child who is unfortunate in their course to suffer from various neurologic conditions. Through practicing humanism, we step outside the restraints of the environmental limitations that a child may be born into but rather focus on the specific and important needs of the individual child. Any child, regardless of where they reside in the world, should be entitled to access appropriate ("gold standard") care to allow them to reach their best state of well-being. This would be inclusive of health, nutrition, education as well as a safe and nurturing living environment.

The editors of this book, Drs. Coulter and Torres, are to be commended for reminding us of our duty and role as clinicians to always follow an approach as exemplified by the concept of humanism. The diverse representation of the contributors to this book permits both a global but also cross-sectional expertise insight. The spiritual and religious narratives enlighten us of the nuances of how child and caregiver interactions can be so much better with relatively simple but sensitive adjustments, as illustrated by the chapter "Tips for the Pediatric Neurologist taking care of Jewish patients." The pragmatic situational texts provide an invaluable resource to aid clinicians in their daily practice. The final section of the focused case stories provides a powerful close and further justify the need for humanism in our daily practice.

These are some important quotes from the text:

Grace Akello. Considerations for humanistic caregiving for neurological conditions in low and middle-income countries.

"In low- and middle-income countries, shifting to humanistic care for neurological conditions invites stakeholders to address availability of medicines, poor staffing, and dysfunctional health systems in tandem with deep-rooted social and cultural beliefs."

Sahar Mohamed Ahmed Hassanein and colleagues. The way to humanism in Pediatric Neurology in Egypt

"A future use of the patients' stories to teach humanism in medical education, medical and non-medical. An empathetic smile on the face, listening to all parents' worries, reassurance, and mutual respect, are the key for humanism."

"Respect their dignity, respect other's rights, respect the parent's worries and always support them, provide your medical care with a smiling face and a reassuring voice, and care for every child as your own kid."

The North American section notes the region's focus on use of high-level technology, which is aimed at definitive cures. But the section highlights how practitioners must still respect the multiethnic, multicultural and multiracial composition of North American society. The reality is that this statement is valid for many regions of the world as technology and medical outcome expectations advance. As such, we need to consider our approach to our patients from our acceptance and openness to being questioned and always telling the truth, admitting when we are wrong or don't know, taking the time to listen, providing periods of silence in the doctor – care – patient space to allow for those unspoken thoughts or questions to come out. To permit the child to stop feeling like a patient but like a child who needs help achieving their life potential.

Victor Alejandro Gaona. Personal reflections on the doctor-patient relationship.

"Heal sometimes, often relieve, always console."

Alcy Torres Catefort. The Latin American perspective on humanism in child neurology.

"In Latin America, great care must be taken not to overwhelm the patient with information that is given to protect the physician from legal ramifications. The paternalistic figure of the omnipotent doctor has disappeared for one more committed to his people, where the patient and their family have more time to ask questions, to inform themselves, and make their own decisions. Young professionals must understand that the patient and their family are at the center of our actions, the reason for being for us, and our mission is not only treating the disease and alleviating pain but comforting and supporting until the end. "

Simone L Ardern-Holmes. Humanism in child neurology: an Australasian Oceania perspective

"...placing the patient at the center, promoting an understanding of the experience of health and wellbeing versus disease and illness, and determining goals and actions based on the values and needs of patients."

Humanism "is respectful and responsive to individual preferences, needs and values, helps to maintain patient dignity and a sense of security. Patient-center care ensures the appropriateness and effectiveness of interventions offered."

Any interface with a child and the family should be culturally sensitive and promotes gaining the trust of the patient. As such it is important to be aware of the basic obligations and taboos in various cultural, spiritual and religious settings to understand certain practices and to avoid inappropriate questions or requests.

Rinat Jonas. Judaism in Pediatric Neurology

"It is important that we as physicians will encourage our patients from diverse religious and cultural backgrounds to feel comfortable expressing their cultural health beliefs and practices. It is our duty to be familiar with and respectful of various traditional healing systems and beliefs and where appropriate, integrate these into treatment plans. When healthcare professionals give humanistic care, patients are more likely to adhere to their medical orders, which results in better health outcomes."

Jaskaran Singh Lamba and Mandeep Rana. Religious perspectives and humanism in child neurology—a Vedantic perspective

"Whether caring for a child on the autism spectrum disorder or a child with cerebral palsy or an intellectual disability, the physician will see the child as more than just an interesting patient or statistic, but as a human being with immense potential, regardless of their race, beliefs, or socioeconomic status. Seeing patients through the window of their beliefs also empowers and supports them."

The third section on humanism in clinical practice is a reality check for us all. From the insight into how to go about communicating with children and caregivers to suggested approaches as illustrated by the 'SPIKES algorithm to give bad news" in the "Pediatric palliative care for children with neurological disorders" chapter by Caley Mikesell and Michelle Grunauer.

When addressing the concept of humanism this extends beyond how we treat our patients and their families, but how we care for ourselves both within and beyond the working environment. If we cannot be kind to ourselves, we will never be able to provide or sustain effective care for others. The chapter on "Child neurologists between burnout and well-being" by Alcy R. Torres addresses this, highlighting how the recent COVID pandemic has exposed the extent of the problem.

The closing section on "Global humanistic stories in child neurology" provides a colorful, emotional rollercoaster through humanism across the world delving into clinician – care – child relationships. The 'F-words' in Childhood Disability: I Swear This is How We Should Think! by P. Rosenbaum and J. W. Gorter is a great section with important points to centre us. The "F-words" of child neurodisability are function, family, fitness, fun, friends and future. The authors state that this framework was compiled to be an appealing way for people to incorporate these concepts into every aspect of clinical service, research and advocacy regarding disabled children and their families. In reality, this whole text should be part of every clinician's practice aid list.

On behalf of the International Child Neurology Association it is an honor that the authors have agreed to this text being included in the ICNA's resources.

Jo Wilmshurst

President of the International Child Neurology Association (2018-202

PROLOGUE
GOALS, OBJECTIVES AND METHODOLOGY

Goals and Objectives

We started this project in 2018 with the goal of exploring the meaning of humanism in child neurology and neurodevelopmental disabilities in every nation, culture and religious tradition in the world. One editor (DLC) had just received the 2017 National Award for Humanism in Medicine from the United States Child Neurology Society and recognized the need for a more global perspective. The other editor (ART) shared similar interests; growing up and training outside the US gave him a dual view about humanism. We created the project together as a joint project between Boston University School of Medicine (ART) and Harvard Medical School (DLC). We named the project "Namaste," which is said to mean, "The divine in me recognizes the divine in you."

The goal of the Namaste project was to realize a global vision of humanism in child neurology and neurodevelopmental disabilities and to share that vision with our colleagues in every country in the world. Practicing child neurology with a humanistic perspective means treating patients and their families with respect. We understood that this could have a very different meaning in other cultural contexts. Thus, we proposed a global effort to learn what humanism in child neurology means in every culture, society and country all over the world. We did not have any preconceived notions about the global aspects of humanism in child neurology. We explicitly rejected any attempt to impose a particular world view (such as an American or European world view) and designed the project to welcome contributions from everyone all over the world. In a global and interconnected world, we hoped to bring all child neurologists together to share the meaning of humanism in every culture, society and country worldwide.

Our first objective was to recruit manuscripts from authors all over the globe who could describe what humanism means from their perspective. Our second objective was to appreciate through these manuscripts the challenges that child neurologists face when trying to bring humanism to their practices and to their lives, and to learn how these experiences affect patients and families. Our third objective was to share all of this information through the publication of this book. We are especially grateful for the continuing support of the International Child Neurology Association (ICNA) which has made all of this possible.

Methodology

We realized that the various perspectives on humanism in child neurology and neurodevelopmental disabilities could be approached from several distinct perspectives. First, we recruited writers who could address the diversity of geographical perspectives in every continent in the world. We also recognized that humanism can also have a religious or spiritual foundation, so we recruited writers who could address the diversity of spiritual perspectives in many of the major religious traditions. We have undoubtedly left out other voices, perhaps especially those who see humanism as secular. The point is that humanism can be either secular or not, so we need to understand and respect all perspectives.

Ultimately, as child neurologists, humanism is a clinical experience of relationships between us and our patients and their families. That is why we also recruited clinical perspectives in which writers explore a variety of clinical topics related to humanism in clinical practice. The chapters in this section are then reinforced by the chapters in the next section, personal stories, where writers share their own experiences of humanism. We are most human when we share our humanity with others, especially with our patients and their families. The stories in this section thereby tie it all together.

Limitations

Our goal was to provide a global perspective on humanism in child neurology and neurodevelopmental disabilities. We have had tremendous support from the International Child Neurology Association. We wanted to be as comprehensive, diverse, nonjudgmental and global as possible. But of course, we know that we have almost certainly left out some powerful worldwide voices. We hope that this book will be the starting point to initiate a global and respectful conversation about the importance of humanism in child neurology and neurodevelopmental disabilities. Our presentation at the joint meeting in 2020 of the International Child Neurology Association and the United States Child Neurology Society is titled, "Humanism: The Time Has Come!" But there is so much more work to be done. As editors, we submit this monograph with the hope that readers everywhere in the world will join us in creating a better and more humanistic world for our patients and their families.

David L. Coulter MD.
Associate Professor of Neurology at Harvard Medical School.
Senior Associate at Boston Children's Hospital.
Boston Children's Hospital.
Boston, Massachusetts

Alcy R. Torres, MD, FAAP
Associate Professor of Pediatrics and Neurology
Assistant Dean of Diversity and Inclusion
Director of the Pediatric Traumatic Injury, International and
Bilingual Programs
Boston University School of Medicine
Boston Medical Center
Boston, MA, USA

PART 1
REGIONAL PERSPECTIVE

1.AFRICA

THE AFRICAN PERSPECTIVE ON HUMANISM IN CHILD NEUROLOGY

Charles K. Hammond
Department of Child Health, School of Medicine and Dentistry, Kwame Nkrumah University of Science and Technology, Kumasi, Ghana

Edward Kija
Department of Pediatrics and Child Health, Muhimbili University of Health and Allied Sciences, Dar Es Salaam, Tanzania

INTRODUCTION

Humanism in medicine employs a respectful and compassionate relationship between physicians, members of a care team, and their patients, and emphasizes physician sensitivity to the values, autonomy and Humanistic of all patients and families (Khilanani, 2020). This model employs thoughts and actions in which human interest, values and dignity predominates and is essential in achieving both physician and patient satisfaction.

In Africa, the practice of medicine, and for that matter child neurology, is undergoing a humanistic revolution. However, the rising pressures related to civil wars and political unrest, famine, poverty, inaccessible healthcare, adoption of new technologies, brain drain, unreasonable restrictions on immigration, separation of children from their families, and the denial of science remain formidable distractions to sustaining humanism in medical practice.

The continent is home to many ethnic groups who have maintained their diverse cultural and traditional beliefs in their understanding of diseases and disabilities in children over many centuries. However, there is a gradual shift to a more modern approach in our knowledge, attitude and practices which places human interest, values and dignity in the center of medical practice rather than an approach that seeks to "please the gods" who were in previous times thought to be the sources of all disease.

In the past, the care seeking attitudes and behaviors of many ethnic groups were largely influenced by their cultural beliefs. There was the tendency to ascribe all misfortunes including disease and infirmities to supernatural forces. In this way, it was justified to seek a supernatural intervention. These beliefs in the supernatural were widespread in Africa and translated into many different practices in different parts of the continent based on the local traditional beliefs and ethnic practices.

For the family of a child with a neurological disorder, there were many unanswered questions and unresolved conflicts ranging from whether an ancestor had offended the gods in one way or the other to whether the disease is the result of a curse or punishment for any wrong committed by the parents. These beliefs drove the search for cure and resulted in many anti-humanism practices such as animal sacrifices and in extreme circumstances human sacrifices.

Despite the more recent introduction of western medical practices on the continent, the traditional beliefs, misconceptions and practices still dominate in many cultures. These are compounded by the limited resources and the wide treatment gap that exist for children with neurological disorders.

In this chapter, we throw some light on the traditional African beliefs and practices for children with neurological disorders and discuss our viewpoint on what the future presents with the gradual shift to a more humanism-centered approach, which seeks to employ science but does not entirely discard the traditional beliefs.

ANTIHUMANISM IN CHILD NEUROLOGY PRACTICE IN AFRICA

The practice of child neurology in Africa in the past was bedeviled with many anti-humanism challenges that bordered on traditional beliefs and superstitions, stigmatization, poorly equipped health infrastructure, lack of human resources and poor social support structures.

In many African cultures, there was poor understanding of the etiological processes leading to neuro-disabilities in children and so families resorted to supernatural factors rather than evidence-based explanations. Among the Ashantis in Ghana, a child with neurodevelopmental delay or regression is said to be suffering from "asram" a term loosely used to describe many chronic diseases in infancy and often believed to be the result of an evil spirit or a spell cast on the affected family by someone with evil intent (Baffoe-Bonnie, 1987; Lefèber & Voorhoeve, 1998; Okyere et al., 2010). There are various types of "asram" named after the clinical manifestations or the traditional/superstitious beliefs associated with the condition. "Asram asensen" (stiffness) may be due to neonatal tetanus or spastic cerebral palsy. "Asram puni" (big head) refers to an infant with macrocephaly usually from hydrocephalus (Baffoe-Bonnie, 1987; Lefèber & Voorhoeve, 1998; Okyere et al., 2010).

"Asram" was thought to be the work of evil spirits. As a result, the treatment rested with the "asram doctor" a traditional specialist who employed herbs, concoctions and incantations as means of treatment. The range of treatments employed included administering herbal enemas, wearing amulets that has powers to ward off the evil spirits, making incisional marks and applying concoctions, and keeping the newborn indoors away from the eyes of evil people, among others (Baffoe-Bonnie, 1987; Lefèber & Voorhoeve, 1998; Okyere et al., 2010). While some of these measures did not influence the natural course of the disease, others impacted negatively and were viewed by some western trained physicians as being unethical (Baffoe-Bonnie, 1987; Lefèber & Voorhoeve, 1998).

In other parts of Sub-Saharan Africa, seizures are considered to be a curse and an individual with this condition is considered to be possessed by evil spirits for the bad things done by the family.

In other occasions, seizures are considered as a method of removing bad spirits or a way in which a person is being asked to accept a calling from the ancestors, and that person will continue to convulse until the calling is accepted (Kija, 2015).

Seizures and some other neurological disorders were considered by traditional beliefs and perceptions to be infectious. Some societies believe if an individual comes into contact with the froth from the mouth of a patient convulsing or smells gas released by a convulsing patient, the individual will also catch the disease. This practice has left many patients convulsing for a long time without assistance and in certain extreme situations people have been left to drown or sustain severe burn injuries for the fear of catching the disease (Kija, 2015).

The superstitious beliefs also had significant negative impact on utilization of orthodox healthcare resources (Okyere et al., 2010; Patel et al., 2017). Once a label of "asram" was placed on the child, the notion was that the condition is "not a hospital disease" The families thus spent a lot of time and resources seeking spiritual help from the "asram" doctor. This delayed hospital visits and the child was often brought to medical attention when severe neuro-disabilities had set in.

Another anti-humanistic element in the practice of child neurology in many African cultures is the issue of stigma, which affects many children with neurological disorders and their families. Families have restrained their children with conditions such as epilepsy, cerebral palsy and autism at home for the fear of being segregated by the local community. A family with a child suffering a neuro-disability is considered to be cursed, thus other community members will avoid interacting with the family leading to poor opportunities for education, lowered self-esteem and an overall poor quality of life for the whole family (de Boer et al., 2008; Goodall et al., 2018).

Basic care for children with neurological disorders in Africa is also affected by the limited availability of healthcare facilities and medical personnel with the expertise in managing these disorders. The primary care for these children is often provided by low skilled personnel who may not have the expertise to make the right diagnosis or offer the appropriate intervention. This results in failure of prevention and a lack of recognition of neurological disorders. In addition, there is poor access to facilities, diagnostic equipment, procedures and medications (J. M. Wilmshurst et al., 2011).

In the last fifty or so years, the continent has experienced unstable political environment through conflicts and frequent military interventions in governance with a resultant macroeconomic difficulty and limited economic growth in many countries. This development further destroyed the already poorly resourced health infrastructure with a return to the cash and carry system of health care financing. While many countries are instituting health insurance schemes, they remain ineffective (Adisah-Atta, 2017). In Ghana, for a child with epilepsy seeking care at a tertiary pediatric center, the National Health Insurance Scheme would cover the cost of consultation, basic laboratory investigations and the traditional anti-epileptic medications. The scheme, however, does not cater for advanced diagnostic procedures such as neuroimaging, electroencephalogram, metabolic and genetic testing. In Tanzania, the team covers neuroimaging and electroencephalogram. However, as in Ghana, newer antiepileptic medications are not covered under both schemes. Thus, the family of the child presenting with epileptic spasms, for example, who would require an electroencephalogram, a brain MRI, metabolic screening and possible genetic testing will have to pay out of pocket to get these investigations done, often from commercial laboratories at high cost. If prescribed with adrenocorticotropic hormone (ACTH) and/or vigabatrin, the family would have to buy from commercial pharmacies from out of pocket.

In many centers across the continent, adult neurologists and psychiatrists provide most of the specialist care for children with epilepsy and other neurological disorders. They often have limited training in pediatric diseases as well as in the interpretation of pediatric neurological investigations. (J.

Wilmshurst, 2017). Many countries on the continent have either one or two pediatric neurologists or none at all. A survey in 2010 identified only 148 doctors who are either formally trained or have a special interest in child neurology, for a population of 927 million (J. M. Wilmshurst et al., 2011). The case is not different for other specialized health personnel such as physiotherapists, occupational therapists, specialist nurses, speech and language therapists, and neuropsychologists who constitute the multi-disciplinary team for the care of childhood neurological and neurodevelopmental disorders.

Specialized training is available in only a few African centers, inevitably leading to the migration to acquire these skills. However, upon completion of their training and return to African environment, these specialized doctors feel disempowered and frustrated with the lack of the most basic of resources. As a result, many do not return but rather remain in the countries where they trained; a phenomenon known as brain drain (J. Wilmshurst, 2017). In addition to the lack of human and material resources, relevant guidelines for the comprehensive care of these children are lacking in most centers on the continent (Donald et al., 2015).

Stigmatization, social exclusion and difficult family relationships have fueled the anti-humanism in child neurology practice globally, and Africa is no exception. There is often a physical and an emotional exhaustion that result from the high financial burden and compounded by difficult family relationships, stigmatization and social exclusion of the child and caregiver (Patel et al., 2017; Zuurmond et al., 2019). In the worst anti-humanism case scenarios, these misconceptions have led to abandonment or infanticide (Allotey & Reidpath, 2001). In many other instances, the father is absent and not involved in the care of the child who is considered a "spirit child" or a source of bad luck. Social exclusions and stigmatizations thrive on the various misconceptions within different cultures. These may include a difficulty in finding placement in mainstream educational facilities or the family's inability to participate in other social gatherings within the community (de Boer et al., 2008; Goodall et al., 2018). These challenges do not only affect the child's health and well-being, but also the health of their caregivers (Hamzat & Mordi, 2007).

THE RECENT EVOLUTION IN CHILD NEUROLOGY PRACTICE IN AFRICA

While admitting that the above anti-humanistic elements are still present in many parts of Africa, it is heartwarming to note that a new trend is emerging in the practice of child neurology on the continent which is more humanistic.

There is a slow reduction in the poverty level on the continent with improved access to education. Hopefully, this will reduce the demonization and the denial of science associated with neuro-disabilities in children. More and more fathers are becoming interested in the health care of their children. Slowly, countries are reviving their social support structures to benefit the child with special needs. The inclusive education policy by the Ghana Education Service allows for children with disabilities to gain placement in the relevant institutions (UNESCO, 2018). This inclusive education concept has been implemented in many countries across the continent (Disability Africa, 2017). In Tanzania, the Government through the Ministry of Education initiated a special needs class in every primary school in the country. This intervention is meant to provide opportunity for children with neurological condition to have access to basic education (Possi & Milinga, 2017).

In Ghana, the Ministry of Gender, Children and Social Protection oversees the Livelihood Empowerment Against Poverty (LEAP) Program. The main objective of the program is to reduce poverty by increasing consumption and promoting access to services and opportunities among the extreme poor and vulnerable. The LEAP program has helped to improve nutrition and increase access to health care services among children below 5 years of age and people with severe disability. The program also seeks to increase basic school enrolment, attendance and retention of beneficiary children between 5 and 15 years of age and to facilitate access to complementary services (such as welfare, livelihoods and improvement of productive capacity) among beneficiary households (Ministry of Gender, Children and Social Protection, Ghana., 2013). Recently, there are many other social intervention programs on the continent, under both governmental and non-governmental agencies (Bateganya et al., 2015; Brenyah, 2018).

The continent is now experiencing some political stability with many countries adopting multi-party democracy with a resultant positive trend in economic growth and political stability which is good for the efforts to reduce poverty and improve health outcomes. There is a slow but steady reduction in the level of poverty and improved accessibility to healthcare and new technologies in many countries. Countries like Ghana and Nigeria have seen a significant reduction in brain drain of doctors with the establishment of the local postgraduate medical colleges. These colleges however do not offer subspecialty training in child neurology yet. The African Pediatric Fellowship Program (APFP) provides a wonderful opportunity for pediatricians from across the continent to have further subspecialty training in child neurology and neurodevelopment in South Africa. The APFP provides a more relevant training in child neurology disciplines in Africa by Africans, equipping and empowering the trainees to implement changes and deliver appropriate health care in settings not so different from where he or she trained (J. Wilmshurst, 2017). Many of these highly trained specialists (including both authors of this chapter) have returned home to established child neurology services in their home countries. They have established and maintained partnerships with global associations such as the International Child Neurology Association, the International League Against Epilepsy, the Child Neurology Society, and the British Pediatric Neurology Association. Through these partnerships, they have acquired newer technologies such as electroencephalograms and implemented training programs targeted at improving the knowledge and skills of non-neurologists such as pediatricians and medical officers who are still key and first point of call for many children with neurological disorders. The Pediatric Epilepsy Training (PET) courses have been rolled in over eight countries in Africa with the APFP trainees contributing to the revision of the course content, training of local faculties and the facilitation of the courses (ILAE, 2018).

A multidisciplinary team (MDT) has been formed to run the neuro-disability clinics at both the Komfo Anokye Teaching Hospital in Kumasi, Ghana and the Muhimbili National Hospital in Dar Es Salaam, Tanzania. These clinics bring together various specialists including a child neurologist, a child and adolescent psychiatrist, pediatricians and various rehabilitation experts such as physiotherapists, occupational therapists and speech therapists as well as social workers and educational experts to attend to the medical, rehabilitation, educational and social needs of children with neurological disorders (figure 1).

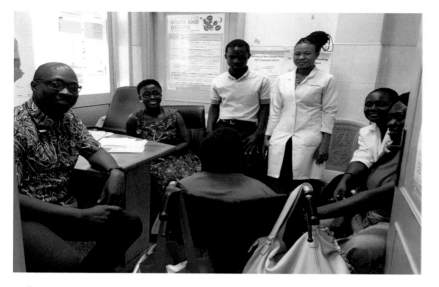

Figure 1: MDT neuromuscular clinic in Ghana showing the patient and his mother, a child neurologist, pediatrician, disability and rehabilitation physician, physiotherapist and occupational therapist. In the adjoining rooms were a dietician and a genetic counsellor.

Advocacy and education by several non-governmental organizations and professional bodies such as the various pediatric and medical associations is a further boost in improving the care of the child with neurological disorder or neuro-disability on the African continent.

CONCLUSION

The practice of child neurology in Africa is undergoing an evolution from anti-humanism practices in the past to patient centered care, which is more acceptable to the child and their families and more satisfying to the child neurologist.

In the past, civil wars and political unrests, poverty, famine, inaccessible healthcare, limited resource, brain drain, demonization of neurological disorders and the denial of science have provided anti-humanistic elements in the practice of child neurology in Africa. In recent times, the continent is experiencing political stability, declining poverty levels, improved education and social inclusion, as well as improved human resources and some technology advancements. These pro-humanism measures are obviously placing the child's interest in the center of the care system and is expected to improve both patient, family and physician satisfaction.

However, there is still a long way to go. Within the African continent the current rudimentary levels of health care must grow through innovative mechanisms to safeguard an appropriate standard of care delivery. In the spirit of humanism, this standard should be comparable to what children with neurological disorders and neuro-disabilities receive in other parts of the world.

REFERENCES

1. Adisah-Atta, I. (2017). Financing Health Care in Ghana: Are Ghanaians Willing to Pay Hig her Taxes for Better Health Care? Findings from Afrobarometer. Social Sciences, 6(3), 90. https://doi.org/10.3390/socsci6030090

2. Allotey, P., & Reidpath, D. (2001). Establishing the causes of childhood mortality in Ghana: The 'spirit child.' Social Science & Medicine, 52(7), 1007–1012. https://doi.org/10.1016/S0277-9536(00)00207-0

3. Baffoe-Bonnie, B. (1987). Asram als spirituelle Krankheitsursache. Der Kinderarzt, 18, 841–843.

4. Bateganya, M. H., Dong, M., Oguntomilade, J., & Suraratdecha, C. (2015). The Impact of Social Services Interventions in Developing Countries: A Review of the Evidence of Impact on Clinical Outcomes in People Living With HIV. Journal of Acquired Immune Deficiency Syndromes (1999), 68(0 3), S357–S367. https://doi.org/10.1097/QAI.0000000000000498

5. Brenyah, J. K. (2018). Implementation of Social Protection Interventions in Africa. Universal JournalofEducationalResearch,6(12),2822–2833. https://doi.org/10.13189/ujer.2018.061216

6. de Boer, H. M., Mula, M., & Sander, J. W. (2008). The global burden and stigma of epilepsy. Epilepsy & Behavior: E&B, 12(4), 540–546. https://doi.org/10.1016/j.yebeh.2007.12.019

7. Disability Africa. (2017). Inclusive education in Africa: Look beyond the school gates. Disability Africa. https://www.disability-africa.org/blog/2017/2/20/z79ogf5cmo0j391ivmurw7tphwptlu

8. Donald, K. A., Kakooza, A. M., Wammanda, R. D., Mallewa, M., Samia, P., Babakir, H., Bearden, D., Majnemer, A., Fehlings, D., Shevell, M., Chugani, H., & Wilmshurst, J. M. (2015). Pediatric Cerebral Palsy in Africa: Where Are We? Journal of Child Neurology, 30(8), 963–971. https://doi.org/10.1177/0883073814549245

9. Goodall, J., Salem, S., Walker, R. W., Gray, W. K., Burton, K., Hunter, E., Rogathi, J., Shali, E., Mohin, A., Mushi, D., & Owens, S. (2018). Stigma and functional disability in relation to marriage and employment in young people with epilepsy in rural Tanzania. Seizure, 54, 27–32. https://doi.org/10.1016/j.seizure.2017.11.016

10. Hamzat, T. K., & Mordi, E. L. (2007). Impact of caring for children with cerebral palsy on the general health of their caregivers in an African community. International Journal of Rehabilitation Research, 30(3), 191–194. https://doi.org/10.1097/MRR.0b013e3281e5af46

11. ILAE. (2018). PETitioning for change: One-day pediatric epilepsy training course becomes worldwide movement // International League Against Epilepsy.

Epigraph, 20(1). https://www.ilae.org/journals/epigraph/epigraph-vol-20-issue-1-summer-2018/petitioning-for-change-one-day-pediatric-epilepsy-training-course-becomes-worldwide-movement

12. Khilanani, A. (2020). Making humanism in medicine more humanistic. KevinMD.Com. https://www.kevinmd.com/blog/2020/01/making-humanism-in-medicine-more-humanistic.html

13. Kija, E. (2015). Traditional Healers and the Treatment of Epilepsy: An African Perspective International League Against Epilepsy. Epigraph,17(1). https://www.ilae.org/journals/epigraph/epigraph-vol-17-issue-1-2015/traditional-healers-and-the-treatment-of-epilepsy-an-african-perspective

14. Lefèber, Y., & Voorhoeve, H. W. A. (1998). Indigenous Customs in Childbirth and Child Care. Uitgeverij Van Gorcum.

15. Ministry of Gender, Children and Social Protection, Ghana. (2013). Livelihood Empowerment Against Poverty. Ministry of Gender, Children and Social Protection, Ghana. http://leap.gov.gh/about-us/objectives/

16. Okyere, E., Tawiah-Agyemang, C., Manu, A., Deganus, S., Kirkwood, B., & Hill, Z. (2010). Newborn care: The effect of a traditional illness, asram, in Ghana. Annals of Tropical Paediatrics, 30(4), 321–328. https://doi.org/10.1179/146532810X12858955921311

17. Patel, P., Baier, J., Baranov, E., Khurana, E., Gambrah-Sampaney, C., Johnson, A., Monokwane, B., & Bearden, D. R. (2017). Health beliefs regarding pediatric cerebral palsy among caregivers in Botswana: A qualitative study. Child: Care, Health and Development, 43(6), 861–868. https://doi.org/10.1111/cch.12490

18. Possi, M. K., & Milinga, J. R. (2017). Special and Inclusive Education in Tanzania: Reminiscing the Past, Building the Future. EDUCATIONAL PROCESS: INTERNATIONAL JOURNAL. http://www.edupij.com/index/arsiv/23/106/special-and-inclusive-education-in-tanzania-reminiscing-the-past-building-the-future

19. UNESCO. (2018, July 9). Ghana: Making inclusive education a reality. IIEP-UNESCO. http://www.iiep.unesco.org/en/ghana-making-inclusive-education-reality-4564

20. Wilmshurst, J. (2017). Paediatric neurology in Africa: Filling the gap. Developmental Medicine and Child Neurology, 59(2), 113. https://doi.org/10.1111/dmcn.13308

21. Wilmshurst, J. M., Badoe, E., Wammanda, R. D., Mallewa, M., Kakooza-Mwesige, A., Venter, A., & Newton, C. R. (2011). Child Neurology Services in Africa. Journal of Child Neurology, 26(12), 1555–1563. https://doi.org/10.1177/0883073811420601

22. Zuurmond, M., Nyante, G., Baltussen, M., Seeley, J., Abanga, J., Shakespeare, T., Collumbien, M., & Bernays, S. (2019). A support programme for caregivers of children with disabilities in Ghana: Understanding the impact on the well-being of caregivers. Child: Care, Health and Development, 45(1), 45–53. https://doi.org/10.1111/cch.12618

CONSIDERATIONS FOR HUMANISTIC CAREGIVING FOR NEUROLOGICAL CONDITIONS IN LOW AND MIDDLE-INCOME COUNTRIES

Grace Akello, PhD
Medical Anthropologist and Associate Professor
Coordinator of Master of Medical Anthropology Program
Gulu University Faculty of Medicine
P. O. Box 166
Gulu, Uganda

Abstract

This essay proposes that humanistic caregiving will substantially improve patients' well-being, especially for neurological and chronic conditions. While sharing experiences in the field, and with reference to epilepsy, I suggest that prescribing antiepileptic medicines is as important for the clients as addressing social and existential experiences like felt stigma, discrimination, ridicule in case of seizures, and isolation. In low- and middle-income countries, proposing humanistic caregiving has various repercussions on cost and human resource investment.

INTRODUCTION

Medical anthropologists examining contemporary biomedical practice (Good 2004, Kleinman 2007, Helman 2007, Farmer 2004, Akello et al. 2010) have discussed the need for humanizing caregiving in clinics as well as improving doctor and patient interaction. While examining the history of biomedicine (Good 2004, Helman 2007) show how disciplinary development and super-specialization meant that clinicians are trained to focus on physical chemical parameters which must be restored in case of illness, thereby aiming at curing individuals. Helman (2007) further gives a distinction between caring and curing. Although caring reflects a more holistic approach in attending to the patient, in contemporary biomedical practice, physicians are pre-occupied with curing and restoring physical-chemical processes the complex whole comprising of social, economic, cultural, environmental and political contexts are depoliticized and ignored.

Yet, for instance (Helman 2007, Kleinman 2007, Akello et al. 2010, Akello 2010, Akello 2013) show how social, economic and cultural factors plays significant role in identifying symptoms of distress, prioritizing health needs and healthcare seeking diagnosis and management. Further, many cross-cultural psychiatrists have alluded to a skewed diagnosis of severe mental illnesses among racial minorities and refugees in the United States (Kleinman 2007, Kirmayer and Pedersen 2014). Whereas there is a growing interest in providing more culturally responsive and effective health care to diverse populations – and the remedy is task shifting and training various specialists in cultural competency courses, the most important missing link in contemporary biomedicine is humane care. Humanistic care invites us to embrace and provide holistic care while problematizing the narrow focus on physiological and bodily processes. To offer holistic care implies paying attention to bodily processes as well as social and existential experience of patient and their caregivers. Humanizing biomedicine, Kleinman(2007) suggests will improve care particularly for chronic conditions and palliative care. The philosophical perspective of humanistic nursing theory (Wu & Volker 2011) resonates with the practice of providing humane care and in management of neurological conditions like epilepsy. Principles proposed in humanistic nursing theory include (1) embodied feeling of helping others, (2) aiming at providing quality care, (3) inter-subjective transaction in nursing (4) demonstrating empathy, (5) compassion, reliability and establishing a good rapport. Nurses are encouraged to reflect on their feelings and biases during caregiving (Wu& Volker 2011). This essay aims to draw clinicians' attention to these parameters in humanistic caregiving. While sharing insights from our I-catch/AAP (2011) project I invite neurologists and psychiatrists to modify contemporary caregiving for neurological conditions. *In low- and middle-income countries, shifting to humanistic care for neurological conditions invites stakeholders to address availability of medicines, poor staffing, and dysfunctional health systems in tandem with deep-rooted social and cultural beliefs.*

STATUS QUO FOR NEUROLOGICAL CONDITIONS IN LOW AND MIDDLE-INCOME COUNTRIES

Whereas there is paucity of data reflecting prevalence, management and prognosis of neurological conditions in low and middle income countries, Peru & Druet-Cabanac (2005) report an African Epilepsy prevalence of 2-58% while Kaiser et al. (1996) survey in western Uganda report an age-specific prevalence of epilepsy at 16.8%. In these settings, epilepsy is experienced as a chronic neurological condition but also as a social, existential, moral and mental health condition. During a fourteen months ethnography in northern Uganda, Akello(2010) documented how epilepsy-related stigma affected children's social, existential and economic well-being.

Other authors (Onodugo et al. 2018) called felt-stigma, the second-epilepsy illness and describe it as major social and psychological problem which people living with epilepsy face. In our settings, mental health departments manage not only organic psychiatric conditions, but also neurological conditions. Epilepsy is one such condition and over 70% of clients who visit psychiatric clinics are people living with epilepsy. In northern Uganda, each client is offered a refill on monthly basis. Adherence challenges with anti-epileptic drugs have been documented (Gurumurthy et al. 2017, Sabate 2003) including forgetfulness, type of epilepsy. Typically people living with epilepsy will not only be confronted with the illness, and challenges of adherence with anti-epileptic drugs but also various social and existential challenges as reflected in the case scenario below:

AN INCIDENT OF AN EPILEPTIC SEIZURE IN NORTHERN UGANDA

In mid-2004 when I conducted an ethnographic assessment of common health problems and quests for therapy among war-affected youths in northern Uganda, it was shocking to observe people's responses to an incident whereby a 15-year old Ocan (not real name to ensure anonymity) had an epilepsy seizure. By observation, children, teachers and other school support staff fled the scene in horror. As I attempted my best to offer first aid and yet Ocan kept jerking, knocking desks, foaming, only a few onlookers moved towards him, though maintaining a safe distance and resignedly reluctant to offer assistance. By the end of the seizure, Ocan was injured, exhausted and bleeding profusely in the limbs. After he regained consciousness, his reaction was even more disturbing. It was one of mixed sadness and shame. Without uttering any words, he picked his school bag and went home, and it was only after two weeks that he resumed his studies. After his departure, one would presume that the source of distress has cleared and things would normalize. Instead, during the entire day, students continued to avoid the scene where the seizure occurred for fear of contagion based on a belief that it was possible to catch epilepsy through stepping on Ocan's bodily fluids. Some students were heard expressing disgust to the school headteachers' decision not to expel Ocan from school as frequently proposed by students together with their parents. The general school atmosphere was that of fear, anxiety and uncertainty. In the meantime, I made inquiries about this strange scenario. Why did all the children yell at me, barring me from moving close and offering help? Why didn't any child or teacher respond to my requests for assistance in offering first aid, removing desks or sharp objects to minimize the seizure-related injuries? And most importantly, how can such a community gripped with fear, stigma and shaming tendencies be humanized so that they will instead offer caregiving when one needs it, particularly during epilepsy-related seizures.

The school headteacher mentioned during interviews how parents are always instructing him to dismiss all children living with epilepsy. For as they argue, "epileptics will infect our children," since epilepsy is contagious. In fact, most headmasters in rural schools do dismiss such children he opined. Similarly all school children avoided, ridiculed and stigmatized children living with epilepsy. They did not want to play with them because all their body fluids were infectious. People living with epilepsy could ignite a serous fight if they touched someone's head as this was viewed as a source of contagion. Many children discussed how in their homes and villages, parents scold them and instruct them to avoid contact with children or close kin of persons living with epilepsy. They prevent them from playing, sharing, or interacting with such children – particularly if they are experiencing seizures. This then is how the culture of contagion and fear for epilepsy is inculcated among populations in many African countries and it is this culture, which impedes caregiving even during critical moments. This anti-social behavior further manifests through stigma and people living with epilepsy therefore face a double burden of the illness and felt-stigma. Similar experiences were discussed by caregivers of children affected by cerebral palsy, neurologically degenerating conditions. Although, there is hardly any statistical data regarding the impact of stigma on such children's social lives, by observation (2011-2014), many school-age children who came for refills at the psychiatric clinic in the regional referral hospital in northern Uganda did not attend school. They described challenges of being accepted in the school settings, irregular dismissals, ridicule, discrimination, stigma and isolation.

In essence, children and families living with epilepsy and other neurological conditions did not only experience the bodily illness and its debilitating symptoms, they also faced social, cultural and psychological stressors in their everyday life.

In Uganda, like in many low and middle income countries, neurological conditions are still managed in psychiatric clinics due to lack of technical staff and diagnostic equipment. Relying on symptomatic presentation, and offering medicines to minimize the recurrence of symptoms including, for instance epileptic seizures characterizes this practice. However, as shown in the scenario above, for children living with epilepsy, after the much needed medicines or surgery, there is still needing to improve patients' comfort while providing compassionate attentiveness.

The approach will necessitate a focus on individual processes, but also the influence of broader disease burdens originating, from cultural and social realms. Meeting the criteria of providing compassionate attentiveness might require forming an interdisciplinary team, with various specialties of care, each team playing a vital role as they are charged with providing care on a regular basis and interact with patients and families regularly. In this way, the management plan embraces a humanistic and holistic approach to patient care (see Wu & Volker 2011).

In (Akello 2013), I discuss an intervention project supported by the American Academy of Pediatrics (I-Catch AAP), which aimed to promote awareness about childhood epilepsy and improve enrolment for anti-epileptic drugs in the communities in northern Uganda. Our approach was through training school children as health workers. The philosophical underpinning followed the biopsychosocial model in mental health whereby the health workers recognize the importance of focusing on the biological, psychological, and social aspects in restoring normality and reinforcing humanistic care in communities. While clinicians in the psychiatric clinic attended to the bodily processes, diagnostics and prescriptions for anti-epileptic medicines trained children played an advocacy role for caregiving. The child health workers promoted awareness about the presence of Anti-epileptic drugs(AEDS), importance of offering first aid in case of a seizure and dispelling local beliefs about catching epilepsy through sharing utensils, being touched by a child living with epilepsy and contagiousness of body fluids.

ADDRESSING SOCIAL AND EXISTENTIAL EXPERIENCES OF EPILEPSY

We employed accessible ways in addressing social and cultural beliefs, which significantly impede caregiving and adherence with anti-epileptic medicines. Through role plays, school children promoted awareness about the importance of social support to address the issue of isolation of people living in sociocentric settings of Africa where people survive through sharing, doing activities together, and being part of a community. In other words, if fear of contagion was an important predictor for offering first aid in case of a seizure our training sessions designed messages to dispel this. For example during our training sessions, we depicted a real scenario where children and adults are terrified at an incident of a seizure. They mention how through helping or offering first aid, they will also catch the disease and prevent anybody who wants to offer first aid from doing so. Because of this belief, a person experiencing a seizure is not rescued from dangerous objects, significantly increasing risk for injury by sharp objects, fires, hot surfaces. In our village outreach activities and training sessions in urban centers, we met many severely injured children due epilepsy seizures. Some families reported seizure related deaths due to drowning when such a child had gone to fetch water from an open water source. Together with Dr. Leila Scourer, we visited a teenage girl who got severe burns, which were disabling because she had a seizure, and nobody offered assistance. She therefore needed multi-pronged care, during the next visit for refill in the psychiatric unit. The severity of scalds, the multiple injuries and disability were further stigmatizing and igniting fear among people who described the extent to which epilepsy causes suffering. In our AAP project, we focused then, not only on promoting awareness but also telling people about how EADS work, the importance of adhering with medicines, the importance of offering first aid and removing any hard objects in the vicinity where one is experiencing a seizure, to promote humanistic care.

Through working with school children, and different health clubs, we disseminated messages through a poem depicting everyday realities of the people living with epilepsy. The poem depicted everyday lived experiences like isolation, discrimination, community stigma in case of a seizure, people's fleeing from the scene of a seizure instead of offering first aid, and availability of free anti-epileptic drugs in the psychiatric clinic. The children were also engaged in a discussion with their audiences who expressed skepticism through asking the persistent question namely: would visiting the psychiatric clinic be a sufficient remedy or as caregivers often asked us:

"is it really true that AEDs cure epilepsy" therefore necessitating one to make a distinction between minimizing symptoms, and curing the disease. In essence AEDs only minimize symptoms. This utterance about managing symptoms is difficult to conceptualize for settings where mostly people engage in quests for therapy – that is seeking for a cure. It could be for this reason that some families having considered the task of enrolling for AEDs only for symptomatic management instead resorted to local herbal remedies. The families argued that if they can use the herbs at home, the effect is not also curing then they did not see a need to change their therapies from local herbs to anti-epileptic drugs. Until the time of writing this article, it is possible to discern that biomedical symptomatic management could resonate with the use of local remedies in only minimizing symptomatic presentation. But our community outreaches were still useful in letting people know about alternative care options. They also learnt that epilepsy is not contagious and were able to engage with the community about the illness.

We preferred teaching the school children through role plays in order to inculcate ideas about first aid in case of seizures in an interaction designed to promote well-being and existential growth in observers, stigmatisers and people who would flee such a scene yet what is needed is first aid. In essence our approach resonates with (WU, Volker 2011) training of nurses to be dependable, be present for the patient. This not only provides the patient with a pillar on which to lean on, but it also encourages positive interactions between patient and nurse. Realizing the cascading effect of this approach, I recommended humanistic care for not only neurological conditions but also other illnesses in low and middle-income countries.

IMPLICATIONS FOR HUMANISTIC CARE FOR EPILEPSY: ALLEVIATING SUFFERING

Inviting super-specialized clinicians to consider humanistic caregiving, particularly for various neurological conditions resonates with the proverbial saying of raising the bar higher for care. I suggest that holistic care will not only end in providing of anti-epileptic drugs and promoting drug adherence but that there is need for compassionate and comprehensive care to include a focus of social, cultural and existential aspects of experiencing this illness.

Promoting awareness about causes of epilepsy

Lay explanatory models about causes of epilepsy and how people can catch this disease significantly contributes to community response in case of a seizure. Whereas introducing biomedical neurological models is one approach through which one can de-stigmatize epilepsy, it is also true that few people readily replace one model with the other. Akello (2013) reports resistance, hybridization of models and many children and adults' ideas about epilepsy causation merged traditional and naturalistic explanations. Where communities imbued and disseminated notions of genetically acquiring epilepsy, and also through ancestral lineage also further caused collective stigma where entire families faced discrimination. Changing loci of stigma made our work tedious, constantly evolving and therefore making it imperative to continuously engage the community. Beyond discourses regarding origins of stigma, types of stigma and how stigma manifests, our overall aim to inculcate empathic response and to encourage the previously fear gripped community to offer first aid in case of a seizure regardless of what one believes in.

Improving epilepsy diagnostic and management processes

Over a four-year period, our (I-Catch/AAP) project documented about 400 new cases of people from East, northern Uganda and South Sudan who were enrolled for AEDS. It is possible that our outreach, which presented people with a likelihood of minimizing frequency of seizure occurrence, influenced their response in seeking care in psychiatric clinics. Outreaches made people hopeful and they were able to see an improvement in their clients' life. But by observation, any re-occurrence of a seizure led to disagreement and questions concerning efficacy of the remedy. Through offering empathic responses and reassurance of clients and families about how anti-epileptic medicines work, it is possible to garner their trust.

De-stigmatizing epilepsy

As seen above, whereas it is difficult to link our current intervention aimed to de-stigmatize epilepsy, when we taught children about the importance of offering first aid in case of a seizure and that epilepsy is not contagious, many people living with epilepsy reported having observed a behavior change particularly in schools. It is this symbolic outcome, of feeling accepted, a change in attitude from fear and fright to caregiving which improved clients' psychological well-being. The confidence that one or two children will behave differently and offer assistance when needed was an important outcome. In essence our intervention enhanced empathetic and supportive interaction, so that the children were able to make other children living with epilepsy more comfortably, improved their self-determination and enhanced their sense of dignity. The humanistic perspective is an approach to psychology that emphasizes empathy and stresses good human behavior, in counseling and therapy.

REFERENCES

1. Akello, G., Richters, A., Reis, R., (2010). Silencing distressed children in the context of war: An analysis of its causes and health consequences. Social Science & Medicine 71(2): 213-220.

2. Akello, G (2010) Wartime children's suffering and quests for therapy in northern Uganda. African Studies Center: Leiden.

3. Akello, G., (2013) Training peer health educators on childhood epilepsy in northern Uganda: opportunities and challenges. American Academy of Pediatrics. December pp 5-6.

4. Good BJ (2004) Medicine, experience and rationality: an anthropological perspective.. Cambridge University Press: Cambridge.

5. Gurumurthy R, Chanda K & Sarma GRK (2017) An evaluation of factors affecting adherence to antiepileptic drugs in patients with epilepsy: a cross sectional study. Singapore medical journal. 98-102. https//doi.org:10.11622/smedj.2016022.

6. Helman, C (2007) Culture, health and illness. Oxford: Oxford University Press.

7. Kaiser C, Kipp, W Asaba G, Mugisha C, Kabagamber et al (1996) The prevalence of epilepsy follows he distribution of oncocerciasis in west Ugandan focus.

8. Kirmayer L & D .Pedersen (2014) Towards a new architecture for global mental health. Transcultural psychiatry51(6):759-76. https://doi.org.10.1177/136346.1514557202.

9. Kleinman A (2007) What really matters: living a moral life amidst uncertainty and danger. Oxford University Press: Oxford.

10. Onodugo, O.O, Ezeala-Adikaibe BA, Ijoma U.C, Achor JU, Onyekonwu CJ et.al (2018) Determinants of felt stigma among patients living with epilepsy attending a tertiary

neurology clinic in south east Nigeria. Open Journal of psychiatry. https://doi.org/10.4236/ojpsych.2018.84029.

11. Preux PM & Druet-Cabanac M (2005) Epidemiology and Aetiology of epilepsy in sub Saharan Africa. The Lancet Neurology, 4, 21-31. https://doi.org/10.1016/S1474-4422(04)00963-9.

12. Sabate W (2003) Adherence to log-term therapies: evidence for action. Report No:WHO/MNC/03.01

13. Wu HL & Volker D (2011) Humanistic nursing theory: application to hospice and palliative care. Journal of advanced nursing 68(2):471-479. Doi:10.1111/j.1365-2648:2011.05770.x.

THE WAY TO HUMANISM IN PEDIATRIC NEUROLOGY IN EGYPT

Sahar Mohamed Ahmed Hassanein, MD, Phd;
Pediatrics department, Faculty of Medicine, Ain Shams University, Cairo, Egypt

Ghada Ahmed Saad Elhawary, MBBch
Faculty of Medicine, Ain Shams University, Cairo, Egypt

Sarah Hisham Hassan Wagdy, BA
Faculty of Al-Alsun Ain Shams University, Cairo, Egypt.

Abstract

Our children deserve a high-quality healthcare and medical services; however, do we provide humanistic medical care to our children with neurologic diseases? Our aim was to explore the perception and factors affecting humanistic approach among Egyptian patients, their families, and healthcare providers.

We conducted 10- to 20-minutes semi-structured individual interviews to 10 parents of children with different neurologic diseases, and for 11 physicians and one recently graduated student from medical school. Participants were asked to describe what humanism means to them. The patients' stories were translated from Arabic to English.

There are barriers in providing humanistic healthcare. These can be financial and healthcare system barriers, culture, attitude, manners and behaviors, religion, faith, and rituals.

This work spotlights the defect in the healthcare providers' humanism. A governmental act is needed to optimize healthcare system and improve healthcare providers' income. Improving work environment and minimizing occupational stress are crucial to have a humanistic care for children with neurologic diseases. A future use of the patients' stories to teach humanism in medical education, medical and non-medical. An empathetic smile on the face, listening to all parents' worries, reassurance, and mutual respect, are the key for humanism.

INTRODUCTION

Asia and sub-Saharan Africa recorded the highest global burden of neurological disorders in children. Many of the disorders occurred during the perinatal period. The burden of living for years with disability in children aged 5-14 years has increased markedly over the last 25 years [1].

Egypt's health challenges affect the rural poor and impact the country's economic growth future, especially in the presence of overpopulation. The quality of medical care has become increasingly important in healthcare system [2]. Socioeconomic inequalities in health with lower-income groups tended to report having worse health levels than higher-income groups [3].

Egypt is in lower-middle income countries with lower - than could be expected - health status [4]. Reaching over 100 million inhabitants, poverty in Egypt has nearly doubled in the last 15 years. Also, Egypt's healthcare system is diverse including both public and private providers. The public system is hindered by continuous underfunding, and low-quality services. The private sector provides higher quality services than public healthcare system [5,6].

The perception of children with disability of themselves is usually a reflection of their caregivers' perception of them, and how their schoolmates, parents, families, and caregivers treat them. Improvement of self-esteem and confidence of children with chronic neurologic diseases should be emphasized, to improve body image and disease acceptance. Humanism describes the attitudes and behaviors that demonstrate interest in and respect for patients' psychological, social and spiritual concerns and values [7].

This is a pilot study aimed to explore the perception and factors affecting humanistic approach among Egyptian children with neurologic diseases, their families, and healthcare providers.

METHODS

A semi-structured interview of 10 to 20 minutes was conducted in-person to 10 parents of children with different neurologic diseases, and for 11 physicians and one recently graduated student from medical school. They were chosen from the university hospital, public insurance hospitals and private hospitals. Participants were asked to describe what humanism means to them. The data is a description of the participants opinion. It is performed face to face or by phone after getting a permission to use their words. Translation was done for the patients'/parents' words from Arabic to English. In Egypt, medical education, medical files and drug prescriptions are in English language, although, Arabic is the main language in Egypt.

STORIES

Patients' stories are considered as a message to the pediatric neurology healthcare providers:

Lessons from the patients, in how to be a humanistic physician?

A mother of a 3-year-old boy with acute necrotizing en-cephalitis. He is treated in a private hospital with a private medical insurance.

First message: Reassure me, I need your support.

"The major issue for us at the beginning was things were am-biguous, and we were feeling that our son was very sick. No one was telling us what was going on so that we would be less worried, that probably was because our son was total-ly normal then lost conscious and became totally unrespon-sive. The pediatric neurologists explained the seriousness of his condition. Despite his poor conscious level at first, early treatment and being beside him talking and hugging, affect-ed his and our psychological condition in a positive way. This resulted in rapid recovery and regained speech, motor, and mental power in few weeks. Having an empathetic reassuring physician with a professional medical care and faith in God is a blessing."

Adolescent with perinatal stroke

Second message: Respect my worries and anxiety.

"When anyone could not find the exact and accurate solution to their problem, devastation, worry and anxiety start to in-vade their heart and thoughts. This might affect health more than the neurologic disease itself. People may utter anything which would affect the recipient in an awful way. This effect makes the life of the affected person more difficult. Therapists should not complicate things for the patient to avoid the dis-continue of therapy."

Adolescent with cerebral palsy patient

Third message: Feel my suffering before bullying me due to my physical disease.

"Each person has their perspective, and thus a certain response to the situation, if the physician is unaware of this and lacks empathy, thus, a mixture of anxiety, worry, lack of confidence and lack of social interaction may affect the patient. During medical checkup to join college, I started to feel as if I am not a human being. I felt that I am treated as a case to prove science by discovering my defects. Same during school years, the healthcare providers were always searching for any physical defect to add to the list, which made my education process very difficult. Bullying by my schoolmates added more social isolation. I could not talk or play with them, felt isolated."

An 11-year-old hemiplegic cerebral palsy patient

Fourth message: get my permission before doing anything related to me, I am not a baby.

"From the first day of my physiotherapy, I felt as if I am not normal and this was a burden for anyone close to me. The stress started to invade my heart and filled it while I was performing my exercises. I felt uneasy and self-rejected. I stopped physiotherapy and any outdoor activities."

A mother of a 6-year-old boy with SMA type2

Fifth message: Learn how to communicate with patients and apply what you have learnt while communicating.

"In my point of view, humanism is being merciful and considerate to the patient and his parents' feelings while dealing with them. I went to a doctor who diagnosed my 16-months old son to have SMA type-1. She told us, that the disease is lethal, and he might not make it to the age of 18-months. We felt desperate and were expecting his death during that month. He is 6-years old now and still alive. Regardless of the disease's burden, physiotherapy centers are psychologically stressful. I hope physicians interact with special needs as if they were their children."

A mother of a 4-year-old child with SMA type2

Sixth message: have a smile on your face, encourage the whole family and give hope.

The mother said: "healthcare providers, whether physicians or physiotherapists, should be caring, merciful, considerate, and treat the child with a smile and empathy. They should provide professional medical care according to the patient's needs, irrespective of their wealth or socio-economic position."

A mother of a 9-year-old boy with Duchenne muscular dystrophy. He is doing checkups in a pediatric neurology clinic of a public university hospital; he has governmental insurance.

Seventh message: Respect my dignity, suffering, and frustration, do not overwhelm me with bad feelings.

He is the eldest of 3 brothers. His mother defined humanity as respecting his social status, his suffering, her concerns, and providing an appropriate free medical care. She brings him to the clinical teaching rounds for the undergraduate and postgraduate medical education sessions. This is a way for financial support as it is a paid session. She felt humiliated by one of the medical staff, he talked to her in a disrespectful way. The students' comments about the death of children with Duchenne and their excitement when seeing a new case, badly affects my boy. He feels worthless just waiting for death. Furthermore, she said "Some doctors are dealing with the patient as an object and not as a human being with feelings."

A mother of a 2-year-old boy with diplegic cerebral palsy due to preterm birth. He is doing checkups in a pediatric neurology clinic of a university hospital.

Eighth message: A unified medical service is needed everywhere, to lessen the family's burden.

The mother said "I tried many physiotherapy centers in public hospitals and private centers. Only one therapist was caring and enthusiastic in improving the child's motor skills. I must travel and the session costs much in an overcrowded governmental health insurance hospital. He teaches me home exercises. I tried a nearby private center, but the therapists were not as good."

A mother of a 16-year-old girl with mild hemiplegic cerebral palsy

Ninth message: Do not increase my psychological burden, a smile on the face is attractive.

The mother said "A child with handicap is not only a family burden, but also causes psychological stress. We do not have time to go out together or to have a normal life. The physiotherapy, occupational therapy, extra effort in doing school homework's and doing daily activities, leaves no time to spend as a family. The tough way the therapist uses to pressure the child to do exercises, leads to refusal of physical therapy. Why do they not smile to the child, even if a fake smile?"

Student's experience

"During our pediatric rotation in medical school, neurologic examinations were on children with cerebral palsy and chronic illness. We should pay money to the mother to allow us to examine her child and practice for our clinical exams. It was very sad to be in this situation and deal with a child as if he was a dummy."

PHYSICIAN'S VIEWS

Physician-1: "Humanism is respecting the checkups, dignity, others' rights, and best interests of the child."

Physician-2: "Humanism is ethical aspects and values of the human being."

Physician-3: "It is a good tool in some cases if the time and settings permit."

Physician-4: "Beside the medical care I have to respect and provide the patient's biological and physiological needs and respect the parents' worries and always support them."

Physician-5: "It means treating the patient not the disease."

Physician-6: "Care for every child as your own kid."

Physician-7: "Provide your medical care with a smiling face and a reassuring voice. I used to encourage the children with chronic neurologic diseases, with the words "you are so sweet, you are very obedient, you can and will be able to do everything soon with continuing training or Gym or swimming." Never used the words "will never be normal"; these are perceived by the children and parents as permanent handicap.

Physician-8: "I keep looking on the face of the parents during clinical interview, to get feedback and assess their satisfaction."

Physiotherapist-9: "The meaning of humanism in dealing with children with neurologic disease is that they are not different from normal children. They are always challenged, and they should win the competition. As physiotherapists we should encourage them to overcome obstacles."

Physiotherapist-10: "I am trying to let the parents feel that I appreciate their perseverance in attending the sessions. Encouraging and engaging the mother during the session to do home exercises improves the child's motor skills. I always look at the face of the child to watch for any pain and intervene immediately if it hurts.

DISCUSSION

In our study we tried to evaluate the perception of humanism among both providers and recipients of healthcare in the child neurology sector. Also, it differs according to the situation. Humanism in clinical practice is a mutual patient-clinician relation.

In our interviews, the patients' perspectives and their expectations differ in acute from chronic neurological diseases. In the story of acute necrotizing encephalitis treated in a private hospital with high insurance, the mother needed to know the final diagnosis and prognosis. In cerebral palsy a chronic disabling disease, humanism was defined as interacting with the patient as a normal person, respecting feelings, and destigmatizing handicaps. Treating the patient in an aggressive or in-humanistic way can be perceived as rejection or disrespect and can result in discontinuing physiotherapy by the patient or the family. Also, the treatment cost and transportation add more burden on the family specially when treated in public hospitals.

The unmet needs, lack of providing disease information and the lack of support were the cause of deterioration in the patients, families, and the medical staff mutual understanding; also, increased stress for the caregiver and lowered quality of life [8]. This is a universal need which should be fulfilled in our Egyptian healthcare system.

The first step in treatment is acceptance of the disease by the patient and family. This can ease the implementation of the management plan. The clinical and communication skill can be the beginning of a humanistic approach in child neurology practice, to do that the treating team should adopt the quotation of "put yourself in other people's shoes." This will build a bridge of confidence between the medical team and the patient.

Healthcare providers should understand the social barriers for those families. In a study done on parents of Greek children with chronic neurological diseases (CND), they were less involved in social and recreational activities, and appeared to be less knowledgeable on the availability of help in emergencies and were less satisfied with rendered medical services [9]. This culture is like the Egyptian one. The Egyptian family of a handicapped child faces; financial, social, psychological, recreational, and schooling problems. In a study evaluating the services provided for Egyptian children with handicap, it is neither integrated nor easily accessible. Children with neurological diseases and intellectual disability, are usually associated with a social stigma and psychological burden on the family [10].

In the present work, the patients are not satisfied with the healthcare provided to their children. Also, in the public system they described being treated in a disrespectful way by some physicians. At the same time the physicians' responses are with humanistic approach, "respect their dignity, respect other's rights, respect the parent's worries and always support them, provide your medical care with a smiling face and a reassuring voice, and care for every child as your own kid." In a way to explore the discrepancy between having the concept of humanistic approach and acting with humanistic approach by the healthcare providers in Egypt, we should search for the obstacles and barriers in Egyptian healthcare system.

First, there are barriers in Egyptian social and healthcare system to reach humanistic healthcare. Physicians, nurses, and other healthcare providers face high levels of occupational stress. They overwork to sustain an adequate living standard. The physicians must continue their postgraduate studies to improve their profession and their income, especially working in public hospitals. They have no time for extra-work in private sectors to earn money.

In developed countries, they continually improve quality of medical-care standards, and quality of the patients' lives. In developing countries, the unmet services and needs differ according to socio-economic positions. In clinical practice it is difficult to provide humanistic medical care to large numbers of patients in public hospitals' outpatient clinics. A study assessed the quality of care provided to Egyptian children with cerebral palsy, there is a wide gap between the actual care provided and the recommended standards. Moreover, the documentation system in the hospital is poor [11].

Egypt faces challenges to implement social justice in healthcare, these can be addressed through 14 short- and medium-term recommendations [12]. Egyptian Ministry of Health effectively increased the number of beneficiaries covered by the Health Insurance Organization (HIO). Political commitment to achieve or accomplish the anticipated health equity enhancements [13]. Targeting the free public care could help reduce the existing socio-economic based inequalities in healthcare coverage in Egypt [14].

In Egypt there are 2 religions: Islam and Christianity. Egyptians are highly spiritual. They have faith in God. The Holy Quran and the Bible encourage mercy and good treatment to others. Humanistic behavior in Egypt as a culture should start from early childhood. Bullying noticeably increased in Egyptian schools in the last few years. The Holy Quran discourages bullying, "O you who have believed, let not people ridicule [another] people; perhaps they may be better than them; nor let women ridicule [other] women; perhaps they may be better than them. And do not insult one another and do not call each other by [offensive] nicknames. Wretched is the name of disobedience after [one's] faith. And whoever does not repent - then it is those who are the wrongdoers." {Holy Quran, Al-Hugurat 11} Studies on the effect of Quran on different psychological and behavioral aspects are reported [15-17].

The second barrier to humanism is cultural attitudes and behaviors, religion, faith, and rituals. The deficiency within the educational system, along with the deficiency of the healthcare system leads to the absence of humanistic attitudes neglecting wellbeing of the patient, parents, and the physician. In an Egyptian study evaluating resident's medical ethics education, more than half described their medical ethics course as ineffective. It was knowledge-based not skills-based [18]. Also, an Egyptian medical ethics curriculum that meets students' concerns, and provides ethical decision making for all medical school years is needed [19]. It has been recommended that incorporating humanism and communication skills to medical education is a must [20]. Role modeling is the primary method to teach humanistic aspects of medical care [21]. Physician's empathetic smile, encouraging words and positive emotion expression touches parents feeling. Humanism public awareness should be a national-based program.

Study limitation

The small number of participants limits the generalization of our findings.

CONCLUSION

This work sheds light on the importance of educating the healthcare providers with the concept of humanism. There are many cultural and environmental factors hindering humanistic medical practice. A governmental act is needed to improve healthcare. Improving the healthcare system and the healthcare providers' finances are crucial to have a humanistic care for children with neurologic diseases. Teaching and training school children and medical students on humanistic attitudes is a must. An empathetic smile on the face, listening to parents' worries, reassurance and mutual respect are the key for humanism.

REFERENCES

1. Newton CR. Global Burden of Pediatric Neurological Disorders. Seminars in pediatric neurology. 2018;27:10-5. Epub 2018/10/09. doi: 10.1016/j.spen.2018.03.002. PubMed PMID: 30293585.

2. Hussein H, Shaker N, El-Sheikh M, Ramy HA. Pathways to child mental health services among patients in an urban clinical setting in Egypt. Psychiatr Serv. 2012;63(12):1225-30. Epub 2012/10/17. doi: 10.1176/appi.ps.201200039. PubMed PMID: 23070112.

3. Elgazzar H. Income and the use of health care: an empirical study of Egypt and Lebanon. Health economics, policy, and law. 2009;4(Pt 4):445-78. Epub 2009/03/04. doi: 10.1017/S1744133109004939. PubMed PMID: 19254431.

4. Gericke CA. Comparison of health care financing in Egypt and Cuba: lessons for health reform in Egypt. Eastern Mediterranean health journal = La revue de sante de la Mediterranee orientale = al-Majallah al-sihhiyah li-sharq al-mutawassit. 2005;11(5-6):1073-86. Epub 2006/06/10. PubMed PMID: 16761679.

5. Gericke CAB, K.; Elmahdawy, M.; Elsisi G. Health System in Egypt. In: van Ginneken E, Busse, R. , editor. Health Care Systems and Policies Springer, New York, NY; 2018. p. 1-18.

6. Mosallam RA, Aly MM, Moharram AM. Responsiveness of the health insurance and private systems in Alexandria, Egypt. The Journal of the Egyptian Public Health Association. 2013;88(1):46-51. Epub 2013/03/27. doi: 10.1097/01.EPX.0000427042.54093.c4. PubMed PMID: 23528532.

7. Branch WJK, D; Haidet, P. The patient-physician relationship. Teaching the human dimensions of care in clinical settings. Jama. 2001.

8. Buzgova R, Kozakova R, Jurickova L. The unmet needs of family members of patients with progressive neurological disease in the Czech Republic. PloS one. 2019;14(3):e0214395. Epub 2019/03/26. doi: 10.1371/journal.pone.0214395. PubMed PMID: 30908542; PubMed Central PMCID: PMC6433266.

9. Tzoufi M, Mantas C, Pappa S, Kateri M, Hyphantis T, Pavlou M, et al. The impact of childhood chronic neurological diseases on Greek families. Child: care, health and development. 2005;31(1):109-15. Epub 2005/01/22. doi: 10.1111/j.1365-2214.2005.00492.x. PubMed PMID: 15658971.

10. Aston M, Breau L, MacLeod E. Diagnoses, labels and stereotypes: Supporting children with intellectual disabilities in the hospital. Journal of intellectual disabilities : JOID. 2014;18(4):291-304. Epub 2014/09/25. doi: 10.1177/1744629514552151. PubMed PMID: 25249376.

11. Khalil M, Elweshahy H, Abdelghani H, Omar T, Ahmed S. Quality of care provided to children with cerebral palsy, Alexandria, Egypt. Eastern Mediterranean health journal = La revue de sante de la Mediterranee orientale = al-Majallah al-sihhiyah li-sharq al-mutawassit. 2018;24(6):522-31. Epub 2018/08/07. doi: 10.26719/2018.24.6.522. PubMed PMID: 30079947.

12. Pande A, El Shalakani A, Hamed A. How Can We Measure Progress on Social Justice in Health Care? The Case of Egypt. Health systems and reform. 2017;3(1):14-25. Epub 2017/01/02. doi: 10.1080/23288604.2016.1272981. PubMed PMID: 31514713.

13. Nandakumar AK, Reich MR, Chawla M, Berman P, Yip W. Health reform for children: the Egyptian experience with school health insurance. Health Policy. 2000;50(3):155-70. Epub 2000/05/29. doi: 10.1016/s0168-8510(99)00073-1. PubMed PMID: 10827306.

14. Benova L, Campbell OM, Ploubidis GB. A mediation approach to understanding socio-economic inequalities in maternal health-seeking behaviours in Egypt. BMC health services research. 2015;15:1. Epub 2015/01/22. doi: 10.1186/s12913-014-0652-8. PubMed PMID: 25603697; PubMed Central PMCID: PMC4307186.

15. Saged AAG, Mohd Yusoff MYZ, Abdul Latif F, Hilmi SM, Al-Rahmi WM, Al-Samman A, et al. Impact of Quran in Treatment of the Psychological Disorder and Spiritual Illness. Journal of religion and health. 2018. Epub 2018/02/28. doi: 10.1007/s10943-018-0572-8. PubMed PMID: 29484510.

16. Ozturk O, Celik AM, Uyar EI. The Relation of Religious Attitudes and Behaviours with Depression in Boarding Quran Course Students. Psychiatria Danubina. 2016;28(4):379-85. Epub 2016/11/18. PubMed PMID: 27855429.

17. Mahjoob M, Nejati J, Hosseini A, Bakhshani NM. The Effect of Holy Quran Voice on Mental Health. Journal of religion and health. 2016;55(1):38-42. Epub 2014/01/15. doi: 10.1007/s10943-014-9821-7. PubMed PMID: 24421119.

18. Mohamed AM, Ghanem MA, Kassem A. Problems and perceived needs for medical ethics education of resident physicians in Alexandria teaching hospitals, Egypt. Eastern Mediterranean health journal = La revue de sante de la Mediterranee orientale = al-Majallah al-sihhiyah li-sharq al-mutawassit. 2012;18(8):827-35. Epub 2012/10/13. doi: 10.26719/2012.18.8.827. PubMed PMID: 23057371.

19. Fawzi MM. Medical ethics educational improvement, is it needed or not?! Survey for the assessment of the needed form, methods and topics of medical ethics teaching course amongst the final years medical students Faculty of Medicine Ain Shams University (ASU), Cairo, Egypt 2010. Journal of forensic and legal medicine. 2011;18(5):204-7. Epub 2011/06/15. doi: 10.1016/j.jflm.2011.02.012. PubMed PMID: 21663867.

20. Montgomery L, Loue S, Stange KC. Linking the Heart and the Head: Humanism and Professionalism in Medical Education and Practice. Family medicine. 2017;49(5):378-83. Epub 2017/05/24. PubMed PMID: 28535319.

21. Weissmann PF, Branch WT, Gracey CF, Haidet P, Frankel RM. Role modeling humanistic behavior: Learning bedside manner from the experts. Academic medicine : journal of the Association of American Medical Colleges. 2006; 81(7): 661-7. Epub 2006/06/27. doi: 10.1097/01. ACM.0000232423.81299.fe. PubMed PMID: 16799294.

2.AMERICA

SEEING THE WORLD THROUGH ANOTHER PERSON'S EYES: A NORTH AMERICAN PERSPECTIVE ON HUMANISM AND NEUROLOGICAL DISABILITY

David L. Coulter, MD
Associate Professor of Neurology at Harvard Medical School
Senior Associate at Boston Children's Hospital

Boston Children's Hospital
Boston Massachusetts

INTRODUCTION AND DISCLOSURES

North America is a continent of Native Americans and immigrants from Europe, Africa and Asia, all of whom blended their own traditions and cultures into what we see today. As a result, humanism in North America has to be approached from a very broad, respectful, multiethnic, multicultural and multiracial perspective. The Native American influence is strong in Mexico and Central America, while the African influence is strong in Haiti and the United States. The European influence is felt everywhere. Asians have been in North America for centuries. A Middle Eastern influence is growing. To be human in North America thus reflects all of these important cultural contributions. The challenge then is to describe an approach to humanism that is consistent with this rich and varied heritage.

I should disclose my own background because it certainly influences what I will suggest in this chapter. My paternal grandfather was born in Ontario, Canada to parents who were from Ireland and Wales. My paternal grandmother was born in New York to French Canadian parents who were from Quebec, Canada. Their family always claimed that my paternal great-grandmother was Native American, which is certainly possible (but unproven) given the proximity of the Mohawk Nation to where they came from. My maternal grandfather was born in Poland to parents who were Jewish. My maternal grandmother was born in Nebraska to Catholic parents who were also from Poland. I was born in Michigan, lived in Texas for a while and now live in New England. My cultural background is thus primarily European, but I will try to speak to the richness of our multiethnic and multicultural North American heritage.

ETHICS AND HUMANISM

Several approaches to ethics can be identified (Coulter 2017) but the most prominent is principlism, which was adopted by the United States Commission on Bioethics (Belmont Report 1978). The ethical principle of autonomy (also known as respect for individual persons) has dominated North American ethical analysis but may feel strange to readers from other cultures in which family and community values are more important. Other ethical principles include beneficence (caring for persons) and justice (providing resources for persons to thrive). So consider my patient CF.

CF is a 19-year-old young man with spastic and dystonic cerebral palsy due to a birth injury. He has normal intelligence and communicates through assistive technology. He nonambulatory. Using his assistive technology, he has communicated very clearly that his goal in his adult life is to be as independent as possible. But his parents do not agree. CF uses whatever resources he can to assert his autonomy, but his parents often override it. How can a child neurologist recognize and support CF's humanity while also recognizing his need for connection with his family and community?

Humanism in a Western or European context derives from the Latin word humanitas ("human nature, kindness and education") and from the Greek word philanthropia ("loving what makes us human"). For example, the great Roman writer Cicero said to his brother that "if fate had given you authority over Africans or Spaniards or Gauls, you would still owe it to your humanitas to be concerned about their comforts, their needs, and their safety" (recovered from the Wikipedia article on the web). Humanism has taken many meanings since that time. It was emphasized by Petrarch and others as the basis of a humanistic education. Humanism in North America can thus be defined as a philosophical and ethical stance that emphasizes the personal value, autonomy and moral agency of individual human beings.

We are most human when we see the humanity of others (anonymous quotation recovered from a church bulletin in 2017), but first we need to see our own humanity. We are then most human when we are able to share our own humanity with others. The challenge is to discover the meaning of humanism in our own lives and then to try to share it with others.

DISCOVERING PERSONAL HUMANISM

Personal humanism can be discovered through answering a series of questions about what it means to be human (Gaventa 2018).

1. Who am I? (personal identity)

2. To whom do I belong? (loving and being loved)

3. Where did I come from? (culture, family and ethnicity)

4. What is the meaning of my life? (values)

5. What is the purpose of my life? (goals)

6. Where am I going in my life? (personal history)

7. Who do I want to become? (future)

Everyone will have their own answers to these questions, so there can be no overarching construct. Sharing our humanism means that each person needs to answer these questions individually and then try to understand how another person would answer the same questions. Deciding how much to share is a personal choice, and every relationship is unique. Part of the art of caregiving is trying to adapt to the humanistic aspects of every clinical relationship.

Rachel Naomi Remen described a trinity of three aspects of patient care which she called fixing, helping and serving (Remen 2012). Surgeons fix, social workers help and chaplains serve. Child neurologists can fix by prescribing medication and therapy, help by supporting children and families, and serve by sharing our humanism. North American medicine has tended to focus on fixing through using the remarkable achievements of scientific research and genetics. Remen (herself a physician and a recipient of caregiving) emphasizes that helping and serving have had the greatest positive impact on her own life. She thus advocates for restoring the balance between the trinity of patient care. Experience teaches that child neurologists can do it all, but we have to adapt the mix to fit each clinical relationship.

HUMANISM IN PATIENT CARE

For the past 40 years, I have had the great privilege to work in public hospitals and clinics in Michigan, Texas and Massachusetts providing free care to poor children with disabilities and their families from African-American, Haitian, Mexican, Central American, Caribbean, African, Asian and Cape Verdean backgrounds. They have taught me a lot about humanism, which I have formulated into what I call the three ways of looking (Coulter 2001-A, Coulter 2001-B). This approach respects the multiethnic, multicultural and multiracial composition of North American society. This approach opposes the institutional racism, Native American genocide and historic discrimination that have plagued North America since the first Europeans arrived. This approach also seeks to move beyond that history and to provide a way to implement the Golden Rule, "Do unto others what you would want them to do unto you."

The three ways of looking can be summarized as follows.

1. The first look is to see the other person as an individual human being, not just as a patient or a case. It tries to see how the other person would answer the previous questions. It is different from empathy or compassion (which see the patient objectively) because it seeks to see the patient's subjective self.

2. The second look is to see the other person as a human being just like myself. It leads me to value for them what I value for myself, and to protect for them what I would protect for myself, including life, liberty and happiness. Erich Fromm wrote, "If I can say I love you, I must be able to say that I love in you everybody, I love through you the world, I love in you also myself."

3. The third look sees in the other person the ground of all being and existence, or the presence of a shared universality of being. It is a rare and unpredictable experience that can happen when we least expect it. It cannot be forced, only welcomed when we are open to it through our experience of the first two ways of looking.

These ways of relating to others can help us to deepen and sustain our relationships with our patients and their families and help us to focus on serving them through a humanistic sharing of who we are. Some people will not want this, which is of course okay.

The United States has a long and troubled history of genocide against Native Americans, institutional racism against people of color, and discrimination against Mexicans, Asians, Muslims and others. Other North American countries have experienced their own challenges to humanism. Some have compared these challenges to a virus that has become pandemic throughout North America and infected the continent ever since 1492. From a humanistic perspective, we can follow this infectious disease metaphor to argue that the sacred Scriptures of our multiethnic, multiracial and multicultural North American heritage can provide a vaccine against racism and hate, and further recognize that the Golden Rule can be the antidote.

A HUMANISTIC APPROACH TO BIOETHICS

Given the varied background of North American society, is it possible to develop an approach to bioethics that would be relevant in every culture, ethnicity and religious tradition present in North America and that would address the ethical challenges of caring for children and youth with neurological disorders? The universality of the approach to humanism described above may provide a way forward. Every human being on earth can consider and answer the seven questions about what it means to them to be human (Coulter 2006). Their answers to these seven questions can also be considered as a description of their individual spirituality, whether they profess a religion or not.

The three ways of looking can be the basis for a humanistic approach to medical ethics (Coulter 2017). This approach goes beyond the stark philosophical concepts such as principles which are derived from Greek, Roman and European traditions. It seeks instead to respect the multiethnic, multicultural and multiracial aspects of North American society. Three precepts can be identified:

Respect in others what I value in myself. This precept is similar to the principle of autonomy but is based on the mutuality of sharing humanism between physician and patient.

Do the most loving thing possible. When we love in the patient what we love in ourselves, we will strive to do that which is best for all. Love—not just duty, convention, rules, or cost containment—is the basis for action.

Seek guidance from the source of my own and the other person's being, through deep reflection, prayer, advice, or sharing. Thoughtful physicians often do this in difficult ethical situations but may not recognize the humanistic nature of these reflections.

These precepts do not appear to depend on any specific religious tradition and should be applicable in all cultures and religions. One need not be religious to apply them to one's practice. They avoid the relativity of accepting cultural practices at face value by providing a general structure for applying differing cultural beliefs to specific clinical situations.

Let's think about how we could apply this approach to my patient CF described above. First, we should try to see him as an individual human being, not just objectively as a young man with cerebral palsy but rather subjectively as a young man with his own personal goals and aspirations. As much as possible, we should try to understand how he would answer the seven questions. Second, we should hold his hand, look him in the eye and say as sincerely as possible, "I hear you. I want to do for you what I would do for myself if I were in your situation." Third, we should try to mediate as clinicians between CF and his family so that we can all share our own humanism with each other. We can try to do the most loving thing possible by trying to appreciate CF's love for his family and their love for him, as well as our love for all of them. Fourth, we can work together with everyone else involved in CF's care, including his primary care doctor, his pastor, his gastroenterologist, his assistive technology specialist and his adult transition planner, to make sure we are all working together to respect CF's humanism and support his goals and dreams for his future.

CONCLUSION

I will conclude this chapter with the following poem, which I wrote to illustrate the humanity of every child with a neurological disorder or disability (Coulter 2017). This poem could also represent the lamentation of my patient CF described above. Every such child can have a personal relationship and a friendship with God. It is up to us as caregivers to recognize and celebrate that relationship and to share our own humanity with them whenever we can.

I had the great privilege to receive the annual national award for humanism in medicine from the Child Neurology Society in 2017. The award is sponsored by the Arnold P. Gold Foundation, whose mission is to "support clinicians throughout their careers, so the humanistic passion that motivates them at the beginning of their education is sustained throughout their practice." And furthermore, the Foundation "strives to ensure that care and respect always govern the relationship between practitioner and patient." When I received the award, I stood at the podium in front of hundreds of North American child neurologists and read this poem to them. The audience, especially the young people who were present, understood and cheered.

JUST TRYING TO FIGURE IT OUT

(Transcribed by a friend)

Hey God, would you mind if I became a Buddhist?
I really like that reincarnation thing they do.
Maybe if I'm a good person in this life,
I'll come back as a movie star, a Pope or a guru.

I mean Jesus, please, just tell me why,
Why did this thing happen, why am I here?
My parents made a perfect little baby,
Gestation going well, no cause to fear,

Then boom! My happy birth gone bad, I had
No oxygen or blood go to my brain---

The doctors said I'd die, my parents prayed,
Somehow I lived, so how can I complain?
But tell me God, was this your plan for me,
To live my entire life within this chair?
I know I shouldn't ask, but I'm confused
(My soul still thinks my CP is unfair).

I really hoped to be a running back
And race for touchdowns for my high school team,
Like all those athletes I'd have liked to be---
I could have been a contender in my dreams.

They say the goals of life are love and work.
You know what God? I can't do either one
(I'd like to date a swimsuit model, though,
Or drive a Lamborghini just for fun).

Wishes won't work, so I have to like what I have:
I like the summer sunshine on my face,
I like my music, my family and my friends
Who help me to enjoy my time and place.

So maybe life is really not that bad
(The alternative of course is not to be);
Sweet Jesus, I just need a miracle---
You healed some folks before, so why not me?

I know I can't expect that it will happen,
Not in this life, maybe in the next.
What I have is all I've ever known,
And what I know is all I can expect.

But when I go to Heaven, or Nirvana,
I'll be the fastest athlete they have seen,
Because I know there won't be any wheelchairs,
And I'll be running for the winning team.

Thank you, God---
We're still friends.

REFERENCES

1. Coulter DL (2006). Presidential Address: Peacemaking is the answer: Spiritual valorization and the future of our field. Mental Retardation, 44: 64-70.

2. Coulter DL (2017). Ethical Issues in Child Neurology. Chapter 164 in Swaiman KF, Ashwal S, Ferreiro DM, et al. (eds), Swaiman's Pediatric Neurology; Principles and Practice, Sixth Edition. New York: Elsevier, pp. 1263-1269.

3. Belmont Report (1978). Ethical Principles and Guidelines for the Protection of Human Subjects of Research. Report of the National Commission for the Protection of Human Subjects of Biomedical and Behavioral Research. Washington, DC: United States Government Printing Office.

4. Gaventa WC (2018). Disability and Spirituality: Recovering Wholeness. Waco TX, Baylor University Press.

5. Remen RN (2012). http://www.dailygood.org/view.php?sid=218

6. Coulter DL (2001-A). Recognition of spirituality in health care: personal and universal implications. Journal of Religion, Disability and Health, 5 (2/3): pp 1-11.

7. Coulter DL (2001-B). Editorial: Three ways of looking: A pastoral approach to clinical care. Journal of Religion, Disability and Health. 4 (4): 1-5.

8. Coulter DL (2017). "Just Trying to Figure it Out," in Disability, Doctoring and Patient Care: Poems from a Life in Medicine. New York: Amazon, pp. 30-3

THE LATIN AMERICAN PERSPECTIVE ON HUMANISM IN CHILD NEUROLOGY

Alcy Torres Catefort, MD
Past President of the Pediatric Ecuadorian Society
Past Ecuadorian Representative of the Latin American Association of Pediatric (ALAPE)
Past President of the VI Course and II Congress of the Iberoamerican Academy of Pediatric Neurology (AINP)1994
Associate Professor of Pediatrics and Neurology
Universidad Central del Ecuador
Carlos Andrade Marin Hospital
Quito, Ecuador

The health perspective for our children in Latin America in the pediatric neurology field lies between the shadows in the frequent crises of our history and the lights in the honest men who have struggled to transform their present in search of a future worthy of children, particularly those affected with neurological problems.

The humanistic practice in pediatric neurology in our region is directly related to historical realities and the educational process through the ages from when we were a society of isolated aboriginal cultures, despite the degree of development that some of these cultures reached. The names of the Aztec, Mayan, and Inca cultures stand out significantly in pre-colonial times. The arrival of Europeans to our region has had an undeniable influence on our language, religion, and traditions, as well as in the socioeconomic distribution during the colonies than in what now is our republic.

Today, we know that approximately one in six children have some neurological problem so it is logical to assume that these ancestral problems have been a challenge for our societies that have had to face the most important thing in a human being, their central nervous system. The central nervous system, which starts very early in the embryonic period and continues throughout life, is what has put us at the peak of evolution; the future of individuals, families, and nations depends on its development.

In pre-colonial cultures, the cause of disease was unknown and were attributed to natural phenomena, such as the eruption of a volcano or the whim of one of their gods, such as the sun or the moon. Diseases were considered as a punishment or a hopeless destiny without the possibility of a cure or even improvement. These populations had extensive knowledge about the effect of herbs that were used to alleviate diseases directly or as part of magical spiritual rites. Pre-Columbian people and in particular, the Aztecs, saw themselves as pawns in the hands of the gods and felt that disease could be considered as punishment for not having obeyed the will of those deities. Another concession of divine intervention was that of predetermined disease. Aztec and Mayan cultures had very advanced knowledge of astrology and even had calendars. Children born on certain days were considered as children who would more easily get sick or who had a noticeably short life expectancy

It is difficult to pin down exactly how complex the practice of medicine was at that time. Most of the treatments were symptomatic. It is surprising to learn, however, that in Peru cranial trepanation for people who suffered from war wounds or epilepsy was carried out since 1000 by the pre-Inca "Paracas" culture. Anesthesia was achieved with coca leaves and alcohol produced from "chicha," with a survival rate of up to 80%.

Rituals to drive away evil and disease consisted of dances with screams accompanied by movement. Inca doctors were a kind of priest and they presided over the healing ceremonies. They were known by the name of "Ichuris," when the "Comascas" populations were entrusted to them and when they were in charge of the "Americas" Inca nobility. These practitioners had specialties; some were in charge of diagnosing a disease, the shamans were in charge of the treatments, and others were concerned with the problems of the soul. Following a review of the numerous treatments based on medicinal plants used by the Incas, a great variety is found for different medical problems; however, except for plants with a calming or hallucinogenic effect, the Incas did not have many resources to treat neurological ailments in children. In many tribes, newborns with malformations were sacrificed at birth. Native diseases in Brazil were more benign than in other regions of Latin America.

The decision of whether someone was cured or not was in some way divine. "Itzanamá," a priest who lived in the year 525 AD, participated in the founding of the city of Maya Chichén-Itzá after gaining fame as a wise man. He is considered the god of medicine, as well as the Lord of the night and day skies. Health and death were considered the product of the will of their Gods. The Aztecs worshiped the God Ope, who protected the newborn, and Xoathicitl, who watched over cribs at night.

At the beginning of the colonial era, there were not many doctors. It is known that a surgeon came on one of Colon's trips but progressively and because of necessity and due to the influence of what was then happening in Europe, the practice of medicine began to have norms. Surely, in those times in many parts of the world, there were many people who had no training who were dedicated to treating the sick. Spain at the head of many European nations created the Protomedicato Tribunal, which functioned in Madrid, and later, when the colonial process advanced, a proteomic was created in New Spain, Mexico, and in Lima.

Universities and schools of medicine were created. The oldest, founded in 1538, is the University of Santo Tomas de Aquino in the Dominican Republic, followed by the University of San Marcos in Lima in 1551 and the University of San Fulgencio in 1586. On June 21, 1578, the first Chair of Medicine was approved, being the oldest in the continent in the Royal and Pontifical University of Mexico, today the National Autonomous University of Mexico. In 1580, Mexico City boasted four hospitals for the Spanish, one for the local population, and others for people of other races. Several groups of nuns and monasteries in the region began to open their doors, reflecting the influence of the Catholic Church on health, as well as in many other activities in our countries. In Brazil, the first official protection measure for the marginalized and abandoned was carried out by the Metropole in Rio de Janeiro in 1693 and years later, in 1738, Romaó de Mattos Duarte was inaugurated the Roda dos Expostos, the first asylum for children.

Pediatric services were inaugurated in general hospitals. The first pediatric hospitals begin to function, following the example of the "Hópital des Enfants Malades," founded in Paris in 1802, which was the first hospital dedicated exclusively to the hospitalization of children and where I had the opportunity to train.

It was not until 1880, however, that Pediatric Chairs began to be created in Latin American medical schools. Subspecialties emerged later, at first according to need but later with more formal training.

In accordance with my academic inclination, upon my return to Ecuador in 1969, I was awarded the position of Professor in the new Chair of Neurological Pediatrics at the Central University of Ecuador in Quito. Simultaneous efforts occurred in Argentina with Natalio Fejerman, who trained at Boston Children's Hospital; in 1965, he began in Monterrey N.L. the first Pediatric Neurology service in Mexico at the IMSS General Regional Hospital, directed by Dr. Raúl Calderón González. Today, there are some training programs, notably in Uruguay, Argentina and Mexico, and dozens of pediatric neurologists, although there are still not enough to supply the demand.

Approximately 193 million children and adolescents live in Latin America, of whom 70 million live in poverty. In 2017, 82% of the wealth created in the world went to the wealthiest 1% of the population. Latin America is the region with the highest economic inequality.

Within this historical, institutional, religious, and cultural framework, it is possible to understand the influences on the practice of humanism in the practice of medicine, in our case of pediatric neurology in modern times. Although communication in the world is extraordinary and access to education is much greater than in past times, there are still many obstacles that go from the process of selecting future doctors, their training, and recognition within a society in survival mode.

There are still myths about epilepsy or intellectual disability. Ancestral stigma about the demonic characteristics of these diseases led to families hiding their loved ones and even depriving them of health care. Many Latin American families still believe in the "evil eye" and put a wool or silk ribbon on the wrists and heels of infants to protect them from disease.

The price of health care makes access to private health services especially prohibitive. Medications such as intravenous lorazepam or intranasal midazolam are not available, and even antiepileptic drugs can disappear seasonally, making care more difficult. Costs also affect health services so that, with few exceptions, many facilities cannot offer 24-hour monitoring with electroencephalography or state-of-the-art imaging systems.

The doctors in our countries have the desire to serve and despite the long hours, the number of patients, and the complexities, they attend their patients with compassion, respect, and professionalism. The modernization of the Faculties of Medicine, health insurance, and hospital centers is responsible for keeping the doctor in that line of service; however, there is still significant variability among professionals.

Families, however, easily recognize dehumanized behaviors. In Latin America, great care must be taken not to overwhelm the patient with information that is given to protect the physician from legal ramifications. The experienced physician finds a balance, but it takes time to develop. Medical schools have been facing this problem for a long time. In fact, there is data that shows a decrease in empathy in medical students from admission to graduation. In contrast, there are still doctors who enter the non-profit profession, who dedicate most of their life to the perfection of the medical art for all who need it.

The democratization of teaching in Latin America has had several effects. On the one hand, it allowed the majority to be trained and to become doctors but on the other, it diminished the power to select the most talented and the best people for this art.

The human demonstrations in the care of children with neurological problems are innumerable in professional practice and are reciprocal. Even in moments of despair and death, the family values the dedication of the professional who, even lacking all the resources, struggles to preserve the visa in all its forms from the resuscitation of the newborn to prevent hypoxic-ischemic encephalopathy, the early diagnosis of meningitis, the care of the traumatized person, the management of the child with seizures or of tumors that cause deformations of the face, or complications that require surgery, such as hydrocephalus.

Our America also has its most frequent diseases, those that are born from unhealthy conditions, poverty, and which are the greatest obstacles not to practicing humanism but to claiming the value of humanity in all our patients.

Our colleagues in Latin America not infrequently do it without monetary compensation, adjusting to the economies of the patient or even taking money out of their own pockets to assist the neediest whom the state does not reach with its programs.

The Latin American family wants to have hope and never forgets those who made bold and erratic predictions only to be exposed years later. It is the patient's right to know the truth, but the time and place must be appropriate.

The paternalistic figure of the omnipotent doctor has disappeared for one more committed to his people, where the patient and their family have more time to ask questions, to inform themselves, and make their own decisions. Young professionals must understand that the patient and their family are at the center of our actions, the reason for being for us, and our mission is not only treating the disease and alleviating pain,but comforting and supporting until the end. This new way of thinking forces the professional to have a complete vision of the patient. It goes far beyond scientific data to understand the individual as a whole and respect the family of our patients as they want to be treated. Our challenge is to decipher it as soon as possible.

The future is promising, however. Pediatric Neurological Societies continue to be founded and there is a growing number of colleagues interested in neurological problems. We have passed from the time of mystery and curiosity and the permanent search for improvement through scientific activities and publications on our specialty.

The Latin American Pediatric Association (ALAPE) and the Iberoamerican Pediatric Neurology Association (AINP), founded by our Cuban colleague Oscar Papazian, have played an important role in this evolution. These organizations are in charge of continuing education for specialists in the region and offer opportunities for scientific exchange.

In the global world we live in now, it is expected that our region will experience significant progress in the next 50 years. One of the obstacles for us has been access to education and with technological advances, we might experience other challenges such as the depersonalization of health care. Thus, it is essential to remember the importance of humanities in education. Quoting Adela Cortina, "The study of humanities promote creativity allowing us to learn from different worlds and empower the attitude of empathy," feeling like our patients and their families. "They help us overcome the trap of individualism and acknowledge the needs of other humans' beings and our interconnection."

To see how a child who suffers from a neurological disorder struggles against disability, to feel the pain of a mother who seeks to do everything possible to help him, to witness the despair of a teacher who tries his best with him to give him equal opportunities in life, are some of the daily experiences of a Pediatric Neurologist.

Pediatric Neurology in Latin America has stood out for facing difficult challenges with fewer resources than many in the world. Although to a certain extent the development of medicine in our region has gained ground in recent decades, the starting point until not long ago was very precarious and incipient. At present, there is still a lack of availability of diagnostic technology, new drugs and lack of access of the population to the health system. For example, it is estimated that half of epileptic children do not receive the treatment they need and only a few have begun to benefit from epilepsy surgery in medical centers in the region. The proportion of children with neurological disorders is greater than in industrialized countries, so, the burden on the health system is greater and with less chance of success.

The Covid 19 Pandemic, unemployment, child malnutrition, little education and a lack of specific awareness of the population aggravate the challenge assumed by a Pediatric Neurologist in the face of these suffocating social problems. These factors accentuate inequalities between more or less favored social groups in societies. The inability of the governments of the countries to equip their public hospitals to promote timely prevention and reduce the avoidable causes of neurological disorders such as infections of the central nervous system, head trauma, perinatal complications, determine a difficult panorama for the practice of the specialty. Increasing vaccination coverage against microorganisms associated with nervous system infections is an imperative in the effort to prevent neurological sequelae.

There are immoral differences between children treated in the public sector compared to the private sector. The access to health resources such as Magnetic Resonance, Tomography, and Electroencephalograms between patients treated in the public sector compared to the private sector. Access to trained professionals and multidisciplinary teams is not yet a general rule for our patients.

This reality of health care in Latin America reveals a lack of leaders and people committed to achieving better indicators of childhood neurological disorders that are at least equal to that of developed countries. The contribution that our region has received from the cooperation of International Organizations such as the American Child Neurology Association, The

American Pediatric Association, AINP, ILAE, ALADE, PAHO and other International Federations in Neuroscience is notable. Many of them have National Chapters in Latin American countries, for example. The incorporation of the International Epilepsy Day that has been taking place in Argentina, Paraguay and El Salvador has allowed to broaden awareness about Epilepsy within their communities.

Heroes and Heroines have achieved great achievements in this field with the creation of several Latin American Epilepsy Centers, the commitment of many social organizations and charitable initiatives have implemented low-cost nurseries for children with neurological problems, such as El Centro de Parálisis Cerebral, Sonrisas para sus niños, Fundación el Triángulo in Quito, Ecuador. There are now programs where boys and girls with Autistic Spectrum Disorders are now practicing soccer with volunteer coaches and American support from the international organizations such as the Wellesley United Soccer Club. In every society, there is good people, and humanism in child neurology can improved by coupling the need with those who can provide.

Latin American Pediatric Neurologists have been pioneers in almost all countries since the rise of the specialty with the training of new professionals, many of them work intensively in their offices in public medical centers, non-profit foundations, religious social initiatives and some contributions of the private company. The effort required to access continuing medical education often involves covering your expenses from your own income. There is still a long way to go, psychomotor, language rehabilitation, special learning and early stimulation have begun to emerge, and there is a need for a greater number of paramedical personnel to complement the care in these care centers.

When medicine cannot offer a remedy for the patient's ailment, our duty is to lighten the burden that these small patients and their families must face, from our Latin American region we recognize the value that international cooperation projects can have for our community.

The potential for the development of our countries depends on the intellectual capacities of future generations but also in their hearts. Throughout my life, and with the active contribution of my wife with the Ecuadorian Pediatric Society and its committee, we managed to get Ecuadorian children some help, as did other former president and the current board of directors; constancy is the basis of success but to achieve it, we must cultivate a creed of humanism every day of our lives.

The Pediatric Societies in Latin-American and its committees work with social conscience and dedicate themselves to work tenaciously, sensitizing young women and raise funds and deliver medical equipment and supplies to those in need. Their silent action by organizing playful acts to partially appease the pain of helpless and sick childhood that, in the face of the imperturbable attitude of the health authorities, cast a shadow over the life of this vulnerable human group, as a consequence of institutionalized injustice in our poor and underdeveloped countries.

IS CURRENT MEDICINE HUMANISTIC? PERSONAL REFLECTIONS ON THE DOCTOR-PATIENT RELATIONSHIP

Victor Alejandro Gaona, MD
Neuropediatrician
President of the Ibero-American Academy of Pediatric Neurology
Professor of Physiology National University of Asuncion
Department of Pediatric Neurology and Neurophysiology
La Costa Medical Center
Asuncion, Paraguay

"Wherever the art of medicine is loved, there is also a love for humanity" - Plato.

I remember the night when I read the list of new students of the medical school at the National University of Asunción, a list that was eagerly awaited by the applicants and their families, who after the demanding and strenuous admission exams were immersed in a sea of anxiety and uncertainty.

When I read my name, the tension, like a long-compressed spring, shot up in uncontrollable joy. The last-year students quickly took the first-year students to a classroom where the traditional "baptism" would take place, a ritual that was repeated year after year with each admission.

Amid my overflowing euphoria, I was struck by a phrase engraved on the platform for the teacher. It said: "Only a good man can be a good doctor" (Nothnagel, 1841-1905). I felt as if my true reception to this school was summed up in that phrase that I imagined was addressed directly to myself. Today, decades after graduating and after years of study, training and work, I continue to evoke that phrase and I wonder if really, and in the depth that it contains, that warning has been fulfilled.Medicine has evolved quickly and the changes that have occurred have, necessarily, had an impact on the people who practice it. It also generated changes in vision and behavior in the doctor-patient relationship - changes that in some cases have been favorable and in other cases counterproductive.

The search for the origins and bases of diseases, to know their pathophysiology, development, and complications, has led us to forget that the true focus of medicine is the patient, and we have insensitively distanced ourselves from them in the drift of our research and progress.

Society as a whole has been changing their opinion about doctors, to the point of not only being suspicious but also judging the medical attitude and its determinations, generating concepts and ideas that may have their origin in ourselves, although later we feel aggrieved by the means to the point of considering ourselves victims of collective misunderstanding.

The patient, the object of our care, exposes and offers his problems to someone he assumes he can trust and whose abilities can bring relief to what ails him. He is exposed not voluntarily but driven by his desire to improve his condition. Unfortunately, the patient does not always perceive empathy in the one whose help he seeks, which makes him helpless, confused and impotent in a situation in which he expected a more warm and effective treatment to generate the bond that allows him to open up in body and mind, allowing a bridge to be built that unites two people in search of the same goal.

As a consequence, society as a whole, by the simple law of reaction, has developed a very rapid loss of the respect that our elders had, making the doctor-patient relationship an exchange of misgivings on both sides, without glimpses of the solidarity, understanding, and respect that should govern human relations in all senses and activities.

Aggravating this situation is the difficulty and inability, climbed to the very high building of our ego, of not understanding the situation or being able to foresee, which derives in a cascade of circumstances that do nothing but make the problem worse by entering an upward spiral whose result does not bode well.

The image for many of our fellow citizens is that of the man in the white coat behind their office desk, who many see as a business counter, giving directions, writing orders or requesting studies, in a cold and impersonal way, not considering the patient at all in their whole dimension, but only as a pathology that must be improved or treated - a tremendous paradox that invades the offices with a cold halo of insensitivity to the sufferer.

It seems that we do not realize, or choose to ignore, that behind the disease there is a person with a whole universe of feelings and needs, family or work relationships, wishes and knowledge, affections and dreams. Forgetting this, we depersonalize patients until they are left without a proper name, transforming them into a mere number or pathology. "Does the 404 have a crisis?" "How's the one in 514?" These phrases are commonly used in medical practice and reflect little affectivity with the patient and his human individuality.

Physicians and patients coincide at one point in space and time, one because of deterioration in their health and the other trying to find the cause, and mitigate or remedy if possible.

This fortuitous encounter establishes a relationship where empathy and trust must be the bases that bring both ends into contact, configuring what is known as the "medical act." When this encounter is carried out in a cold and impersonal way, on the part of the doctor, it is inevitable that the patient loses its confidence and delusion and instead, insecurity, apprehension and doubt grow in him, complicating the necessary fluidity in the treatment to reach a good outcome and to restore the health of those who come to us.

More and more voices are raised accusing and pointing to doctors as insensitive and dehumanized people, indolent and indifferent to the pain and suffering of their patients, and more and more we close ourselves off, ignoring comments that we consider inappropriate and unfair.

But I think that we should stop and analyze whether these accusations and trials, which we consider to be wrong, have any basis in reason and to consider when, or for what causes, this distancing leads to situations that are antagonistic to doctors and patients.

I think we must first know what medical humanism means, since patients are accusing us of lacking it, and thus try to understand what happens by rectifying what we have forgotten or abandoned.The idea of humanism encompasses a wide range of concepts that include respect and appreciation of the human being as a whole and therefore is related to feelings of generosity, compassion, respect for the attributes and individuality of each person, and the cultivation of interpersonal relationships.

Seen from this perspective, the practice of medicine is the practice of humanism itself, since it requires the involvement of the doctor with the patient, where feelings that make up the very essence of that activity are combined.

The doctor immerses himself in the patient's intimacies, in his doubts and concerns, in his fears and hopes, trying to restore the lost balance and motivating his search for help, placing his trust in the person from whom he hopes for a long-awaited solution to what ails him.

It must be created, by necessity itself, a current of affinity between the two in such a way that the problem that accompanies one can be understood in its entirety by the other person, establishing the link that must unite them in the search for a solution or at least to an improvement in the patient's situation.

This current of sympathy needs to consider the patient as a whole in which the biological and the emotional, their social and cultural individuality, their aspirations, and their possibilities that are in a personal balance and whose rupture is what we consider the presence of an illness or loss of health.

We must be aware of the fact that restoring that balance correctly or trying to return it to its initial state of perfection will not always be possible, since in some cases the impossibility will be insurmountable despite the efforts and knowledge that we apply to it.

Despite the above, the doctor who uses affection still has a lot of work to do if he considers that not only is there a suffering body but also an emotional being that suffers, in equal parts, from the impact of the disease. This gives rise to a phrase that summarizes and says much of what is expected of a doctor who assesses a human being in all the breadth of its components: "Heal sometimes, often relieve, always console." This statement has been attributed to various authors, including the French physician, Adolphe Gubler, and Claude Bernard (considered to be a great physiologist and the father of so-called experimental medicine).

Despite the great technological advances in medical engineering, genetics, laboratory studies and other advances that have allowed us to search the depths of the interior of the human being and make available to the examiner from images of the interior of the body to the complex DNA, the very essence of medicine has not changed from its origin. The essence that was installed at the precise moment in which a human approached his equal in search of relief, establishing a link that, despite the ups and downs of history, persists to date under the name we call the "doctor-patient relationship."

This relationship, mentioned above, acquires another dimension when we place it in the practice of the field of Pediatrics, in all its specialties, since a sick child is equivalent to a sick family and this broadens the spectrum of anxieties and expectations, often already present before the first contact with the specialist: an amalgam of fears about the possible result of the consultation and medical evaluation.

These causes can be found within the time limitations due to the numbers of patients, the deterioration of the fabric of society as a whole, the exploitation of the doctor by public or private institutions, the demand of an increasingly intolerant clientele eagerly searching for successful results or the economic demands of a growing consumer market. Each one of these situations mentioned, or all of them together, have managed to crumble what has long required construction.

A reason for this may have been the inability to maintain the development of the proper empathy that must exist in each event, that attitude that leads us to try to understand what people's feelings and emotions try to transmit to us. This allows us to objectively and rationally understand what patients or families transmit to us and to locate ourselves in the universe of their emotions.

Empathy, whose origin is Greek ("empatheia"), emphasizes the bond between the emotions of people, generating feelings of love and concern for others, constituting the engine of the need for help to others and approaching them with the desire to exercise or offer the required support, following the moral principles that govern human conduct.

The empathic person develops common points or affinities with others by practicing the almost forgotten art of listening, establishing an immediate and affective connection, allowing the interlocutor to expose their most intimate emotions and/or concerns.

With this, we can understand and perhaps foresee the reactions, behaviors, and decision-making of those with whom we interact, according to the information, good or bad, which the medical examination generates.

We see that empathy is necessarily a vital component of medicine and a tool that builds the bridge that unites people, achieving greater openness, collaboration, and the necessary understanding to try to restore the physical and emotional balance of those who come to us.

It is very evident that empathy is a fundamental component and whose absence can jeopardize the emotional bond and interfere with the expected result.

We should ask ourselves: Are we establishing channels of empathy with our patients and their families? Do we feel identified and affectively related to them? Do we understand them and "put ourselves in their place, " as mentioned above?

If our answer is negative, I think that we are not following a good standard and we will not develop stable and lasting emotional ties with patients; at the same time, as a consequence, they will retract and distance themselves, not allowing us to scrutinize in all the depth and magnitude necessary to understand their problems and thus, be able to give them the help they seek.

We must not forget the time factor, that tyrant who cannot be stopped and who constantly runs, since it is also an indispensable element to take into account in the medical act. The patient comes with a baggage of doubts, information, or questions that he wishes to share, such as his contribution to the search for the solution to his problem or that of his family member. In short, he wants to be listened to, giving perhaps minor details but considered of the utmost importance from his perspective, and he expects the maximum attention and interest from his interlocutor.

That desire collides, many times, with the scarce time that we dedicate to patients, having to interrupt them when trying to orient the data more consistently and logically to obtain a possible diagnosis quickly. In our eagerness, on many occasions, the patient perceives what he interprets as lack of interest, carefreeness, or lack of sensitivity on the part of the medical provider, not allowing the proper foundation of affectivity to be built.

This is particularly notable when the doctor is caught in the tangle of large corporations, public or private, which demand high productivity from him to the detriment of the efficiency necessary in his practice. This required productivity drastically cuts the time dedicated to patients, reducing it to just a few minutes and generating a kind of "mechanization or automation" of the medical act itself.

Obviously, patients and family members do not know or perceive the tremendous pressure the doctor is under, forcing situations that generate friction and misunderstanding, increasing the resentment between the patient, who is mistreated and misunderstood, and the doctor, who feels abused and exploited.

In a small survey carried out with colleagues working in various public institutions, the daily hours of consultation and the number of patients attended in that period were obtained to have a clearer picture of the use of time. The answers are shocking to the highest degree that, although we intuited them, we did not imagine the magnitude of what we would discover. The average time dedicated to the patient is less than 10 minutes, from their entry and exit, for taking a medical history, examination, diagnostic guidance, study requests, prescriptions, and indications with the consequent and necessary explanations that are always required.

Is this the way to practice good medicine? It seems to be an assembly line destined to injure and further degrade the already deteriorated relationship that exists between the doctor and those who come to him, losing the required amount of humanism. Therefore, it is also our task, as medical professionals, to fight for the rights of patients to quality care and for the respect that we deserve as people and as professionals.

Adding to this is the tremendous profusion of medical schools with a production of colleagues without clear studies of the needs that exist in each medium and of the capacity of the system to absorb, train and specialize in the various disciplines, appropriately both in the professional as in human aspects.

On the other hand, in these same schools, the disease is studied more deeply than the patient. The approach to the person as a whole is not practiced or taught, rather everything is directed to the pathology that he presents, without considering his emotions or feelings that make him unique.

We need to teach how to define the difference between disease and patient. The first is the reason that has led the patient to seek help and that is presented as a sign or symptom constituting a pathology; the second is the one who suffers, with their fears, anguishes, and other feelings.

Regarding the first reason, technology and great advances have provided us with many effective tools that allow us increasingly accurate and effective diagnoses and treatments, correcting pathologies and restoring organic balance. However, for the second reason, that is the patient or family who suffers, the doctor continues to have the same elements that he had from the very beginning of medicine: interest in the patient, respect, and appropriate treatment established by a pattern of confidence that calms, comforts and relieves.

Finally, we believe that a new form of medical ethics is required, something that is already in line with the current situation and that focuses on an adequate doctor-patient relationship that is the most exact manifestation that represents the very essence of medicine.

To do this we must become the engines of change, starting within ourselves and then transmitting it to others both in words and in acts and deeds. and humane.

3.ASIA

HUMANISM IN CHILD NEUROLOGY: A CONUNDRUM IN INDIA

Rekha Mittal
Additional Director (Pediatric Neurology)
Madhukar Rainbow Children's Hospital,
New Delhi, India
President, Association of Child Neurology (India)

Vishal Sondhi
Associate Professor
Department of Pediatrics,
Armed Forces Medical College,
Pune, India

INTRODUCTION

Humanism, as defined in, "Attitudes and habits of highly humanistic physicians," is the combination of "scientific knowledge and skills with respectful, compassionate care that is sensitive to the values, autonomy, and cultural backgrounds of patients and their families" [1]. The authors also add that this concept has "foundered as medicine (has) evolved into an increasingly analytic, biomedically focused field." Humanism, though variedly defined, succinctly implies a rational philosophy of life that is informed by science, inspired by art, motivated by compassion with the aim of asserting the dignity of each human being. It is the ethical life stance that stands for building a more humane society.

The following experience by the second author during his residency period represents the different perspectives of humanism, right from the period of residency. As a Pediatric Neurology Resident of a busy government hospital, working in Pediatric Neurology OPD meant seeing nearly 400 patients divided among 7-10 residents in a period of 6 hours; this meant completing the evaluation of each patient within 9-10 minutes. Despite the scarce time, all residents shared stories of their cases at the end of the day. That afternoon, my "story of the day" was a family of four that had travelled more than 1500 km, after a 30-hour train journey. The father was a daily wage earner, with an average daily income of Rs 60-per-day (less than a dollar-per-day). They had with them, an alert four-months floppy infant in the lap with tongue fasciculations, hypotonia, and areflexia; a floppy infant, with a likely diagnosis of spinal muscular atrophy. Genetic testing was advised and would cost them INR 500 (~USD8) – after concession. However, the father refused the test; he was forthright about it – he could not afford it. His only question was how long the child would survive; and what could be done to ease suffering of the child.

The four resident doctors discussing the family had different perspectives. One saw the tragedy of a helpless infant, destined to die early, no matter what the treatment; the second saw a complacent family letting their child die from a terminal disease without putting in enough effort; the third saw a culture, values and disparity that he felt were hard truths in an unequal and immoral world; and I thought of the recent article on the success of Nusinersen, which was far away from the child, literally and metaphorically; the family would never even know of its existence. This discussion filled me with conflicting thoughts. The family seemed devoted, but was just financially incapable of taking care of the infant, the way "we" wanted them to; should we sit on judgement on them? Should they be considered uncaring or immoral because of a financial limitation?

This incident reflects daily conflict in medical practice and reverberates with most pediatric neurologists in India. Humanism, just like the four residents sitting in the consultation chamber, has many viewpoints and every individual is entitled to his or her own perspective.

PEDIATRIC NEUROLOGICAL DISORDERS: CHANGES AND CHALLENGES

The Global Burden of Disease Study in 2015 estimated that neurological disorders ranked as the leading cause-group of global disability-adjusted life-years (DALY) in 2015 (250·7 million, comprising 10·2% of global DALYs) and the second-leading cause-group of deaths (9·4 [9·1 to 9·7] million, comprising 16·8% of global deaths) [2]. A significant proportion of this affliction is either the pediatric population, or patients who have transitioned into adulthood, but the disease started in childhood. Thus, the burden of Pediatric neurological disorders is large and increasing, and poses a challenge to the sustainability of health systems

Certain characteristics of pediatric neurological disorders make them inherently difficult to manage, necessitating extraordinary humanistic skills. These include the following:

1. Most pediatric neurological disorders are chronic. Almost all of them result in varying degree of physical and intellectual impairment and disability, often requiring assisted living, not only as children but through adulthood [3].

2. Many disorders are progressive, and regression in a normal child, with possible early death, can be more devastating, both emotionally and financially, than the sudden loss of a child due to a catastrophic CNS insult.

3. Intellectual disability and behavioral problems are often associated with many pediatric neurological disorders. This may impair the interaction between the child and family members, resulting in a cycle of detachment, neglect, guilt and emotional distress.

4. The etiology of many of the neurological disorders remains unknown despite extensive investigations. Till the diagnosis is resolved, parents remain occupied with finding the cause, rather than working on better care of the child [4].

All of this translates into children and families vulnerable not only because of medical condition itself, but the financial and social repercussions as well. They are thus in particular need of solace and a humanitarian approach.

INDIAN PERSPECTIVE ON HUMANISM IN CHILD NEUROLOGY: A TANGLED WEB

India is a vast country with a present population of over 1.38 billion and nearly 30% of these are children below 15 years. The uniqueness of India lies not only in the number of people but also in its cultural diversity, the financial disparity, incongruent literacy, inadequate rehabilitation facilities and skewed doctor-patient ratio.

Patrick French in his book, India: A Portrait, which the author calls an "intimate biography of 1.2 billion people," admits that India "with its overlap of extreme wealth and lavish poverty, its mix of the educated and ignorant, its competing ideologies, its lack of uniformity, its kindness and profound cruelty, its complex relationships with religion, its parallel realities and the rapid speed of social change—is a macrocosm, and may be the world's default setting for the future" [5].

In addition, like other developing countries, India is passing through a phase of epidemiological transition wherein a significant burden of diseases related to infections/ infestations (meningo-encephalitis, tuberculosis, neurocysticercosis), adverse perinatal conditions (cerebral palsy) and malnutrition coexist with an increasing affliction with traumatic, neoplastic, metabolic, vascular, neuroimmunologic and genetic disorders [3-6]. Thus, India has practically more than twice the burden of disease, and less than half the healthcare facilities as compared to the western countries.

Additionally, medical guidelines are mostly driven by western researchers working in advanced medical systems, where nuances of the local cultural values of different regions are not understood. The Pediatric Neurologist on ground has to adapt to the socio-cultural and financial circumstances of each individual patient.

The most prominent areas where the humanistic skills of practicing Pediatric Neurologists are brought to the fore in India include:

CULTURAL DIVERSITY

The cultural diversity of India manifests with 22 languages and six main religions that are practiced in the country [7].

Within each religion, there are multiple castes, tribes and sects that are based on traditional social and occupational divisions. The net result is that the national population of over 1.38 billion comprises some 50,000 to 60,000 endogamous sub-populations. This impacts several management aspects of pediatric neurological disorders, ranging from the ways in which health/ disease is perceived to health seeking behavior and attitudes of parents.

Hechanova and Waeldle suggest that there are five key components of diverse cultures that have implications for mental health professionals [8,9]. While the authors make their arguments in the specific context of mental health and disaster situations in Southeast Asia, their comments provide a framework for cultural diversity in the context of neurological disorders among children.

The first element that they identify is emotional expression [9]. In context of Indian setting, an affluent family may be boisterous, loud and impatient with regard to disease and management; while another family from an underprivileged section of society may feel almost "guilty" of coming to you. Similarly, pain may be exaggerated in the former and may go unexpressed in the latter. Gauging the actual situation is imperative for correct medical management as well as for appropriate emotional and moral support; it requires patience and empathy, a skill often honed by many years of medical practice.

The second element is shame [9]. This element plays a significant role in disorders of cognition, learning and behavior, e.g. children with autism spectrum disorder, learning disabilities and attention deficit hyperactivity disorder. This shame stems from the notion that society would think the child is "crazy," and in an attempt to protect family reputation and personal dignity, parents may end up delaying management. The stigma attached to some of the disorders (including epilepsy) is huge and may even lead to family being ousted from the village. Denouncing the family for delay in seeking appropriate medical help serves no purpose; it only results in guilt, or family members blaming each other, which is counter-productive. Shame can also result from information to the family about the inheritance patterns; there may be ostracization of the carrier or affected parent, especially in case of maternally inherited disorders. Extreme tact is required to manage genetic counseling in such families. The Pediatric Neurologist in such cases may choose to reveal the genetics only to the mother, if it appears that she might become an outcast in the family.

The third is power [9]. This involves two aspects: first, the power hierarchy within the family and second the power conflict between the doctor and the patient. Though the mother is usually the pivot of history taking in a child with a neurological disorder, providing antenatal, perinatal and developmental details and other minute clues which only she might have noticed, the child neurologist in India may end up with the daunting task of taking history from grandmother/ grandfather of the child, because she may have been rendered powerless in a patriarchal system (Figure 1). Sometimes the parents may completely surrender to doctor admitting that they know nothing as to what happened to child. In both these scenarios, the neurologist has to move on without historical details.

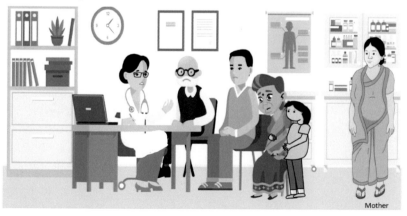

Fig 1. Family counseling. The mother, a silent bystander in the process.

Fourth, they discuss the nature of collectivism [9]. In some collectivist cultures, especially in some tribes and religions in India, the society is resilient and takes care of the disabled child. This is a tool that can be game changer and is especially useful when dealing with Buddhist families from Ladakh and Christian families from north-eastern India. The complete village is a family, is ingrained in some of them and is important while chalking therapeutic path.

And the fifth aspect they discuss is spirituality and religion from the point of view of attribution as well as in terms of coping with disease [9]. Due to this factor many families initially resort to traditional medicines (including homeopathic and ayurvedic medicine). This may not only delay the appropriate treatment but also lead to treatment related adverse effects (like heavy metal poisoning).

In addition to aforementioned elements, there are other major implications of cultural diversity in India. For example, there is a long tradition of uncle-niece marriage and unions between a man and his maternal uncle's daughter (mother's brother's daughter) in South India [10]. Also, consanguineous marriage is common among Muslim communities [11]. On the contrary, Hindus in the northern states avoid marital unions between biological kin, because of a prohibition on consanguineous marriage believed to date back to approximately 200 BC [10,11]. Thus, while enquiring about consanguinity is imperative among a Muslim family and a South Indian Hindu family, the same will spark hostility and loss of trust for the doctor examining a child from a North Indian Hindu family; extreme tact is required to elicit this aspect of the history. Furthermore, the food habits and taboos vary between this diversified population. While non-vegetarian food is staple for Muslims, it is unimaginable for some Hindu families. Also, some orthodox Hindu families abstain from cooking or eating onion and garlic [12]. These factors have to be considered when drawing up diet plans e.g., ketogenic diet, and special diets and supplements.

These cultural barriers are further compounded by linguistic impediments. Biomedicine in India exists almost solely in the realm of English. Students, at all levels of healthcare related education (doctors, nurses, paramedical workers) read medical textbooks written in English and are expected to write their examinations in English [7]. Consequently, their technical understanding of biomedical conditions is in the English language. In addition, health workers are often not completely fluent in languages that are not their mother-tongue, which results in non-English-speaking patients receiving very simplistic messages or crude translations, free from nuances essential for a patient to make a genuinely informed decision [7]. Furthermore, the internal migration of individuals frequently leads to situations of language discordance in clinical setting for example, a Telegu speaking individual living in Kerala, where Malayalam is the mother tongue. Thus, the patients who are more likely to experience language discordance in the clinic such as members of linguistic minorities and illiterate migrant laborers are also more likely to access care in overcrowded, understaffed public hospitals and clinics where health workers cannot spend much time with each individual and the power differential between doctors and patients is greater. Additionally, all the medicines have labels and strengths in English, which the parents are often unable to read. It is common practice in India for the patient to buy all the medicines in the prescription, and return to the doctor who, no matter how busy they are, often goes over each medicine with dose and timing. The prescription often has a diagrammatic representation of the doses, which the patients find easier to understand (Figure 2).

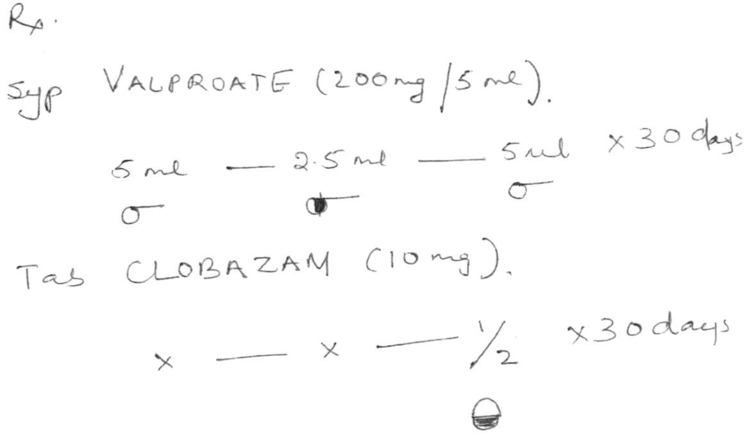

Fig 2. A sample hand written prescription, showing doses

Thus, a child neurologist in India overcomes discordance at multiple echelons of culture, language and family structure in order to improve familial satisfaction and quality of care of children with neurological ailments.

ECONOMIC DISPARITY

The landscape of Indian healthcare system ranges from the glitzy steel and glass structures of state-of-the-art corporate hospitals to ramshackle outposts [13]. The private sector is the dominant player in the healthcare arena in India; the public healthcare system, though offering care at low or no cost is perceived as unreliable and not sought if one can afford private system. In addition, apart from the recently launched national insurance scheme (Ayushman Bharat), only ~10% of the Indian population are covered by any form of health insurance. Thus, >75% of healthcare expenditure comes from the pockets of households, and individuals who are poor are most sensitive to the cost of health care and effect of health expenditures are greater in rural areas. In 2004–05, about 39·0 million (30·6 million in rural areas and 8·4 million in urban areas) Indian people fell into poverty every year as a result of out-of-pocket expenditures [14]. These estimates do not take into account the effects on people already living below the poverty line who are pushed further into poverty or those groups who are forced to forego health care as a result of the costs. These financial health-care constraints do not include the additional costs associated with seeking care, such as costs of foregone wages, transportation, childcare, or the loss of earnings due to ill health [14]. Moreover, many disorders in child neurology require frequent follow-up, repeated investigations (like neuroimaging, EEG), long-term pharmacotherapy (like anti-seizure drugs), rehabilitation protocols (like speech therapy, occupational therapy); and despite these efforts a proportion of children may have lifelong disabilities of varying magnitude. Thus, the economically challenged and socially marginalized individuals have to make a "humane" but seemingly harsh choice between spending their limited resources towards educating the apparently healthy child or on a child who may or may not be able to achieve full potential. The onus again is on the neurologist, to chalk a path that conforms with finances of the family and also does not deviate from the "evidence-based recommendations" made by experts. An example would be prescribing a drug of second choice, which is cheaper (phenytoin), rather than an expensive drug of choice (carbamazepine / oxcarbazepine) in focal seizures.

Many pediatric neurologists (in fact, many practitioners) with stand-alone practices, actually bill the patients after the consultation is over. This gives them a chance to assess the economic status of the family, and charge accordingly, so that no patient remains bereft of medical advice.

ACCESS TO HEALTHCARE

In India, individuals with the greatest need for health care have the greatest dificulty in accessing health services and are least likely to have their health needs met. Beyond the socioeconomic domain, there are two more factors that affect the accessibility to healthcare in India: gender and location. A recent study from North India demonstrates that male: female ratio in pediatric outpatient was 1.8:1, and the authors concluded that female patients, especially younger females, who reside further away from the facility are less likely to visit the facility [15]. Distance is another important non-monetary barrier that impedes access to health care, especially in rural areas. This physical reach of healthcare is defined as "the ability to enter a healthcare facility within 5km from the place of residence or work" [13]. A recent study assessing institutional delivery in rural India reported that only ~58% of the women in rural India live within 5km of health facility [16]. Most of the textbooks mention a "multidisciplinary approach" for management of child with chronic neurological disorder and majority of rural setups are inadequate for the same. Hence, for a large majority of Indian population, the "multidisciplinary approach" is usually several kilometers and some hours away. As a result, there is a delay in deciding to seek care; delay in reaching an adequate healthcare facility and delay in follow up. Hence, it is essential that the management plan is individualized focusing on these aspects. This may mean deviating from established protocols, for example, starting of antiepileptic drugs even after a first unprovoked seizure if the child resides in place where healthcare facilities are not easily accessible.

HUMAN POWER CRISIS

India's health workforce is made up of a range of health workers. The workforce includes many informal medical practitioners, generally called the registered medical practitioners (RMP). For a large proportion of population, especially the poor and those in rural setting, the RMP are often the first point of contact. They usually have strong professional links with qualified allopathic doctors, neuroimaging facilities, pathology laboratories, and corporate hospitals to which they refer patients in return for commission [17]. Results from one study suggest that 25% of individuals classified as allopathic doctors (42% in rural areas and 15% in urban areas) have no medical training [17].

A 2011 study estimated that India has roughly 20 healthcare workers per 10,000 population: allopathic doctors (31%), nurses (30%), pharmacists (11%), AYUSH (indigenous medicine) practitioners (9%) and others (9%) [13,17]. A child with the neurological disorder requires care beyond allopathy, and nursing; involving speech-, occupational-, physio-therapist, genetic counsellor, and nutritionist. And going by the above data, these constitute less than 2 per 10,000 population. In addition, this workforce is not distributed optimally, with most preferring to work in areas where facilities for family life are superior. Thus, the Pediatric Neurologist often ends up advising on this aspect of management as well, if he feels this would be inaccessible to the child.

The patients routed through the networks of RMP and other alternative channels frequently reach the neurologist late; they may be on wrong management principles or on inadequate drug doses and would have spent substantial financial resources before the optimal treatment is envisaged. Often the RMPs command great respect and faith in the family's residential area, and they may also have to be taken into confidence before starting treatment.

The neurologist, therefore, has to navigate through these issues before the child can be helped. Thus, the key to a humane pediatric neurology practice in India lies in adapting it to allow for social, cultural, economic, educational and residential differences, instead of a "one size fits all": in effect, a form of personalized medicine, to bring about best results not only for the affected child, but the family and health providers as well.

CONCLUSION

Despite the above-mentioned challenges, practicing child neurology in India is exciting; probably the challenges make it more fulfilling. The last two decades have witnessed a deepening interest in Child Neurology. Structured training courses, including DM and fellowships in child neurology and epilepsy, are now available at multiple centers in the country. These will improve the physical doctor-patient gap. Foundation courses that stress communication skills and the economics of medicine have been made part of medicine curriculum in an attempt to bridge the meta-physical doctor-patient gap.

Back to the "story of the day" narrated earlier:

The next day, as I walked to work, I wondered what I would come across next. My eyes fell on the family sitting by the roadside, with the younger infant in the lap of mother. The elder sibling ran to me and presented me with a drawing made with the limited crayons that she had: a drawing of sunrise. Was it a new dawn around the corner? I thanked the child, patted the cheeks of my little patient, and wished good luck to family. I turned around, feeling confident there were many facets to a situation.

As Michael Shermer puts it, "The goal of scientific humanism is not utopia but protopia—incremental improvements in understanding and beneficence as we move ever further into the open-ended frontiers of knowledge and wisdom" and tenacious protopia is what we aim for here in Incredible India [18].

REFERENCES

1. Chou CM, Kellom K, Shea JA. Attitudes and habits of highly humanistic physicians. Academic medicine. 2014;89(9):1252-8.

2. Group GBDNDC. Global, regional, and national burden of neurological disorders during 1990-2015: a systematic analysis for the Global Burden of Disease Study 2015. Lancet Neurol. 2017;16(11):877-97.

3. Mohamed IN, Elseed MA, Hamed AA. Clinical Profile of Pediatric Neurological Disorders: Outpatient Department, Khartoum, Sudan. Child Neurol Open. 2016;3:2329048X15623548.

4. Popp JM, Robinson JL, Britner PA, Blank TO. Parent adaptation and family functioning in relation to narratives of children with chronic illness. J Pediatr Nurs. 2014;29(1):58-64.

5. French P. India: A portrait: Vintage; 2011.

6. Sahu J. Child neurology in India: challenges and opportunities. Journal of the International Child Neurology Association. 2017.

7. Narayan L. Addressing language barriers to healthcare in India. National Med J India. 2013;26(4):236-8.

8. Gopalkrishnan N. Cultural Diversity and Mental Health: Considerations for Policy and Practice. Front Public Health. 2018;6:179.

9. Hechanova R, Waelde L. The influence of culture on disaster mental health and psychosocial support interventions in Southeast Asia. Mental Health, Religion & Culture. 2017;20(1):31-44.

10. Krishnamoorthy S, Audinarayana N. Trends in consanguinity in South India. Journal of biosocial science. 2001;33(2):185-97.

11. Bittles AH. The impact of consanguinity on the Indian population. Indian Journal of Human Genetics. 2002;8(2):45-51.

12. Meyer-Rochow VB. Food taboos: their origins and purposes. Journal of ethnobiology and ethnomedicine. 2009;5(1):18.

13. Kasthuri A. Challenges to healthcare in India-The five A's. Indian journal of community medicine: official publication of Indian Association of Preventive & Social Medicine. 2018;43(3):141.

14. Balarajan Y, Selvaraj S, Subramanian S. India: towards universal health coverage 4. Health care and equity in India Lancet. 2011;377:505-15.

15. Kapoor M, Agrawal D, Ravi S, Roy A, Subramanian S, Guleria R. Missing female patients: an observational analysis of sex ratio among outpatients in a referral tertiary care public hospital in India. BMJ open. 2019;9(8):e026850.

16. Kumar S, Dansereau EA, Murray CJ. Does distance matter for institutional delivery in rural India? Applied Economics. 2014;46(33):4091-103.

17. Rao M, Rao KD, Kumar AS, Chatterjee M, Sundararaman T. Human resources for health in India. The Lancet. 2011;377(9765):587-98.

18. Shermer M. The Case for Scientific Humanism. Scientific American. 2019;320(1).

SOCIAL AND CULTURAL FACTORS IN MEDICAL C.ARE OF CHILD NEUROLOGY IN JAPAN; FROM A PHYSICIAN'S PERSONAL EXPERIENCE

Masanori Takeoka MD, FAES
Department of Neurology
Boston Children's Hospital
Harvard Medical School
Boston, Massachusetts

INTRODUCTION

When providing medical care of child neurology in Japan, there are many factors that need to be considered. While there are many differences in the medical system, factors associated with such systems and linked economic factors will not be discussed here. We will focus on the factors involving humanism, social and cultural factors that play a major role.

I will present my view based on personal experience growing up in the Japanese culture, with a family of physicians, attending medical school, and clinically practicing at academic and community medical facilities in Japan. Currently practicing child neurology at an academic institution in the United States with many international referrals, I have had the opportunity to see the clinical practice of child neurology in Japan from an outside view, and allow comparing to other various cultures.

Japan has been accepting more immigrants from overseas over the past few decades although the overwhelming majority of the population is still those born and brought up in Japan; I will not discuss here about factors relevant to providing medical care for immigrant children in Japan.

CULTURAL BELIEFS

The predominant religions in Japan are Shinto and Buddhism, with Shinto being the older religion.

Shinto is polytheism focusing much on nature; although not clear, the religions has been in Japan for around 2000 years or even longer.

Buddhism was introduced in Japan in mid sixth century. Later Shinto and Buddhism have undergone syncretism of the two religions, which has become the overwhelming majority belief in the country. Other religions such as Christianity and Islam are minority.

Understanding the beliefs in Shinto and Buddhism, in the syncretism form in Japan, is important when trying to understand the cultural and religious background while providing medical care in Japan.

Japanese people in general relatively accepts events that are associated with nature more than in other cultures, including natural cause of death and even natural disasters. They commonly share very high levels of love, fear and respect to mother nature. Similar beliefs may be seen in other cultures such as in within Asia, although this may be more extreme in Japan.

As a part of that belief, they tend to believe in and respect life in all forms without hierarchy (plants, animals, insects etc.). There is also belief in second life after death, and reincarnation which may potentially take place as different form of life, not as a human being.

Considering such background in beliefs, they often are able to accept the natural course of illnesses much more as inevitable, compared to other cultures. Not intervening and accepting the natural course, is a more acceptable option to medical care in many cases.

On the other hand, human intervention is considered more optional, and they are less likely to accept treatment related risks and adverse reactions. In general, mortality and morbidity associated with human intervention is less accepted, compared to having the same consequence as a part of a natural course.

EXPECTATIONS VS. TRUE FEELINGS

I often find that I need to show I share their common background and beliefs before patients and families open up to communicate.

There is the concept of "tatemae" and "honne," the first representing socially expected comments and behavior, while the latter representing true feelings, intentions and beliefs.

When interacting with patients and families in the clinic setting, they often start at the initial encounter with expressing their "tatemae," with expectations of how the communications will go at the visit and expectations of the outcome (e.g. receiving the expected type of prescription medications, or having diagnostic evaluations they had in mind).

The "honne" part often is not shown in the initial encounter; patients and families will take time to build belief and trust in their providers before they open up and express their "honne."

Overall, Japanese people have a general belief that there is "less variation" in ethnic background among Japan people, sharing common ancestry, cultures and values of life; this is likely not true, as there are likely many geographic origins from where the human race migrated and settled in the Japanese Islands. These include areas from the Northern Asian continent and the islands from the South.

Either way, it takes time through many conversations, often mentioning and discussing non-medical topics, to demonstrate that I share common culture, beliefs and values before patients and families open up and share their "honne."

PERSONAL TRUST AND PRIVATE DISCUSSIONS

Because of such issues in trust and beliefs, patients and families are less open about discussing personal information; it takes time to discuss issues that they may not feel directly involved with the medical care they are seeking.

The "team approach" meetings with multiple medical providers, are not accepted in Japan in general; they could be viewed as "bullying" patients with families, forcing the medical opinion with a large number of specialists. This view may be stronger in Japanese people in particular, as they are not comfortable to freely express their true thoughts when multiple people are present.

There is also a culture of feeling "shame" when patients and families express something that is against specialists such as medical providers, in particular when there are multiple such specialists at the same time.

When there are multiple providers, also the degree that patients and family feel trust, may greatly differ from one provider to another.

Based on such factors, when attempting "team meetings" with multiple medical providers, patients and families will shut down and only mention their "tatemae" not their "honne."

In general, the only way to hear their "honne" is spending time to build trust and have highly private conversations often by one provider at a time.

Families also like to have high level of control of the distribution of personal or private information.

For similar reasons, patients and families do not like cross coverage of medical care; often they only accept such coverage only for emergencies and temporary care; the cross covering physicians often will get access only to their "tatemae" and not to their "honne," in regards to longer term care. They like to keep information limited to primary medical provider and limit information to others; however, each patient and family member may have their own standards for such level of communications.

On the other hand, there are also times when patients and families may shop around without telling their primary medical provider. This often happens when patients and families are not able to obtain their desired outcome, and before there is a firm trust built between the primary provider and the patients and/ or families.

There may be the factor of "shame" on both sides regarding second opinions; the expectation is not to openly seek a second opinion, unless openly admitting there is lack of full trust. Once such lack of trust is admitted by the provider, patient and/or family, this may be interpreted as "disrespect" (could be to various degrees), and it is much more difficult to repair in Japan.

CULTURE OF RESPECT AND EXPECTATIONS, IN GENERAL

Generally Japanese people show respect to accomplished people, in regards to their role or position in the society (teachers, professors, physicians, etc.) more often that as an individual person.

In the medical field, most patients and families respect physicians and medical staff, and do not like to disagree and make them unhappy; also Japanese people expect that such behavior may not help obtain the service and care they are seeking.

This also comes from expectations of generally being polite and kind to each other in the "public" (they are more open to family members), resulting in expressing their "tatemae," not their "honne."

Such concept regarding expectations and adjusting communications may be a factor contributing to their tendencies and preferences, of avoid taking share of responsibility in medical decision making.

They tend to trust and expect their medical providers to take care and be responsible of the outcome.

In general, patients and families have more difficulties dealing with negative outcomes, when they are associated with expected risks involved in medical interventions. As above, they will accept such outcomes better if the medical provider explains that the outcome was associated with the inevitable natural course of the illness.

However, they are less likely to accept errors in diagnosis, which is no different than in any industrialized society/culture.

CONCEPT OF RIGHTS AND RESPONSIBILITIES WITH DEMOCRACY IN JAPAN

Historically, democracy was not a part of Japanese culture and was brought into Japan with modernization, but likely in fragmented forms. Japanese politicians and educators often discuss human and political rights without the concept of accompanying responsibilities.

Long before democracy there have been the concept of responsibilities without rights, thus most Japanese have been educated that they are totally independent.

Because of such misconception, Japanese patients and families do not feel that consent and agreement to treatment is accompanied by sharing responsibility in decision making and outcomes.

The approach from patients and families is highly variable, regardless of educational level. Some may show extreme interest in self-learning to be involved in medical decisions, while others will have no interest and have the medical provider take total responsibility.

COMPLEXITY OF THE LANGUAGE AND WRITTEN COMMUNICATIONS

The complexity of the Japanese language is another factor when trying to communicate with patients and families.

Verbal and non-verbal communications are both major components.

Regarding the Japanese language, there are many ways of expressions, based on social factors including hierarchy.

"Keigo" is the form of Japanese expressions adjusted by hierarchy and social situations. "Sonkeigo" is one of its forms expressing respect by modifying and elevating descriptions of acts associated with the opponent of the conversation. Oppositely, "kenjogo" shows respect by modifying and lowering descriptions of own acts, thus showing humbleness. Finally, "teineigo" is used for more general use, without adjusting to hierarchy and whether the acts relate to self or the opponent.

In general, "sonkeigo" and "kenjogo" are considered more formal.

Without social experience, many younger adults who even grow up in the Japanese culture may mix up "sonkeigo" and "kenjogo"; appropriate usage needs years and decades of experience. When uncertain, many younger adults may mostly use "teineigo" and avoid the more formal other two forms to avoid humiliation from improper use.

Separately, Japanese young adults like to create their own abbreviations, regardless whether they are accepted outside of Japan or not. The younger generation adults and adolescents often are quick in adopting, and once they become widely used, these abbreviations may become publicly accepted words in the language (e.g. Japanese "Anime").

Awareness of such variable expressions, some that are traditional and some that are changing, is a great challenge when trying to learn to communicate with others in Japan, even in the clinical setting.

In regards to the written Japanese language, through grade 9 Japanese students are mandated to learn over 2000 characters that are necessary to read newspapers and official printed documents. For medical documentation, there are a few hundred additional special characters for medical use only that need to be learned.

English is a mandatory subject in school; however, the focus of learning is on reading and writing in English, not on oral communication. Providing medical discussions with patients and families in English, is not an option for the clinics in Japan. When desperate, most Japanese adults may be able to read written English and look up words as necessary; however, verbal discussions in English are extremely difficult for most Japanese adults, unless they have spent time living overseas.

NON-VERBAL COMMUNICATIONS AND PERSONAL EXPECTATIONS

Non-verbal forms of communication play a major role when communicating with Japanese people. There is a great amount of information communicated through nonverbal cues.

They also like to often use "indirect expressions," avoiding "direct expressions and communications" in many situations in particular when not in agreement with the opponent.

Generally, Japanese patients and families also expect medical providers to acknowledge and even know how to interpret nonverbal cues and "indirect expressions." This is often encountered when they want to gently sent messages of disagreement to their medical provider, in particular to those that they trust.

CULTURAL EXPECTATIONS AND SOCIAL / COMMUNITY PRESSURE

Overall, it is expected by many Japanese patients and families that the medical providers follow general expectations commonly shared by people grown up in the Japanese society, to gain their full trust. They may show respect to their specific role as providers but do not show full trust or tell their "honne," when they do not feel they share the same beliefs and cultural expectations.

Historically in the past, local community leaders without global knowledge and understanding, have misinterpreted and taken initiatives on their own, tried to develop and enforce their own rules and values. This often happened with good intent, but without the guidance from regional or national leadership, and at times were uncontrolled and forceful. These local leaders often have provided social pressure on others within the local community, to follow such local beliefs and standards. Generally Japanese people tend to fear isolation from such local communities with common beliefs, and also tend to strongly discriminate those that resist.

Many people who have grown up in the Japanese culture do not realize this problematic and potentially dangerous tendency, unless they experience living in communities and societies outside of Japan, involving other cultural beliefs. Such tendencies of social pressure from the local level were often likely contributing to tragic historic events in the past, at times involved in various socioeconomic discrimination and conflicts. Such tendency is still currently seen with tragic events regarding Social network services (SNS).

It is important to acknowledge such tendency for expectations and beliefs when dealing with Japanese patients and families in the clinic. While the Japanese society is realizing the potential danger, the general public in Japan is still in the immature state, in understanding the responsibilities of accepting and protecting those with other opinions and values; this applies to cases even within the traditional Japanese community, and not just for others with various cultures and beliefs from outside of Japan.

SPECIFIC FACTORS RELATED TO CLINICAL CHILD NEUROLOGY IN JAPAN

Neurological illnesses are a common reason for seeking care in children in Japan, with seizures, developmental delay and motor weaknesses being common reasons for seeking medical care.

As febrile seizures are common in Japanese children, seizures in the setting of fever is generally accepted without discrimination; in general, symptoms associated with acute illnesses that are likely transient (such as convulsions with infections or trauma), are better accepted by families and society, compared to chronic and hereditary conditions.

Historically, children with intellectual disability and epilepsy have been stigmatized, which has improved over time; in rural areas, residual stigmatization may still exist. There is social discrimination to children who are physically and mentally "different" from others. Such social stigmatization could still interfere with access to medical care.

The barriers to establish relations and building trust with the patients and families, are no different in child neurology compared to other pediatric subspecialties, although the discrimination factor may be more common for the epilepsy and developmental or intellectual issues as above.

In recent years, adults with epilepsy have come more open to disclose their illnesses; however, it is still common that families may resist disclosing family history of neurological and psychiatric disorders.

Similarly, illegal drug use in children and adolescents is socially stigmatized and subject to discrimination, thus often such history in patients or family members are often not disclosed.

OTHER SOCIAL FACTORS

Japanese pharmacies have a long tradition and experience in dispensing medications in powder form using sachets, in particular for children. While tablet forms are available, patients and families are not expected to split, cut, or crush tablets at home. If crushing is necessary, pharmacies are expected to crush and prepare in sachets when dispensing.

Such practices also likely stems from the concept that patients and families are not expected to need taking additional steps with their prescribed medications.

Likely associated with expectations of patients and families, they expect having local providers be able to provide most high-level care, and they are not willing to travel long distances for medical care.

This issue with physical access and travelling may also be associated with the unwillingness in many cases, to take responsibility and take the initiative to seek desired medical providers for their care, or to be involved in medical decision making.

They also expect easier access to medical care, preferring frequent visits locally, and used to walk-in visits or scheduled with minimal waiting time (e.g. within the week).

CONCLUSIONS

Overall, there are many psychosocial and cultural factors to consider when providing care for children with neurological disorders in Japan.

Dealing with issues with verbal and nonverbal communications may be the initial step; afterwards, showing the acceptance of common beliefs and values, also personal and social expectations, are critical to build trust.

In clinical care, such steps are very important for Japanese patients and families to feel comfortable to open up and express their true feelings. They are very resistant to open discussions, needing more privacy, even more so than in other industrialized societies.

Overall, such delicate communications involve politeness, being formal, and sensitive to culture, beliefs and expectations.

Table 1. Psychosocial factors to consider (when taking care of children with neurological conditions in Japan)

Expected responses vs. true beliefs and feelings ("tatemae" vs. "honne")

Complexity of Language

Nonverbal cues / communication

Shared beliefs and cultural background

Respect factor

Personal expectations

Social / community expectations

THE BASIS OF CHINESE MEDICAL ETHICS: ANALYSIS OF ANALOGIES AND DIFFERENCES WITH MEDICAL ETHICS IN THE WESTERN HEMISPHERE

Edgard Andrade- MD, MS, FAAP & FAES
Pediatric Neurologist and Epileptologist, Institute of Pediatric Neurosciences, Ocala, FL. USA

Zhao Liu, MD, PhD
Division Head, Pediatric Neurology, Department of Pediatrics, University of Illinois, Peoria, IL. USA

I. Introduction

II. Fundamentals of ancient Chinese biomedical ethics

III. The four principles of ancient Chinese medical ethics

IV. Conclusion

V. References

INTRODUCTION

The four principles of modern biomedical ethics---justice, beneficence, non-maleficence and respect for autonomy---were originally described by Beauchamp and Childress in America and by Gillon in Europe in the 1970's [1]. Such principles have been popularly accepted in most of the Western hemisphere medical field as universal and unequivocal guidelines in the medical decision-making process [2]. As a consequence, this viewpoint has led to the conclusion that any personal preferences such as philosophy, religion, beliefs, moral theory or stance towards life situations can be adapted to the aforementioned four moral principles and their scope of application. This universal approach to biomedical ethics and the four ethical principles are assumed to be transcultural and utilize a similar language that can be applied in a cross cultural context worldwide [3]. However, this approach is sometimes challenged in Eastern societies such as China or Middle Eastern countries. The basis of this criticism is that ethical issues are a manifestation of a specific local culture so the four ethical principles cannot be applied in every situation worldwide. In addition, the fact that the ethical theory is developed from an American common morality suggests that it may not be generalizable, transferable or applied universally to other societies [4].

The aim of this manuscript is to describe past and current principles of Chinese medical ethics and how the four basic principles of Western biomedical ethics might apply to Chinese society based on the Chinese foundation of such principles and to evaluate the feasibility of a transcultural application of the principles into a different non-western cultural context. Then, the chapter will discuss the basis of Chinese medical ethics and will test if the four principles exist in Chinese culture and if they are comparable to Chinese medical standards. In the chapter's second half, we describe the universality of virtue ethics and how Chinese teaching has focused on this aspect of medical practice in comparison to its role in Western bioethics. Finally, the chapter will describe the current Chinese medical bioethical principles and the need to join right virtue to right action and contrast them with the four principles of Western biomedical ethics and summarize the applicability of Chinese ancient bioethical principles in the modern era.

FUNDAMENTALS OF ANCIENT CHINESE BIOMEDICAL ETHICS

The most representative author of medical ethics in China was the physician and Taoist Sun Szu-miao who appeared in the medical literature in the seventh century with the book On the Absolute Sincerity of Great Physicians. The principles promulgated in that book continue to be the main drivers of the current Chinese practice of medicine [5]. Szu-miao underscored the necessity of extensive education and rigorous self-discipline. In addition, he highlighted the importance of compassion and human kindness as the basis of medical practice. Sun Szu-miao described the current principles of medical ethics in five areas:

Area 1: The purpose of medical practice

1.The goal is to help not to gain material goods.

2.Save lives and do not kill the living.

3.Avoid seeking fame.

Area 2: The requirements of a good physician

1.Master the foundations of medicine, working energetically and enthusiastically.

2.Be calm and firm in disposition: do not compromise your integrity to selfish wishes.

3.Commit to save every living creature with great compassion.

Area 3: The manner of medical practice

1.Possess a clear mind and maintain a dignified appearance.

2.Avoid excessive talking, provocative speech, or bullying others.

3.Do not consider self-interest and personal fortune. Rather, sympathize and help the needy.

4. Examine and diagnose carefully, prescribe accurately and cure effectively.

Area 4: Attitude towards patients

1.Treat others as you would want them to treat you, no matter if the person is poor or rich.

2.Do not reject patients with difficult to treat diseases. Be compassionate and kind.

3. Do not abuse the kindness offered in the patient's house while he/she suffers the pain of the illness.

Area 5: Attitude towards other physicians

1.Do not undermine another physician to exalt your virtue.

2. Do not speak badly of others or criticize their behaviors.

The moral principles discussed by Szu-miao emphasize the need to help and the character required of a physician , based on the Confucian influence as the utmost paradigm, with other schools of thought, like Taoism and Buddhism also contributing to such values [6]. After this seminal work, other publications related to bioethics and physician moral character appeared sporadically in Chinese medical literature. Some other important authors include Chu Hui-ming in the fifteen centuries with the book Medical Cures Learned by Heart, Kung Hsin in the sixteenth century with Exhortation for Enlightened Physicians, Kung Ting-Hsien with Ten Maxims for Physicians and Ten Maxims for Patients, Chen Shih-kung in the sixteenth century with Five Commandments and Ten Requirements for Physicians and Chan-Lu in the sixteenth century with Ten Commandments for Physicians. The authors' main take home messages can be summarized as follows:

1. To appreciate the value of life and practice medicine with compassion and humaneness

2. To learn Confucianism prior to practicing medicine.

3. To improve medical knowledge by following reliable resources.

4. To improve the clinical skills and maintain a high professional decorum.

5. To be productive, not greedy for money and fame.

6. To treat patients equally as they were your relatives.

7. To be truthful and selfless in treating patients.

8. To treat female patients only in the presence of an attendant and respecting their privacy and confidentiality.

9. To be modest and prudent towards other colleagues and not to criticize them.

Careful review of these manuscripts demonstrates the influence of ancient Chinese medical ethics in the foundation of the following principles:

1. Ancient Chinese medical ethics is established on the basis of Confucian ethics. For more than twenty-five hundred years, the Confucian scriptures were essential to teach medical students. The ethical principles developed by Confucius were the dominant moral philosophy and ideology of Chinese culture. Most scholars trained in the Confucian school of thought, practiced medicine, and formulated their professional ethics on such principles [7]. Medical practice was regarded as a main lifelong duty. The moral standards for a physician were the same as if it was

of a Confucian alumnus, also known as the "superior man". It was well accepted that a physician saving the patient's lives and promoting welfare was equal to be considered a Confucian scholar's, realizing that their moral and political aspirations was to bring peace and prosperity to people [8]. A good reflection of this concept is the well-known saying that "the achievement equals that of a good prime minister" frequently used by Chinese citizens to recognize a successful physician [9].

2. Humaneness is the cornerstone of Chinese medical ethical principles. Confucius commented that the concept of humaneness is bidirectional. It is a virtue that means love and benevolence and is the general virtue of morality which is the basis of all virtues. The practice of medicine should be based on humaneness [10]. The Chinese culture exalts the merit of good physicians by calling them the heart of humaneness, because is the inherited aspects of humaneness that gives value to the practice of medicine.

3. Chinese medical ethics reveals the obligation of a duty – based ethics that emphasizes the physician's responsibility to care for their patients and not seek profit and fame nor compromise their integrity with selfish wishes and desires, making Chinese medical ethics a strong deontological system [7].

4. Chinese medical ethics is a virtue based Confucian ethics. Confucianism describes the morality of an individual as the cornerstone to the achievement of social order and the basis for the blossoming of human kindness. If physicians cultivate this virtue, it will guarantee the ethical aspects of their medical practice. Personal traits like wisdom, selflessness, restraint, modesty, sincerity, compassion, humaneness, righteousness, trustfulness, frugality, diligence and determination are key aspects of Chinese medical ethics [11]. Only a physician who practices such

virtues is considered a good physician. Also, the fact that physicians with both skills and virtues are considered admirable and praised is a reminder of the indispensability of medical virtue.

Since the seventh century, after the time of Szu-miao, ancient Chinese medical ethics was based in the Confucian theory. Chinese physicians and other medical providers were frequently compared with Confucian-oriented politicians who were able to accomplish goals of bringing peace and prosperity to people [12]. They were also expected to be virtuous and to achieve the moral standards described in Confucian theory. Consequently, medical virtue has been the focus of Chinese physicians in their daily practice and the maintenance of humaneness has become the main virtue.

THE FOUR PRINCIPLES OF ANCIENT CHINESE MEDICAL ETHICS

RESPECT FOR AUTONOMY

Autonomy means self-governance and implies that one can act freely according to one's own chosen plans. The basis of respect for autonomy involves a respectful attitude and respectful action. It is also implicitly acknowledged that everyone has the right to have an opinion, make choices and make decisions based on their own believes and values. The autonomous actions of an individual should not be constrained by others when no harm is inflicted to other persons.

The concept of autonomy is the youngest medical principle of modern medical ethics. American medical ethics has incorporated the autonomy principles primarily in the last 30 years [13]. Therefore, there are not many bibliographic resources exploring issues such as the respect for autonomy in ancient Chinese medical ethics. This is especially true when we recall that the ancient Chinese Empire was a society of aristocracy, patriarchy, social classes and paternalistic views. With careful examination and avoidance of hard interpretation, however, documentation of respect for autonomy can be discerned.

The concept for autonomy in Chinese medical ethics is related to Kant's principles of moral justification. In that theory, one of the most important laws describes that no person should be treated as a means to an end but rather always as an end [14]. Kantian philosophy indicates that persons are free, rational human beings and possess absolute moral value. The unconditional self-determination and capacity for freedom is the basis for a person to be respected. Kant believed that autonomy of will was the distinctive feature of a person and it was through acts of rational choice that individuals state their own dignity, making it the highest feature of human nature. Violation of personal autonomy prevents them from pursuing their goals and influencing their destiny by treating them merely as means to an end desired by others rather than as an end to themselves [15].

John Harris also supported the notion of distinctive self-consciousness, capability to value a person's own life and the intrinsic rationality that a person has and that makes that person's life valuable [13]. That life should be respected is the strongest point for morality and includes two essential elements:

1.Concern for the welfare of others

2.Respect for the wishes of others

As a consequence, respect for autonomy is the way in which one acknowledges the value of human life expressed rationally and self-consciously by others as it is for oneself and entitles others to make decisions and choices to determine their own destiny [16].

Sun Szu-miao also described an implicit requirement in all physicians to demonstrate a respectful and devoted attitude towards the patients under their care and towards the medical profession. Physicians should hold high ethical principles, maintain self-integrity, avoid selfish desires, and be concerned with their own behavior and with the patient's welfare. In other words, similarly to the Kantian school, physician should regard patients as ends and not means. In general, physicians are required to carry a strong will and self-discipline, comparable to the Kantian self-legislation and autonomy. Physicians should maintain an unconditional, categorical, and imperative duty towards patients. They should act as if they were thinking for themselves [17]. Physicians should not ponder their own fortune but rather preserve life and have compassion. Physicians should look at their patients who come for help as if they would for themselves and sympathize with their griefs. Physicians should help their patients wholeheartedly.

Sun Szu-miao also recommended not using living creatures, not even a hen's egg as medications. This approach was influenced by the Buddhist school that all living creatures are created equally and deserve respect for life [18].

Albert Schweitzer also said that the fundamental principle of morality is that human beings should approach all life with the same reverence they have for their own [13]. The basis of the ethics should be that the individual should practice the same reverence for life towards all forms of life as if it were towards their own.

Chu Hui-ming (AD 1590) physician and Confucian disciple described the virtue of veracity and telling the truth. He encouraged physicians to learn consciously from each case and avoid engaging in false practices. Hui-ming advised that physicians should be forthcoming from the beginning of the physician-patient relationship and if the medical prognosis is poor, physicians should disclose such information as soon as possible [10], to prevent shame or reproach at the end for withholding such information.

Chen Shih-kung (AD 1605) highlighted the concept of female patients' confidentiality. Physicians should not visit a female patient alone and should do so only in the presence of a witness. Female disorders should be examined with the highest discretion, kept in secret and not revealed to anyone.

The principle of respect for autonomy in Chinese medical ethics holds doctors responsible for a respectful attitude toward all patients and for assisting them to the point of their own self-sacrifice. Other qualities of Chinese medical ethics that are representative of respect for autonomy includes veracity, trustfulness, and sincerity. Chinese respect for autonomy is thus comparable to the Kantian principle of treating persons as ends and not as means.

However, in modern life, limitations on respecting patient's autonomy are multifactorial. Patient autonomy is not explicitly mentioned in ancient Chinese medical ethic principles nor in certain Western documents and codes [19]. This may be because traditionally patients come to their doctors for a cure.

Maintaining a respectful attitude towards patients is the cornerstone of an interpersonal relationship and the basis of a good doctor-patient relationship. However, this concept does not always lead to the conscious awareness of a physician respecting the autonomous choices of the patient [18]. Furthermore, in ancient Chinese medical ethics, physicians and caregivers did not always respect their patient's choices. An understanding of cultural factors and local variations of social practice may have contributed to such perception.

NON-MALEFICENCE

This principle states that a human being is not to inflict evil, harm or risk to others. Healthcare providers pursue non-maleficence through their medical training, diligent care, and competent skills. Chinese medical ethics states that mastering medical knowledge, studying reliable resources, maintaining clinical acumen, expanding one's base of knowledge and demonstrating high professional standards are the pathways to reach the standard of non-maleficence [20]. The basic requirement for all physicians to preclude doing evil and harm is to be friendly, frugal and avoid greed for wealth and fame.

Sun Szu-miao described in his publications the principles of saving life, respecting living creatures and showing devotion and diligence in medical care. Physicians should not enjoy themselves while the patient is suffering. Chinese medical ethics specifically recommends avoiding delighting while a patient is suffering [7]. The physician should not enjoy beautiful scenes nor enjoy peaceful sounds while visiting a sick patient.

Chan – Lu (AD 1627-1707) documented a set of rules for physicians that describe the practice of non-maleficence. The rules state how to maintain the standard of care, clinical competence, medical skills and prudence [21], and at the same time prevent the risk of harm to patients by avoiding the following situations:

1.Evil habits

2.Over self-confidence

3.Prejuice

4.Lack of initiative

5.Careless diagnosis

6.Magic healing

7.Treating noble and common people differently

8.Neglecting patients

9.Obtaining high compensation

10.Criticizing other physicians

BENEFICENCE

This principle refers to actions done for the well-being of others and is exemplified by mercy, humanity, love, altruism, charity, kindness, and benevolence. The cornerstone in both ancient and modern Eastern and Western medical ethics is to promote the welfare of their patients. The main area of focus in Chinese medical ethics is the moral doctrine of beneficence and compassion to humanity. Sun Szu-miao said that the main role of a physician is to help, not to gain material goods [13]. Medical doctors should commit to the care of every living creature with compassion and respect.

Kung Hsin (AD 1556) described that a good physician reflects righteousness and humaneness. Doctors should relieve pain and suffering among all the patients under their care and not focus on their own glory [10]. Physicians should treat those who are ill and restore health.

Kung Ting-Hsien (AD 1615) described the ten command-ments for physicians including the rule that they should adopt a disposition for humaneness and assist every individual with effort and good will. Ancient Chinese medical ethics expects physicians to first learn Confucianism prior to medical knowl-edge and practice medicine with compassion and humane-ness [5]. Medical practice must be regarded as a career of philanthropy, selflessness and acting with generosity to help the sick. Both ancient Chinese medical ethics and Confucian ethics thus emphasize the principle of beneficence.

JUSTICE

This principle is defined by appropriate, equitable and fair treatment in what is due or owed to other persons. Injustice is the opposite and is defined as a wrongful act or omission that denies due benefits to persons or lacks fair distribution of the burdens [22].

Gillon has described justice in the field of medical ethics as a fair distribution of scarce resources (also known as distributive justice), respect for people rights (also known as rights-based justice), and respect for morally accepted laws (also known as legal justice). In terms of ancient Chinese medical ethics, justice implies that physicians should treat the patients under their care righteously, equally and fairly [2]. Chinese medical ethics implies that physicians should provide medical care without regard to the patients' background and treat all who seek medical care. Patients should have equal access to medical care for all in need and special help should be provided to the indigent and poor.

Sun Szu-miao described that if an individual seeks medical care for illness or another difficulty, a physician should not pay attention to the social status, wealth, age, physical qualities, nationality, or level of education [8]. Doctors should treat everyone equally.

Kung Hsin (AD 1556) described that a good physician should display qualities like humaneness, appropriateness, justice, and righteousness. Medical practitioners should aim to do the right thing and do things right. The concept of justice implies appropriate treatment towards people [14].

Chen Shih-kunk (AD 1605) described the idea of treating everyone whether rich or poor the same way. He described, for instance, that prostitutes should be treated the same way as daughters of wealthy families, to exemplify characters like respect, justice, and equality [22]. He advocated for giving medicine free of charge to the poor and for facilitating financial help to the unemployed. The basis of this concept is that without food, the medicine alone cannot relieve the distress of the

illness. Along this line, Rawls defined the differential principle of justice, in which inequality should not exist at all. The
concept of justice in medical ethics requires that doctors treat
patients equally and to be compassionate with the poor and
to extend free of charge services. In terms of physician's relationships, Chinese medical ethics recommends that medical
providers be modest and prudent towards other physicians
and not criticize their colleagues [8].

UNIVERSALITY OF VIRTUE ETHICS AND CURRENT CHINESE MEDICAL ETHICS

With the influence of Western medicine, China's medical
structure has experienced rapid changes and medical professional ethics standards began to be more valued. China's medical and health care system has moved from the traditional
individual practice to the group practice in large public hospitals, which brings new moral requirements for physicians'
behavioral standards. Under the new system, the sense of responsibility of medical doctors lies not only in the sense of
responsibility for patients, but also in the sense of social responsibility, sense of responsibility for the employed hospital,
cooperation with peers, and openness to technology.

The rapid development of medical technology has revolution-
ized medicine by bringing new hope for diagnosis and treatment of human diseases, but also carries a heavy economic
burden. Ethical problems caused by medical high-technology
itself have become increasingly prominent, such as dealing
with brain death, organ transplantation, quality of life and
so on. These ethical problems cannot be solved solely by the
ancient principles. Therefore, it is necessary to establish new
and more specific moral standards that incorporate the need
to join right virtue to right action and to adapt to social developments and to medical and health services. China's Health
Ministry promulgated the medical ethics standards and implementation measures for medical personnel, which became the

first nationwide professional ethics standard with universal binding force. The norms put forward specific requirements for the behavior of medical personnel on several aspects. The first criterion is to save the dying, heal the wounded and implement socialist humanitarianism. At the same time, the code emphasizes respecting the personality and rights of patients, showing sympathy, concern and consideration for patients, not seeking personal gains through medical treatment, not divulging patients' privacy and secrets, and respecting the moral standards that medical staff of the same profession should abide by. The standard embodies the combination of traditional medical ethics and modern medical ethics. From the perspective of cross-cultural comparison, there are extensive similarities between Chinese and Western early medical ethics in the description of medical professionalism. These can be found for example in Aristotelian virtue ethics as in his Nicomachean Ethics and Eudemian Ethics as well as the Magna Moralia with its implications for medical practice. With the risk of falling into oversimplification, medical virtue ethics may be defined as a set of fundamental rules, principles or character traits that define a moral life consistent with the ends, goals and purposes of practicing medicine. Virtue ethics provided the conceptual foundation for professional ethics. Being virtuous is not sufficient itself. Right virtue has to come with right action in order to be ethical [23]. Throughout the years, however, virtue ethics has been overshadowed by principle-and rule-based ethics.

Medical ethics has experienced a process of evolution from prognosis to behavior, and then to value judgment. With the development of professionalism and the establishment of medical systems, as well as under the influence of different religions and philosophies, the development of Chinese and Western medical ethics shows their own characteristics. With the cultural background of Confucianism as the main source, "medicine is benevolence" has become the basic principle of

Chinese medical ethics. Ancient Chinese medical ethics did not emphasize the establishment of a unified moral code of conduct. With the introduction of Western medicine and the establishment of modern medical systems, however, the Chinese medical community has begun to attach importance to the construction of universal professional ethical standards based on traditional medical ethics. Especially in the current stage of social and economic transformation, it is important to strengthen professional ethics standards and to join right virtue to right action in order to be ethical [23]. In the end, whether responding to the rapid development of medical technology or to the continuous change of medical and health service systems, the fundamental Chinese standard of "medicine is benevolence" must remain vital as the essence of medicine.

CONCLUSION

The four concepts of modern western medical ethics [24], justice, beneficence, non-maleficence, and autonomy are well exemplified in Chinese medical ethics. Beneficence and non-maleficence are the corner stones in Chinese medical ethics, demonstrated by humaneness as the central theme in Confucian philosophy and the foundation of Chinese medical ethics. Justice is exemplified in Chinese medical ethics with righteousness and equal treatment towards persons and extended help to the less fortunate [1]. Autonomy is explicitly demonstrated in Chinese medical ethics through respect for patients, the requirement that they be treated as ends and not as means, and with a devoted, decorous, sincere, selfless attitude towards fair medical practice. It requires physicians to value all life with respect. One observed difference is respect for the patient's autonomy which is not mentioned explicitly in Chinese medical ethics [18].

The defined four principles provide a binding duty for physician's behavior but do not provide a strategy for conflict resolution when the competing principles clash. However, it is possible to develop justifiable and coherent answers to ethical dilemmas through overriding, balance, and specification of the principles [12]. At the same time, the process is influenced by cultural values and social conventions since medical practice is based in the doctor-patient relationship. In the typical Chinese culture, the emphasis on family values and the common good may cause individuals to sacrifice their autonomy for decision making in favor of social values or preferential family choices [17]. The public interest before individual rights may lead to the interpretation of justice, non-maleficence and beneficence in a socially oriented way which likely will suppress the concept of individual rights and autonomy. In addition, a paternalistic or patriarchal tradition may affect the doctor-patient relationship and influence the decision-making process towards medical paternalism. Therefore, a beneficence approach as oppose to an autonomy approach may be well entrenched in medical practice in the Chinese culture [10]. In the Western hemisphere, medical ethics has a propensity to benefit the value of individualism and underscore the principles of autonomy, privacy, individual rights, and self-determination. Both Chinese and Western medical ethics share the same principles. However, the outcome of balancing and overriding is dissimilar due to several reasons, among which , Chinese medical ethics chooses the principle of beneficence as the predominant principle as oppose to the autonomy principle more frequently observed in Western cultures [2].

Chinese medical ethics uses humaneness as the cornerstone value and emphasizes its importance in medical practice and in personal responsibility to the common good of society. Chinese medical ethics has learned that individual rights and autonomy cannot be sacrificed [3]. Beneficence and social common good should be balanced keeping in mind autonomy and individual rights.

For Western cultures, where autonomy is the cornerstone value, the core values of Chinese medical ethics such as compassion, physician duty to care, humaneness, sincerity, selflessness, and devotion might be perceived as unrealistic and old fashioned [9]. However, it also seems that the medical profession today has become driven by profit making in a consumer driven society or by the lure of maintaining an institutional medical job in which physicians fulfill their responsibilities and avoid giving personal opinions that can be negatively seen as paternalistic or manipulative.

Chinese medical ethics reminds us to accept humaneness as a method to stop alienation, overextended autonomy and individualism, and as a way to make the physician-patient relationship more meaningful and durable, [15]. It is a currently forgotten skill described centuries ago in the ancient healing art that is needed today.

REFERENCES

1. NIE, J. B. The plurality of Chinese and American medical moralities: toward an interpretive cross-cultural bioethics. Kennedy Inst Ethics J, v. 10, n. 3, p. 239-60, Sep 2000. ISSN 1054-6863 (Print)

2. ZHANG, M. X.; LIU, S. [A comparative study on the ethics of Western and traditional Chinese medicine]. Zhonghua Yi Shi Za Zhi, v. 38, n. 4, p. 209-13, Oct 2008. ISSN 0255-7053 (Print).

3. RAPOSO, V. L. Lost in 'Culturation': medical informed consent in China (from a Western perspective). Med Health Care Philos, v. 22, n. 1, p. 17-30, Mar 2019. ISSN 1386-7423.

4. AKSOY, S. [Ancient Indian and Chinese medical oaths and the comparison of their medical rules]. Yeni Tip Tarihi

Arastirmalari, v. 7, p. 65-76, 2001. ISSN 1300-669X (Print) 1300-669x.

5. FAN, R. Towards a Confucian virtue bioethics: reframing Chinese medical ethics in a market economy. Theor Med Bioeth, v. 27, n. 6, p. 541-66, 2006. ISSN 1386-7415 (Print) 1386-7415.

6. LI, E. C. et al. Chinese ethics review system and Chinese medicine ethical review: past, present, and future. Chin J Integr Med, v. 17, n. 11, p. 867-72, Nov 2011. ISSN 1672-0415 (Print) 1672-0415.

7. HO, M. J. et al. A tale of two cities: understanding the differences in medical professionalism between two Chinese cultural contexts. Acad Med, v. 89, n. 6, p. 944-50, Jun 2014. ISSN 1040-2446.

8. QIU, R. Z. Medicine--the art of humaneness: on ethics of traditional Chinese medicine. J Med Philos, v. 13, n. 3, p. 277-99, Aug 1988. ISSN 0360-5310 (Print) 0360-5310.

9. QIAN, Y. et al. Insights into medical humanities education in China and the West. J Int Med Res, v. 46, n. 9, p. 3507-3517, Sep 2018. ISSN 0300-0605.

10. WANG, X. Y. et al. Principles of ethics review on traditional medicine and the practice of institute review board in China. Chin J Integr Med, v. 17, n. 8, p. 631-4, Aug 2011. ISSN 1672-0415 (Print).

11. TSAI, D. F. Ancient Chinese medical ethics and the four principles of biomedical ethics. J Med Ethics, v. 25, n. 4, p. 315-21, Aug 1999. ISSN 0306-6800 (Print) 0306-6800.

12. JIANG, L. et al. Subject, function, and trend in medical ethics research: a comparative study of Chinese and non-Chinese literature using bibliometrics. J Evid Based Med, v. 5, n. 2, p. 57-65, May 2012. ISSN 1756-5391.

13. MICOLLIER, E. (ETHNO-)MEDICAL ETHICS IN GLOBALIZ-
ING CHINA: TRACING LOCAL KNOWLEDGE AND ADAPTA-
TION OF BIOMEDICINE. J Int Bioethique Ethique Sci, v. 26,
n. 4, p. 101-16, 157-8, Dec 2015. ISSN 2608-1008 (Print)
2555-5111.

14. LEONARD, R. A. Chinese medical ward: an American's observations. Perspect Biol Med, v. 55, n. 2, p. 299-317, 2012.
ISSN 0031-5982.

15. BOWMAN, K. W.; HUI, E. C. Bioethics for clinicians: 20. Chinese bioethics. Cmaj, v. 163, n. 11, p. 1481-5, Nov 28 2000.
ISSN 0820-3946 (Print) 0820-3946.

16. IP, P. K. Developing medical ethics in China's reform era.
Dev World Bioeth, v. 5, n. 2, p. 176-87, May 2005. ISSN
1471-8731 (Print) 1471-8731.

17. CHEN, X.; FAN, R. The family and harmonious medical decision making: cherishing an appropriate Confucian moral
balance. J Med Philos, v. 35, n. 5, p. 573-86, Oct 2010. ISSN
0360-5310.

18. CONG, Y. Doctor-family-patient relationship: the Chinese
paradigm of informed consent. J Med Philos, v. 29, n. 2, p.
149-78, Apr 2004. ISSN 0360-5310 (Print)0360-5310.

19. ZHANG, X. et al. Attitudes of Chinese medical students toward the global minimum essential requirements established by the Institute for International Medical Education. Teach Learn Med, v. 16, n. 2, p. 139-44, Spring 2004.
ISSN 1040-1334 (Print)1040-1334.

20. GUO, Z. Chinese Confucian culture and the medical ethical tradition. J Med Ethics, v. 21, n. 4, p. 239-46, Aug 1995.
ISSN 0306-6800 (Print)0306-6800.

21. HU, L. et al. Chinese physicians' attitudes toward and understanding of medical professionalism: results of a na-

tional survey. J Clin Ethics, v. 25, n. 2, p. 135-47, Summer 2014. ISSN 1046-7890 (Print)1046-7890.

22. ZHAN, T.; YAO, Y. [A preliminary study of Dao gao yao huang shi shu (Oath of Praying for the King of Medicine), a Chinese version of Hippocratic Oath]. Zhonghua Yi Shi Za Zhi, v. 48, n. 6, p. 342-345, Nov 28 2018. ISSN 0255-7053 (Print)0255-7053.

23. PELLEGRINO, E.; THOMASMA D. The virtues in Medical Practice.(New York: Oxford University Press 1993) ISBN 0-19-508289-3 .Chapter 1 p. 3-17, Chapter 2 p 18-30 and Chapter 14 p. 175-182.

24. BEAUCHAMP T, CHILDRESS J. Principles of Biomedical Ethics , 3d ed. (NewYork: Oxford University Press, 1989) ISBN 9780195059021

4.EUROPE

THE PRACTICE OF HUMANISM IN PEDIATRIC NEUROLOGY IN EUROPE

Dídac Casas-Alba
Pediatric Neurology Service, Hospital Sant Joan de Déu (University of Barcelona)

Jaume Campistol
Assistant Professor in Pediatrics at the University of Barcelona
Barcelona, Spain

Index:

INTRODUCTION

The concept of humanism in Medicine is a key theme in the clinical practice of this discipline from its origins. The term humanism was coined in the 19th century to designate a philosophical trend that developed in the Renaissance with the aim of claiming anthropocentrism as opposed to medieval theocentrism. The dignity and autonomy of the person were exalted, as well as the importance of reason to respond to the questions of man, taking up the classic legacy of thought of Greco-Roman culture. In this context, the Hippocratic Oath is popularized in many medical schools, a text that has an ethical content and that guides the doctor in the exercise of his profession, highlighting the duty to act for the benefit of the sick and especially protect them from injustice [1].

William Branch defines humanism as the doctor's attitudes and actions that demonstrate an interest and respect for the patient and address the patient's concerns and values, with psychological, social and spiritual dimensions [2]. According to Jordan Cohen, humanism is understood as a way of being, a set of convictions including altruism, duty, integrity, respect

for others, and compassion for the sick [3]. The term professionalism is closely related to humanism. Professionalism is a
way of doing, a set of behaviors that meet the expectations of
the patient; therefore, humanism is also the starting point of
the Charter of Medical Professionalism, which establishes the
fundamental principles of primacy of patient well-being and
autonomy and of social justice [3,4].

HISTORY

Medicine encompasses multiple branches, one of which is Pediatrics. Within Pediatrics, the neurological diseases of children have special relevance. Neuropediatrics is the medical
specialty that analyzes and studies the child in their development process and deviations. Some of the pathologies treated
by the neuropediatrician, such as epilepsy, autism, intellectual disability, and infantile cerebral palsy, have been causes of
significant inequality throughout history.

Attitudes towards patients with neurological deficits have
changed significantly throughout history. Plutarch in ancient
Sparta recorded the infanticide of newborns with some defects [5]. The spread of Christianity in the Middle Ages introduced the concept of charity, which led to the condemnation
of infanticide and the creation of hospices, homes, and hospitals for the care of children with functional diversities that
parents had abandoned, or society had rejected. Although this
was an advance, on the other hand, it was linked to a negative
element of marginalization that has been perpetuated until
the beginning of the 20th century [6]. The doctor and philosopher John Locke (1632-1704) was one of the first to defend
the education of children with intellectual disabilities [5].
Edouard Séguin (1812-1880), a French doctor and educator,
was also one of the pioneers on the subject, developing and
putting into practice his own method of education for children with intellectual disabilities. Even in the middle of the
20th century, we should not forget the atrocities committed

by the German National Socialist Regime toward this population [5]. After the Second World War, there was a revaluation and better acceptance by society of children considered "disabled" [5]. Pearl Buck (1892–1973), who was awarded a Nobel Prize in Literature, was one of the first to describe the lives of children with disabilities and their families, as a result of her own experience with a daughter who had phenylketonuria [5].

HUMANISM IN PEDIATRIC NEUROLOGY IN EUROPE

In this framework, we propose to analyze/review the practice of humanism in Pediatric Neurology in contemporary Europe, a field in which there have been notable advances, but which still faces important challenges.

The Resolution of the United Nations Convention on the Rights of the Child, approved by 140 countries in 1989, has been an engine for the humanization of pediatric care in Europe [7]. With the aim of implementing the principles of this Resolution, in 2000 the Child-Friendly Health Care (CFHC) Initiative was launched, promoted by Child-Health Advocacy International in collaboration with UNICEF and WHO [8]. This Initiative highlighted that even in developed countries where pediatric care can offer the latest technological and therapeutic advances, efforts must continue to be made to minimize the fear, anxiety, and suffering of children with neurological problems, along with those of their families [8]. The CFHC became part of health policy in the CFHC Guidelines approved by the European Council in 2011 [9], which also made

reference to the recommendations of the European Association for Children in Hospital (EACH) [10].

These recommendations represent the ideal framework for pediatric care in Europe today. As basic principles, all children should be considered and treated as holders of human rights, requiring special attention without discrimination based on sex, race, color, language, religion, origin, or other status [9]. Likewise, all children must be treated with care, sensitivity, justice, and respect through a careful process, with special care for their personal situation, well-being, and specific needs, with full respect for their physical and psychological integrity [9]. All children should have equitable access to quality health services, with special attention to the most vulnerable, such as those with motor or mental disorders [9]. In all actions concerning the medical care of the child, the interest of the child must be taken into account first [9]. It is recommended that children should only be admitted to a hospital when the care they require cannot be offered in an outpatient setting [10]. Children should be treated with tact and understanding, always respecting their privacy [10]. It is argued that children should be able to be accompanied by their parents or care-givers at all times [10]. This idea has favored the presence of parents not only in hospitalization in the neuropediatric ward but also in the neonatal and pediatric intensive care units, and even in the case of pediatric emergencies [11]. There should never be restrictions on visiting a hospitalized child [10].

Measures must be taken to mitigate physical and emotional stress [10]. For example, work is being done to create spaces with child-friendly designs and the presence of clowns or entertainers in the hospital environment is becoming more common (Figure 1) [12]. In line with the above, in recent years, animal-assisted neurological rehabilitation therapies, especially with dogs, have become popular [13]. Neurological rehabilitation is crucial in children and adolescents with disabilities, but it is generally a long-term process that can generate stress, negative feelings, and lead to the abandonment of treatment due to lack of motivation. Interactions with animals, generally dog or horses, has been shown to decrease anxiety, depression, behavioral problems, and to improve self-esteem and communication skills (Figure 2) [14]. Evidence has also been gathered in recent years in favor of animal-assisted interventions (dogs, horses, dolphins) in patients with autism [15]. Preliminary data suggest that these types of interventions promote verbal and nonverbal social behaviors, and simultaneously may decrease aggressive behaviors [16].

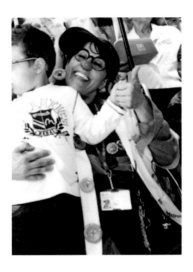

Figure 1. Clowns at the hospital environment

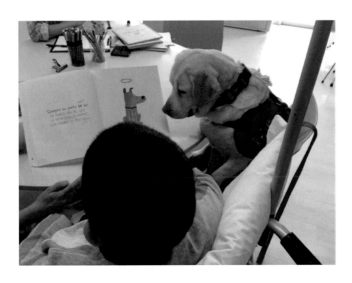

Continuing with the recommendations for more humane pediatric care, in order to be involved in the care of their child, parents or caregivers must receive and understand all relevant clinical information that concerns their child and they must be a very active part in the decision-making process [10]. Children also have the right to be informed and take part in decisions regarding their health, always in a way that is appropriate for their age, their ability to understand, and their maturity [10]. In a survey carried out by the European Council of children from different countries in Europe, it was found that a greater effort of listening, respect, and dialogue with the child in the field of medical care is required [17]. Some studies aimed at analyzing the causes of this problem point, among others, to a deficit in the training of health personnel in communication skills with the pediatric patient [18].

It is the physician's duty to protect the patient with a neurological disease from unnecessary medical treatment or research [10]. Modern medicine boasts of being very scientific; therefore, it tries to be as objective as possible and leans on technological bases. Analyzes, measure, quantifies, relates the signs of the disease, and somewhat leaves the symptoms or much of the information that can be offered to the patient and his family. But we must be aware that these elements are essential pillars in the diagnosis. This medicine arouses feelings of wonder and fear. In amazement at their ability to arrive at the final explanation of each disease and at the development of increasingly sophisticated diagnostic and therapeutic techniques.This is an aspect of special interest in the daily clinical practice of Neuropediatrics, a discipline that addresses many diseases considered rare that often lead to very complex and expensive explorations, as well as treatment in the framework of research studies, where the risk and the benefit for an individual patient has to be weighed.

It is highly recommended that children be cared for in pediatric emergency services and hospitalization facilities, by health personnel specialized in Pediatrics and especially by pediatric nurses [10]. The same concept applies to the care of the most complex or serious neurological pathologies that affect children, and who should be attended by specialists in Neuropediatrics. Scientific societies have been developed in Europe with the aim of promoting training and increasing the scientific level of this medical specialty, such as the Société Européenne de Neurologie Pédiatrique, founded in 1970, and the European Paediatric Neurology Society, established in 1999.

According to the report of the Better Health, Better Lives: Research Priorities of the WHO European Delegation, children in Europe with intellectual disabilities experience a wide range of inequities, largely unfair and avoidable [19]. This document highlights the determining factors of greater vulnerability and issues a series of recommendations for the protection of this group. First, children and young people with intellectual disabilities must be protected in a special way, since compared to the general population; they have a higher rate of exposure to toxins in the prenatal and postnatal periods. Furthermore, they are more frequently exposed to adverse socioeconomic circumstances, bullying, and abuse, and therefore have a higher risk of developing mental health problems [19,20]. This last element is of special relevance in the case of intellectual disability of genetic origin that associates behavioral alterations with greater vulnerability in developing psychiatric pathology.

The growth and development of children with intellectual disabilities in a family environment should be encouraged [19]. When biological families are not able to offer a minimum level of basic care, efforts should be made to find foster or adoptive families [21]. Despite the fact that parents are the main caregivers of a child with a disability, the impact of siblings and their invaluable contribution in care and in promoting school and social adaptation are also relevant. They seem to have a greater impact on the parents' health, the child's behavioral problems, or the socioeconomic condition of the family seems to have a greater impact on the parents' health than the degree of intellectual disability [22]. Currently, a model is also being worked on that aims to include adults with intellectual disabilities in the community, avoiding their institutionalization as far as possible [19]. Protected group homes are being organized, under the supervision of a house manager and work is being done on the labor and social integration of people with physical or mental disabilities.

Caregivers who care for children with complex and chronic neurological pathologies are at increased risk of developing physical and mental health problems [19], due to multiple factors, including cultural background, socioeconomic conditions, and characteristics of the caregiver and the patient. For example, there is significant variability in strategies for coping with adverse situations, acceptance capacity, resilience, or expectations for improvement. To protect the caregiver's health, it is important to ensure that they have understood the relevant information about their child's diagnosis and prognosis, the objectives pursued, as well as the care required, thus anticipating situations of avoidable anxiety or frustration. In line with the above, it is important to maintain a close communication channel between the neuropediatrician, the family, and any caregivers, often by phone or email, always respecting confidentiality in the framework of the doctor-patient relationship.**Specialized care**

It is necessary to be vigilant in caring for and protecting children with chronic and rare neurologically-based diseases against the dangers that may affect their rights. Specialized care for a patient with a chronic neurological disease may require a large number of hospital visits, which generate additional indirect costs for families in terms of days not worked and travel, which is why the role of the nurse manager is very helpful. Social workers are also very important, in order to make socioeconomic and other useful resources available to families. Psychological care is essential, either individually or with groups of parents. In recent years, a large number of associations of parents of children with rare diseases have emerged at local, national, and supranational levels in Europe [23]. These associations have become key in facilitating contact between patients and parents with medical professionals and researchers. In this way, mutual support can be achieved from shared experiences, while raising awareness in society to publicize the disease and to work on multidisciplinary projects, with multicenter studies supported and encouraged. These associations can assist in projects and help raise funds for rare disease research.

PALLIATIVE CARE IN NEUROPAEDIATRICS

Pediatric palliative care was recognized as a specialty in 2006, and since then, specific programs have been developed in multiple pediatric hospitals in Europe. Three types of care are offered: in the hospital setting, in the outpatient setting, and in the home setting. In the EAPC report Atlas of Palliative Care in Europe 2019, it was reported that 21 countries have established palliative care programs for hospitalized patients, 27 countries have programs in the outpatient setting, and 29 countries work with programs for the patient at home [24]. Perinatal palliative care represents a high percentage of the care offered [24]. Fourteen countries reported including palliative care training in the curriculum of Pediatric residents [24].

One of the most recent milestones in the humanization of the clinical practice of Neuropediatrics has been the professionalization of palliative care for the neurological patient. The objective of palliative care is to offer patients and families facing disabling or life-threatening illnesses a better quality of life, attending to the physical, psychosocial, emotional, and spiritual aspects. Neuropediatric patients with severe or terminally ill conditions are often candidates for palliative care because they have pathologies with few therapeutic options and a very uncertain prognosis. In a multicenter study that analyzed the most frequent diagnoses in 515 patients in follow-up for palliative care, it was observed that 41% had genetic or congenital pathologies, 39% neuromuscular pathologies and 50% had associated severe intellectual disability [25].

Most authors agree that pediatric subspecialties must learn to apply the principles of palliative care to routine clinical practice, referring children to specialized units in situations of greater severity or complexity, although the identification of this turning point can be particularly difficult.

One of the areas of shared work between neuropediatricians and pediatric palliative care specialists is the neurological patient admitted to the Intensive Care Unit [26]. In this scenario, the communication of bad news and decision-making regarding the limitation of therapeutic effort especially relevant. In a review article on the parents' perspective in decision-making regarding the end of life of a child with neurological pathology, most wanted to actively participate [27]. Although most of the literature is focused on the end of life, families need support as early as the first months following the diagnosis [28]. Neglecting this demand for care in periods of some stability can lead to feelings of loneliness and helplessness on the part of families.

UNIVERSITY EDUCATION

Work is also being done at the university level to improve the training of medical students. Medical training must be comprehensive; the medical curriculum should include aspects related to the humanities to allow students to become competent professionals of ethical conduct and adequate sensitivity. In order to become people who not only meet the demands of society but who contribute to its improvement, and in Pediatrics enhance the child's comprehensive health and minimize disability.

For this type of medicine, teaching has necessarily had to be modified with curricular changes that favor understanding and the ability to analyze and capture new elements over the memorization that is more typical of traditional teaching. The goal is to prepare for the future, which can sometimes be confused with training for the medicine of "success," with new technological achievements and acceptance of new ethical postulates capable of altering the course of patients' lives. In practice, these concepts have meant depersonalization of patient care. To be fair, the latter is not only due to technology but to the prevailing currents of thought that disfigure the doctor as a person who always has definitive results in hand. With things set out like this and with doctors being part of this disenchanted universe, the deterioration of the doctor-patient relationship, the cornerstone of good medicine, is easily understood. Our western culture forces us to prioritize the objective and the more technical, and to belittle the subjective. Brilliant solutions are proposed from the scientific point of view, but the humanity that must surround all medical acts is forgotten. Dialogue is therefore not established and this is essential and must always prevail in the conduct of all medical activities and even more so in the practice of Neuropediatrics.

Conclusion

Throughout this chapter, we have reviewed some of the advances and challenges of the humanistic practice of Neuropediatrics in Europe. Neuropediatrics is a medical specialty that cares for the developing child often facing serious and disabling pathologies, which are often the cause of inequity. That is why the clinical practice of this specialty requires a humanistic perspective, to put the patient and their family at the center and to attend to all aspects of individual, physical, psychological, spiritual, and social needs. In Europe, much work is being done and much progress is being made in the comprehensive care of children with various chronic pathologies, especially with disabilities of neurological origin. Neuropediatrics is not an exception, but rather a vanguard in this field, working with the child, their family, their educators and with other services (pediatricians, palliative care providers, social workers, educators, animators, in a multidisciplinary way to try to improve the comprehensive health of the child and their family. Many neurological pathologies of the child are considered rare diseases and the role of associations of parents of children with rare diseases is emphasized in giving visibility to the disease and promoting research. Finally, the formative role of university teaching in the practice of humanistic medicine is analyzed.

REFERENCES

1. Miles SH. The Hippocratic oath and the ethics of medicine. Oxford: Oxford University Press; 2004.

2. Branch WT, Kern D, Haidet P, Weissmann P, Gracey CF, Mitchell G, et al. Teaching the human dimensions of care in clinical settings. J Am Med Assoc. 2001;286(9):1067–74.

3. Cohen JJ. Viewpoint: Linking professionalism to humanism: What it means, why it matters. Acad Med. 2007;82(11):1029-1032.

4. Medical Professionalism Project. Medical professionalism in the new millennium: a physicians' charter. Lancet. 2002;359(9305):520-522.

5. Williams AN. Chapter 22: a history of child neurology and neurodisability. Handb Clin Neurol. 2010;95:317-334.

6. Velarde-Lizama V. Models of Disability: a Historical Perspective. Empresa y Humanismo. 2012;15(1):115–36.

7. The United Nations Convention on the Rights of the Child. Adopted and opened for signature, ratification, and accession by General Assembly resolution 44/25 of 20 November 1989.

8. Southall DP, Burr S, Smith RD, Bull DN, Radford A, Williams A, et al. The Child-Friendly Healthcare Initiative (CFHI): Healthcare provision in accordance with the UN Convention on the Rights of the Child. Child Advocacy International. Department of Child and Adolescent Health and Development of the World Health Organization (WHO). Royal College of Nursing (UK). United Nations Children's Fund (UNICEF). Pediatrics. 2000;106(5):1054–64.

9. Council of Europe guidelines on child-friendly health care. Adopted by the Committee of Ministers on 21 September 2011 at the 1121st meeting of the Ministers' Deputies.

10. European Association for Children in Hospital. The EACH charter with annotations. EACH European Association for Children in Hospital; 2016.

11. Parra C, Vidiella N, Marin I, Trenches V, Luaces C. Patient experience in the pediatric emergency department: do parents and children feel the same? Eur J Pediatr. 2017;176(9):1263–7.

12. Karisalmi N, Mäenpää K, Kaipio J, Lahdenne P. Measuring patient experiences in a Children's hospital with a medical clowning intervention: a case-control study. BMC Health Serv Res. 2020;20(1):360.

13. Hediger K, Boek F, Sachs J, Blankenburg U, Antonius-Kluger E, Rist B, et al. Dog-Assisted Therapy in Neurorehabilitation of Children with Severe Neurological Impairment: An Explorative Study. Neuropediatrics. 2020;10.1055/s-0040-1708545.

14. Purewal R, Christley R, Kordas K, Joinson C, Meints K, Gee N, et al. Companion animals and child/adolescent development: A systematic review of the evidence. Vol. 14, International Journal of Environmental Research and Public Health. MDPI AG; 2017.

15. Ávila-Álvarez A, Alonso-Bidegain M, De-Rosende-Celeiro I, Vizcaíno-Cela M, Larrañeta-Alcalde L, Torres-Tobío G. Improving social participation of children with autism spectrum disorder: Pilot testing of early animal-assisted intervention in Spain. Heal Soc Care Community. 2020;28(4):1220-1229.

16. O'Haire ME. Animal-assisted intervention for autism spectrum disorder: A systematic literature review. J Autism Dev Disord. 2013;43(7):1606–22.

17. Kilkelly U. Child-friendly health care: the views and experiences of children and young people in Council of Europe member States. Strasbourg: Council of Europe; 2011.

18. Damm L, Leiss U, Habeler U, Ehrich J. Improving care through better communication: Understanding the benefits. J Pediatr. 2015;166(5):1327-1328.

19. Emerson E, Barron DA, Blacher J, Brehmer B, Clinch S, Davidson PW, et al. Better Health Better Lives: Research Priorities. 2012 .Available from: [last accessed June 21, 2020] http://www.euro.who.int/__data/assets/pdf_file/0018/174411/e96676.pdf?ua=1

20. Emerson E, Hatton C. Mental health of children and adolescents with intellectual disabilities in Britain. Br J Psychiatry. 2007;191:493–9.

21. Glidden LM. Adopting Children with Developmental Disabilities: A Long-Term Perspective. Family Relations. 2000;49:397–405.

22. Saloviita T, Itälinna M, Leinonen E. Explaining the parental stress of fathers and mothers caring for a child with intellectual disability: a Double ABCX Model. J Intellect Disabil Res. 2003;47(4–5):300–12.

23. European Rare Disease Federations. Available from: https://www.eurordis.org/content/european-disease-specific-federations [last accessed June 21, 2020]

24. Arias-Casais N, Garralda E, Rhee JY, Lima L de, Pons JJ, Clark D, et al. EAPC Atlas of Palliative Care in Europe 2019. Available:https://dadun.unav.edu/handle/10171/56787%0Ahttp://dadun.unav.edu/handle/10171/56785 [last accessed June 21, 2020]

25. Feudtner C, Kang TI, Hexem KR, Friedrichsdorf SJ, Osenga K, Siden H, et al. Pediatric palliative care patients: A prospective multicenter cohort study. Pediatrics. 2011;127(6):1094–101.

26. Knies AK, Hwang DY. Palliative Care Practice in Neurocritical Care. Semin Neurol. 2016;36(6):631–41.

27. Zaal-Schuller IH, Willems DL, Ewals FVPM, van Goudoever JB, de Vos MA. How parents and physicians experience end-of-life decision-making for children with profound intellectual and multiple disabilities. Res Dev Disabil. 2016;59:283–93.

28. Davies H. Living with dying: families coping with a child who has a neurodegenerative genetic disorder. Axone. 1996;18(2):38–44

5.OCEANIA

HUMANISM IN CHILD NEUROLOGY: AN AUSTRALASIAN PERSPECTIVE

Simone L. Ardern-Holmes, MBChB, PhD, FRACP
Senior Clinical Lecturer
University of Sydney Faculty of Medicine and Health
Staff Specialist Neurologist
The Children's Hospital at Westmead
Westmead, NSW
Australia

INTRODUCTION

Australasian child neurologists proudly contribute to international efforts to optimize the health and wellbeing of children and families with neurologic conditions. We embrace the challenge and thrill of expanding scientific knowledge through anatomy, physiology, radiology, pharmacology, molecular biology and genetics. As such, neurology is an intensely scientific and reductionist discipline, but due to the 'carative' in addition to the 'curative' responsibility, our specialty stands to benefit immensely from a humanistic and person-centered approach. Alongside applying the science, the exercise of providing care for the patient and family is fundamental.

In this chapter, indigenous cultural perspectives on health and wellbeing in Australasia are introduced. These concepts emphasize shortcomings of the western dichotomy of mind and body, which is untenable in child neurology. Attention is focused on the importance of social context including family and community, and a spiritual dimension identified. Following on from this holistic view of health, several personal narratives illustrate the relevance of indigenous models of healthcare and the principles of humanism in child neurology in Australasia.

ON "BEING HUMAN" AND HUMANISM IN MEDICINE

In 2008, BBC Earth presented the documentary series "Being Human." Jon Farrar's introduction stated "To be human is to be at the center of our own universe, to experience life in all its colours and all its potential" [1]. The aim of the series was to examine who we are, why we behave the way we do, to understand our past and our future, and how to live better. This emphasized the individual within a bigger sphere and the act of experiencing life within a rich diversity of possibilities. Being human impacts on our experience of disease and illness, our conception of health and wellbeing, and our various needs to achieve optimal healthcare.

Recently, in his invited commentary on why humanism in medicine is more important than ever, George Thibault chose the Webster's Dictionary definition of humanism as "Any system or mode of thought or action in which human interests, values and dignity predominate" [2]. He described the principles of placing the patient at the center, promoting an understanding of the experience of health and wellbeing versus disease and illness, and determining goals and actions based on the values and needs of patients [2].

Humans experience life in different environments and cultural contexts, through the senses of vision, hearing, taste, touch, smell, and through our responses via cognition, emotion, movement, communication, and participation in community. These very senses and responses are compromised in the presence of neurologic disorders facing children, families and health care providers. What does this mean for any particular child and family, and for the health professional? While curing disease and restoring complete health is the goal of every physician for every patient, this goal is only sometimes achievable in child neurology. On the other hand, our caring responsibility is to relieve suffering, and always to provide comfort [3-5].

Humanism through patient-center care requires physicians to comprehend the patient's narrative and emotion [4]. It is respectful and responsive to individual preferences, needs and values, helps to maintain patient dignity and a sense of security. Patient-center care ensures the appropriateness and effectiveness of interventions offered [4,6,7].

CULTURE

Australasia is a region of significant cultural diversity, recognizing indigenous people from different islands, including the Māori from New Zealand, Aboriginal people from different communities around Australia, and Torres Strait Islanders who are geographically part of the state of Queensland in the north. We recognize the significance of culture, language and the land for the wellbeing of indigenous people. Understanding indigenous health perspectives informs the practice of humanism in medicine in our region, and must continue to shape policy and delivery of health care services.

A model of health developed to represent the values of New Zealand Māori is particularly instructive. This model was first explained in 1985 by Professor Sir Mason Durie [8], following findings of research conducted by the Māori Women's Welfare League in response to declining health status and barriers to health care experienced by Māori people. Hauora, the Māori philosophy of health and wellbeing, includes recognition of four dimensions, which must be in balance. Hauora is represented as the walls or sides of a house or whare, Te Whare Tapa Whā (Figure 1) as follows: Taha Whānau Family Health, Taha Hinengaro Mental Health, Taha Tinana Physical Health and Taha Wairua Spiritual Health [8].

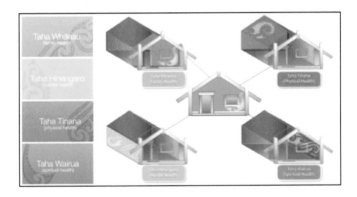

Figure 1. A New Zealand Māori Model of Health Te Whare Tapa Whā based on the explanation provided by Professor Sir Mason Durie (8).

In addition to physical health, recognition is given to social wellbeing and self-esteem within the context of family, emotional wellbeing and self-confidence in the context of mental health, and personal beliefs regarding spiritual wellbeing.

179

Spirituality concerns the search for meaning, sense of purpose and connectedness in life, understandably means different things to different people, and as a consequence, is difficult to define. It is most relevant during times of illness, crisis and transition, key periods requiring interaction with health professionals [6].

Whilst western medicine predominantly focuses on physical health, medical curricula include teaching on the biopsychosocial model, which recommends a more holistic approach. These aspects are included in Te Whare Tapa Whā. Similar dimensions are endorsed among Aboriginal, Torres Strait Islanders and other cultural groups.

For many indigenous patients and families, delivery of health care is most effective with input of indigenous workers, in a traditional community setting. As this is seldom possible in child neurology, it is imperative to develop an awareness of differing values and customs. The following section outlines important cultural principles for Māori and Aboriginal and Torres Strait people taken from health care guidelines [9,10].

Indigenous educators emphasize the investment of time to establish a relationship between patients and health care workers is essential to an effective partnership. Respect for a narrative style of communication is important, along with recognizing and exercising contemplative silence as a routine.

In Māori culture, the head is considered tapu or sacred. Māori understand that examination of the head is necessary in medical care. In turn, health care providers appreciate that touching the head must be done with care and respect, asking permission and monitoring response with sensitivity.

Māori and Aboriginal people along with Torres Strait Islanders tend to avoid eye contact as a mark of respect. Lack of eye contact should not be interpreted as rudeness or disinterest. Similarly, direct eye contact from health care providers may create a barrier. Avoiding cross-gender eye contact should be considered. It is advisable to take the lead from the patient/ family and where appropriate, to ask about preferences.

Men's and Women's business remains a fundamental part of cultural practice in many groups. Furthermore, how decisions are made in families varies between cultures.

The place of the individual alongside extended family in indigenous communities may contrast substantially with that in other cultures. In addition, the process of checking understanding of the patient and family requires more than a simple affirmation, as answering "yes" may hold different meaning to an indigenous person, such as "we've spoken enough today, my family are waiting."

Interpreters and cultural advisors can provide particularly helpful guidance at times of major stress, such as communicating a new diagnosis, recommending treatment or supporting families through palliative care experiences. The use of traditional prayers, or Māori karakia, may be valuable alongside medical procedures to establish balance in significant health care encounters.

An openness and curiosity about patient and family experiences, values and preferences includes and extends beyond cultural awareness, and is at the core of humanism in medicine the Multidimensional Impact of Neurologic Disorders on Children and Families

We know from the work of Varni et al. involving 2500 pediatric patients from the US, Europe and Australia, versus 9,500 controls, that chronic health conditions impact significantly on physical and psychosocial health, emotional, social and school functioning, domains reflecting health related quality of life (HRQOL) [11]. Across 10 disease groups including cerebral palsy, psychiatric conditions (attention deficit, disruptive behavior disorders, anxiety, mood disorders and pervasive developmental disorders), cancer, rheumatologic disorders, diabetes, obesity, asthma, gastrointestinal, cardiac disorders, and end stage renal failure, both children and parents in the cerebral palsy cluster reported the lowest HRQOL. Other than for physical health, patient and parent reported HRQOL for those with psychiatric disorders ranked lower than most other conditions, with a notable negative impact of anxiety on emotional wellbeing [11].

The associations recognized by child neurologists in practice between neurodevelopmental, neurologic, and psychiatric co-morbidities and how they impact on QOL are increasingly evident in the published literature. Neurodevelopmental disorders represent a significant proportion of referrals for child and adolescent mental health services. In over 400 Norwegian children with affective disorder and schizophrenia, 55% had associated neurodevelopmental disorders (attention deficit hyperactivity disorder, tic disorder or autistic spectrum disorder; 70% boys), with anxiety the most frequently occurring psychiatric comorbidity [12].

Similarly, the coexistence of neurologic features of epilepsy and movement disorders, and psychiatric symptoms has recently been highlighted [13,14]. As underlying genetic and immune-mediated mechanisms of disease are identified, it is becoming increasingly evident that the patient's various symptoms derive from the same disease process [14]. It follows that comprehensive care must draw on the expertise of neurologists and psychiatrists together, in a coordinated way. The traditional western dichotomous view separating mind and body is becoming less and less informative.

Large population based studies now provide robust evidence of the complexity of childhood epilepsies and associated co-morbidities. Data from the Norwegian Patient Registry (2008-2013) included over 1,125 million children born aged 0-17 years at the end of follow up [15]. Epilepsy affected 6,635 individuals (0.6%), and nearly 80% of those had more than one comorbid condition (medical disorders 55%, neurologic disorders 41%, neurodevelopmental and psychiatric conditions 43%). Risk of comorbidity was present even in uncomplicated epilepsies [15].

On a personal level, families of children with epilepsy experience extreme distress at the time of seizures - disconnection from the child with altered awareness, and fear of loss of life during seizures with respiratory and motor manifestations. The impact of the epilepsies extends well beyond experiences during and around management of seizures alone. The high frequency of functional problems across multiple domains and associated reduction in HRQOL for Australian children with various epilepsies was described in 2003, identifying a two to three times increased rate of behavioral problems versus the background population [16]. Although increased epilepsy severity predisposes to social difficulties in Australian children and adolescents [17], poor psychosocial outcomes occur in North American children even after epilepsy remission [13]. This speaks to the need to support the wellbeing of family and community participation, Taha Whānau.

The substantial negative impact of specific epileptic encephalopathy such as Dravet syndrome on HRQOL is now recognized, in excess of other milder epilepsy syndromes. In 162 children from Glasgow, increased epilepsy severity, motor disorder, learning difficulties and behavioral problems were all clearly associated with reduced HRQOL [18]. Comorbidities were common, including conduct problems (35%), hyperactivity and inattention (66%) and difficulties with peer relationships (76%) [18]. Not surprisingly, the humanistic and economic burden on families is significant but is poorly understood. Efforts to characterize are underway, with a view to developing interventions to improve outcomes of comorbidities and HRQOL for affected children and families [19].

Hopefully once effective strategies are established, these will be generalizable to other severe epilepsies.

Recent recommendations outlining comprehensive care for neurologic disorders such as Dravet syndrome [18], and tuberous sclerosis [20], reflect increased understanding of the multidimensional clinical problems experienced by patients.

PATIENT AND FAMILY NARRATIVES: REFLECTIONS

The following patient and family narratives are included with permission and sincere acknowledgement (Figure 2).

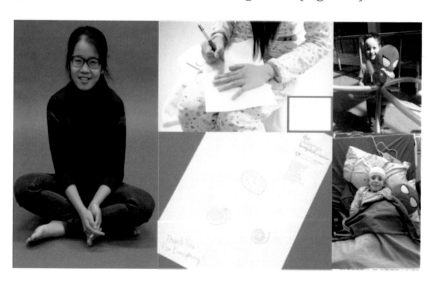

Figure 2. Human Faces in Child Neurology

A 2-year-old boy with unilateral exotropia and mild speech delay, child of Caucasian parents, was referred for diagnostic evaluation of paroxysmal motor asymmetry (flexion of the right arm when running) and staring spells, with EEG showing bursts of high amplitude spike and wave followed by slow waves in the left posterior frontal region. An underlying structural brain lesion was suspected but not identified on magnetic resonance imaging (MRI). Although staring spells in early childhood were non-epileptic, the EEG remained remarkable for frequent sleep potentiated generalised discharges. Education was provided regarding the potential for epileptic seizures, and surveillance established to monitor and support possible behavioural, cognitive and psychiatric comorbidity of a presumed genetic generalised epilepsy. Despite investigations, a definite underlying aetiology was not established. The experience of hospitalisation in the presence of other children and families with greater disability was distressing. Could this be what their future might hold?

Despite the child's pleasing ongoing progress and lack of clinical seizures, his parents experienced significant anxiety around uncertainty of the future, and worked hard pursuing every avenue to optimise outcomes. At the age of 9 years, an episode of non-convulsive status epilepticus occurred, which readily settled with anti-epileptic medication. Throughout this journey, the child and family required not only technical expertise and information relating to childhood epilepsies, they also cite effective communication including the sense of genuine care for the health and wellbeing of their son as crucial. The combined science and art of medicine facilitated a sense of safety and comfort required to cope, and in fact to flourish.

The second narrative concerns a creative 13-year-old girl with a two-year history of hand tremor, dysarthria, swallowing difficulties with poor control of oral secretions, which had been increasing over several months. The predominant problem identified by the child concerned the significant impact on peer relationships. Originally from Vietnam, she had emigrated to Australia 4 years earlier with her mother. As such, family support was limited, cultural differences including language were significant, and the family were hampered by socioeconomic disadvantage. The motor, behavioral and neuropsychiatric manifestations of disease including impulsivity, emotional lability with pseudobulbar affect and anxiety, were impressive compared with the relatively bland appearances on MRI showing T2/FLAIR hyperintensity in the caudate and putamen consistent with Wilson's disease. A multidisciplinary team of medical, nursing, allied health professionals and interpreters worked with the child, family and community agencies including education. Dietary and medical therapy was instituted to control the disease process preventing further decline. A comprehensive plan was devised to ensure safety, and ongoing rehabilitation to restore functioning and community participation. The child and family were grateful for the disease specific clinical treatment provided, along with the passion that animates professionalism [21], which constitutes the humanistic approach essential in her care.

The third narrative involves a 2-year-old girl of parents from Afghanistan, resident for 10 years in Australia. The child had been well until two left sided focal motor seizures associated with Todd's paresis occurred. Epilepsy partialis continua developed within two weeks of seizure onset, with a dramatic decline in language, and increasing functional limitation due to seizures and progressive left sided hemiparesis. The EEG showed right sided slowing with multifocal epileptogenic activity, and right-sided seizures. Progressive right-sided atrophy was evident on MRI without any definite underlying brain malformation, consistent with a diagnosis of Rasmussen's encephalitis. The epilepsy was refractory to treatment with antiepileptic medication and immunotherapy. The child's parents and extended family were deeply distressed by the evolution of her symptoms and decline, doubted the diagnosis, and were frustrated by the ineffectiveness of treatment. The child lost the ability to mobilize independently and was at daily risk of injury from frequent tonic seizures causing falls. Ongoing seizures overshadowed every opportunity to sense and respond to her surroundings.

Hemispherectomy was recommended to the parents. They felt overwhelmed, later describing the experience of a complete "shutdown," unable to think clearly after hearing possible surgical risks, unable to proceed, honoring their duty to prevent harm. Over subsequent months, recognizing their child's progressive decline, and being given time to learn more, they consented to surgery. Time was required to absorb additional information, to discover hope for the future that lay in the potential benefits of surgery. They learnt from the experience of other Australian families that surgical treatment offered the opportunity for improvements in cognitive, social, emotional, behavioral and physical domains even in the presence of hemiparesis, and particularly if rendered seizure free [22]. In retrospect, they identify the trusting relationships established with the treating team as fundamental in satisfying their confidence that surgery could be undertaken safely. It is a joy to parents, extended family and the health care team alike, to see this child smiling and playing, manipulating toys purposefully with her strong hand, making eye contact as she exclaims with pleasure at the discoveries now before her.

Through patient-center care and effective communication, health professionals can effectively engage patients in forming preferences and taking decisions, even in the face of uncertainty [7]. The emphasis on care, rather than cure, puts the individual and their family first, rationalizing treatment.

THE CHILD NEUROLOGY TEAM AND AUSTRALASIAN PROFESSIONAL PRACTICE FRAMEWORK

Child neurology practice in Australasia is governed by professional associations including the Australian and New Zealand Medical Associations, the Pediatrics and Child Health Division of the Royal Australasian College of Physicians (RACP), and the Australian and New Zealand Child Neurology Society (ANZCNS). In accordance with the Professional Practice Framework of the RACP, our goal is to serve the health of patients, communities and populations. In doing so, we acknowledge the need for excellence in diagnosing and treating disease, recognition of diverse experiences of illness and values regarding health and wellbeing, and the principle of patient center health care, i.e. both the science and the art of child neurology. Core competencies in professional skills include communication, teamwork and cultural competence.

Exercising humanism in child neurology recognizes not only the patient and family, but also healthcare providers. The importance of team members including nursing, and allied health professionals alongside the physician must be genuinely acknowledged. Child neurology is a demanding field due to complexity, chronicity, and intractability of clinical problems. While exercising a humanistic approach provides enormous professional reward, it can be wearing and provoke strong emotions. Consider the example of intensive care rounds with end of life issues facing the family of a previously well child rendered unconscious due to intracranial injury, perhaps a child the same age as your own, or that of a close friend.

Advocating for adequate resourcing of patients and families and evolving clinical services is essential at this time. Appropriate expansion of multidisciplinary teams is crucial to keep pace with the scientific advances we are fortunate to enjoy in child neurology, without outstripping our capacity to also provide humanistic care.

Figure 3 shows a word map of the principles behind humanism in child neurology. The content of this figure is drawn from the literature [23], and keywords from the value statements of the ANZCNS, RACP, Australian and New Zealand Medical Associations.

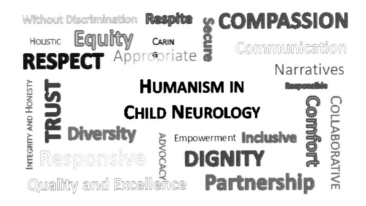

Figure 3. Principles behind Humanism in Child Neurology drawn from value statements of the professional associations in Australasia and Martimianakis et al. [23]

CONCLUSION

Disorders affecting the nervous system impair the ability of children and families to experience life in all its fullness. Clinical skills utilized in diagnosis and treatments are aimed at restoring functioning and participation. A humanistic approach honors the caring responsibility in health, acknowledges variable patient values and preferences, and directs health care interventions to be most appropriate, effective and to maintain human dignity.

Child neurology is not a "one size fits all" business. Ideally, health services should be flexible, coordinated and multi-dimensional, consistent with the philosophy of indigenous people of Australasia. Allied health management, behavioral and psychiatric expertise alongside medical and surgical sub-specialties including neurology, genetics, radiology and neurosurgery are crucial, together with appropriate family supports (including interpreters, cultural and spiritual advisors) to meet the specific needs of children with neurologic disorders. Such collaborative efforts in partnership with patients and families are at the heart of humanism in child neurology and are the foundation of excellence in clinical care [12,18].

Ps. Dr. Ardern-Holmes acknowledges Connor C. Holmes' efforts in revising earlier drafts of this manuscript.

REFERENCES

1. Farrar J. What does it mean to be human? wwwbbcearth-com. 2008.

2. Thibault GE. Humanism in Medicine: What Does It Mean and Why Is It More Important Than Ever? Acad Med. 2019;94(8):1074-7.

3. Gordon J. Medical humanities: to cure sometimes, to relieve often, to comfort always. Med J Aust. 2005;182(1):5-8.

4. Schattner A. The silent dimension: expressing humanism in each medical encounter. Arch Intern Med. 2009;169(12):1095-9.

5. Gold A, Gold S. Humanism in medicine from the perspective of the Arnold Gold Foundation: challenges to maintaining the care in health care. J Child Neurol. 2006;21(6):546-9.

6. D'Souza R. The importance of spirituality in medicine and its application to clinical practice. Med J Aust. 2007;186(S10):S57-9.

7. Epstein RM, Peters E. Beyond information: exploring patients' preferences. JAMA. 2009;302(2):195-7.

8. Durie MH. A Maori perspective of health. Soc Sci Med. 1985;20(5):483-6.

9. Aboriginal and Torres Strait Islander Patient Care Guideline. State of Queensland (Queensland Health). 2014;May.

10. Best practices when providing care to Maori patients and their whanau-Practice Standard. Dental Council of New Zealand. 2008;May.

11. Varni JW, Limbers CA, Burwinkle TM. Impaired health-related quality of life in children and adolescents with chronic conditions: a comparative analysis of 10 disease clusters and 33 disease categories/severities utilizing the PedsQL 4.0 Generic Core Scales. Health Qual Life Outcomes. 2007;5:43.

12. Hansen B, Oerbeck Beate, Skirbekk Benedicte, Petrovski Beata and Kristensen Hanne. Neurodevelopmental disorders:prevalence and comorbidity in children referred to mental health services. Nordic Journal of Psychiatry. 2018;72(1-8):285-91.

13. Baca CB, Vickrey BG, Caplan R, Vassar SD, Berg AT. Psychiatric and medical comorbidity and quality of life outcomes in childhood-onset epilepsy. Pediatrics. 2011;128(6):e1532-43.

14. Peall KJ, Lorentzos MS, Heyman I, Tijssen MAJ, Owen MJ, Dale RC, et al. A review of psychiatric co-morbidity described in genetic and immune mediated movement disorders. Neurosci Biobehav Rev. 2017;80:23-35.

15. Aaberg KM, Bakken IJ, Lossius MI, Lund Soraas C, Haberg SE, Stoltenberg C, et al. Comorbidity and Childhood Epilepsy: A Nationwide Registry Study. Pediatrics. 2016;138(3).

16. Sabaz M, Cairns DR, Bleasel AF, Lawson JA, Grinton B, Scheffer IE, et al. The health-related quality of life of childhood epilepsy syndromes. J Paediatr Child Health. 2003;39(9):690-6.

17. Stewart E, Catroppa C, Gill D, Webster R, Lawson J, Mandalis A, et al. Theory of Mind and social competence in chil-

dren and adolescents with genetic generalised epilepsy (GGE): Relationships to epilepsy severity and anti-epileptic drugs. Seizure. 2018;60:96-104.

18. Brunklaus A, Dorris L, Zuberi SM. Comorbidities and predictors of health-related quality of life in Dravet syndrome. Epilepsia. 2011;52(8):1476-82.

19. Jensen MP, Brunklaus A, Dorris L, Zuberi SM, Knupp KG, Galer BS, et al. The humanistic and economic burden of Dravet syndrome on caregivers and families: Implications for future research. Epilepsy Behav. 2017;70(Pt A):104-9.

20. Curatolo P, Moavero R, de Vries PJ. Neurological and neuropsychiatric aspects of tuberous sclerosis complex. Lancet Neurol. 2015;14(7):733-45.

21. Stern DT, Cohen JJ, Bruder A, Packer B, Sole A. Teaching humanism. Perspect Biol Med. 2008;51(4):495-507.

22. Sabaz M, Lawson JA, Cairns DR, Duchowny MS, Resnick TJ, Dean PM, et al. The impact of epilepsy surgery on quality of life in children. Neurology. 2006;66(4):557-61.

23. Martimianakis MA, Michalec B, Lam J, Cartmill C, Taylor JS, Hafferty FW. Humanism, the Hidden Curriculum, and Educational Reform: A Scoping Review and Thematic Analysis. Acad Med. 2015;90(11 Suppl):S5-S13.

PART 2

RELIGIOUS PERSPECTIVE ABOUT HUMANISM IN CHILD NEUROLOGY

AMERICAN NATIVE PERSPECTIVE APPLES VERSUS ORANGES

Contrasting Paradigms of Definition and Options for Persons Identified as Developmentally Disabled, within Western Post-Industrial Societies and Native American Indian Societies. Identifying the Spiritual and Social Connotations of Each Worldview.

Candace Cole-McCrea Ph.D
Professor Emeritus
Great Bay Community College
Portsmouth, New Hampshire

It was his third birthday when I took him for the first time to a Native American Indian gathering, a Pow Wow. Though he was three years old, he was quite small and developmentally at about age ten months, just beginning to walk and talk. I took him in a stroller. I walked around with him, undisturbed, until a trader asked about him. When I mentioned that he was a mestizo, half Native American and half Mexican, our whole day changed. Leaders and drummers of the Pow Wow came over to meet us. People gave him gifts, to include a handmade Native doll. An honoring dance was performed with all dancers following us within the Pow Wow circle. The treasured final gift of the only honoring blanket was given to him by the Eldest elder. It was a fine day of glorifying the life of this child, struggling so hard to grow and develop. He was respected for being the person himself; the gift he was, recognized and honored, no matter what his developmental issues were.

Thereafter, we went home, back into the dominant culture of America. The week followed with phone calls from clinical professionals and medical staff who wanted to do assessments, early intervention people who were determined to help him progress as much as he could, though it had already been determined by them that he would never catch up to his peers.

Two worlds. Two belief systems. Two zeitgeists.

How to make sense of it all...

I begin by looking at the effects of the two cultures on my own life. I am half Mohawk and half the grandchild of an immigrant Scottish Highlander, raised in small town, New England. I am the child of both worlds. My spiritual reality has been strongly groomed by both.

To see with the mindset of the dominant American culture, I begin by considering Georg Simmel, a nineteenth century sociologist, who authored the essay, "The Stranger". He discussed the experiences and consequences of people who, generally, did not fit comfortably, like a correct puzzle piece, within cultural expectations. He theorized that while these "strangers" did not fit conveniently into roles and statuses, that they held unique social positions. Since their thinking, attitudes, and behavior did not fit the norms, they could be perceived as brilliant and as genius, or as inferior, morally criminal or sick by the defining dominant culture. I found myself as a child, born with a significant "impairment" to be given an assumed status as an inferior, developmentally disabled person, and thus also a stranger. I was not included; I existed "alongside". I was not asked what I thought about anything. I was not accepted into our religious community, although I could attend services with my parents. I sat "alongside". It was assumed that religion was too complicated for me to understand. I was not accepted within our educational system; I went to school but existed "alongside" the real students. I was a deviant; I was ostracized, but somehow at the same time, I was perceived as an Innocent.

Today, I am still that stranger; however, now I cherish my identity. I have been allowed to see with more than one cultural lens. I have been able to discern what suits my life-world best. I have spent over 40 years counseling and teaching others, guiding them through spiritual and cultural crises. I have been blessed.

A tool that has helped me understand the spiritual and cultural challenges of both the Native and the dominant American culture is an ideal type, as defined by Max Weber, and specifically theorized by Ferdinand Tonnies. Weber defined ideal as classification types that have clear and separate demarcations; he emphasized that while ideal types do not truly exist, they allow for an analyst to clearly see the extremes of multiple views.

Tonnies used ideal types to describe and define two types of societies, allowing us to be able to see connotations of economic, social, psychological and spiritual assumptions of each. He titled these two types of society gesellschaft and gemeinschaft. Understanding the differences between these two ideal types is critical to understanding the differences in religious and spiritual perspectives, personal identity formation, and statuses for persons within each culture, to include those who do not fit into averages. Each of these types see and experience deviance differently.

TONNIES IDEAL TYPES OF SOCIETIES

(Characteristics abbreviated and modified to fit the focus of this paper)

GesellschaftGemeinschaft

Modern industrialTraditional (pre) industrial

Instrumental rolesUniqueness valued

Rational/IntellectualTraditional/Spiritual

Contractual bondsCommunity solidarity

Persons as meansPersons as ends

IndividualismSocial Identities

Innovation valued. Old Ways Respected

Individual freedomKinship bonds strong

Individual choices Group influences behavior

Pride of self-accomplishmentPride of responsibility to group

Individual ethicsMutually shared ethics

Individualized religion"Religion" socially grounded

In the gesellschaft society, persons are respected and valued according to their abilities to perform expected pre-existing economically vital roles. In the gemeinschaft society, persons are respected and valued for being true to their "being", while participating in the spiritual well-being of the whole, in common or unique ways. (Remember that these are ideal types. Societies can exist anywhere along the spectrum on or between these two extremes.)

Each society affects persons in different ways. Current western society is a gesellschaft society; a society that more easily adapts to social upheaval and change, though persons within the society experience increased stresses and anxieties as their own selves are always vulnerable to failure, loss, even abandonment. Tribes typify gemeinschaft societies, which do not adapt easily to change, but whose members are deeply rooted in relationships to peers, clans, tribes, land, animals and nature in physical, social and spiritual ways. When those bonds hold, like roots of a tree, the person remains grounded. This summarizes the differences between individualism and tribal identities.

At this point, we comprehend Hillary R. Clinton's book on child rearing, in which she explains that it takes a village to raise a child. The child, in traditional cultures, learns their identity as a member; not as an individual. "We are our relations" is a common Native American aboriginal phrase. This carries extremely significant connotations.

I will give one example from my own life. My maternal grandfather was a Baptist minister; my paternal grandparents were traditional Long House Iroquois. I grew up being pulled to both extremes. My maternal grandfather wanted me baptized and was concerned that I needed to conduct my life in ways that would get me to Heaven. My paternal grandparents spoke of no such things. They spoke of needs of our peoples so all could thrive, so all could advance in the afterlife. In one religion, I was to save myself, even if family and loved ones were not saved; in the other, I could not separate my concerns from the well-being of others.

I remember hiking in Alaska, climbing a small mountain, praying for clearness. My heart was torn. Finally, after days and nights alone, I made the only decision I could make. I, at the young and naïve age of eighteen, spoke to the God of my maternal family. "God, if you are there, please, understand that I cannot commit to Christianity wherein I may be saved and those around me condemned to a hell. I could never be happy in a Heaven while others are suffering. I would have to leave the Heaven and go into the hell to comfort them. God, I must choose to spend my life committed to the well-being of others. I do not want to ever be in your Heaven unless all others are welcome. I pray that you do not force me therein."

I left that mountain, grew and became more sophisticated through the years and yet, that declaration has remained forefront in my life. As a result, most of what is taken for Christianity in the dominant culture holds no attraction for me. Many sects of Christianity, including Baptists, Methodists, Catholics, Mormons, and others have been disappointed or disgusted with me as their missionary work has failed to hold me.

Comparing the two types of societies, then, note that in the gesellschaft society the child is raised to fit expectations and roles. The culture trains the child to be a good citizen and worker. In the gemeinschaft society the elders will question who the new child was created to be. The child, it is assumed, is unique and will fit into the culture in a way that is perfect for who they are born to be, even if that way has never been known previously. It is the duty of elders to help that child find their unique importance to the tribe. Thus, in a gesellschaft, the child learns to find value of self as an economic and functional cog in society; in a gemeinschaft, the child discovers themselves a True Self, a source of the continuing life and blood of community.

Now, it becomes possible to define the concept of "developmental disability" within the two types of societies. Within the gesellschaft society, a person with developmental disabilities is one who does not meet functional and economic role expectations. Within a gemeinschaft, a person has a developmental disability, if one wants to borrow the term, if that person is individually centered and irresponsive to their relations. A person performing trigonometry may be seen developmentally disabled while a person careful not to disturb moss on the ground may be viewed as developing respectfully, and thus "more normally". As a unique theorist of American society, George Herbert Mead, explained, a person does not become fully human until they are considerate in their actions and behaviors of the entire social world. To Mead, self-centeredness is a sign only of undeveloped human potential.

I will close with two examples. One, when training prospective teachers who are choosing to teach on native reservations, I advise them to throw out the Bell Curve. Often, they ignore me. They have been taught to reify this judgmental tool of standard education. They teach in elementary schools on reservations and try to evaluate the little ones using the curve. They soon discover that reservation children who catch on to studies quicker than others, perform slower testing would predict. Nothing can be done to get them to perform faster or to advance.

Time and again, I get a phone call or an email from teachers, frustrated by this apparent lack of ambition. I remind them of my admonishment. I remind them that the children's first responsibility is a bond with their peers; that bond will hold them securely throughout their lives. They will not compete with their in-group. They perform at the level of the slowest among them. To raise their achievement, group tasks will have to be created wherein all succeed or all fail. These children value the unique spiritual consciousness within their in-group as their true identity. For them, "We Are" becomes inseparable from "I Am".

My second example is even more telling. During the 1960's, I volunteered with Vista, an American aid organization, to help Alaskan Native Americans adapt to a 20th century culture, after oil pipelines began destroying their traditional food sources and habitat. My task was to interface between villages and state governments with oil company interests. Often, conferences to explain the dominate culture's economic needs were held in Fairbanks, a central city. Native leaders were invited to attend. I was to go along and to somehow bridge the gap of understanding between cultures.

I would attend, thereafter, to try to interpret and explain what and why the American culture was doing what it was doing, and to clarify what options that left for the native community.

The "chief" I was responsible to would listen to me, question me until he could recite the words I was saying, then ask for no further discussion from me.

Back at the village, I would go around with him as he went from home to home, telling villagers what had been said. He asked villagers in every home to come back to him and to tell him what they thought he should do. Never would he make up his own mind or come to a decision. He could not.

It took me a long time to understand why he was chief, since he could not come to a decision or even comprehend much of what had been said. Slowly I realized why he was so valued and so respected. This "chief" was what westerners would call "developmentally and intellectually disabled". He was not capable of making strategic or corporate decisions. This was exactly why he had been elected "chief". He depended on the voices of his people to determine the course of action for his village. He had to listen and follow their lead. As he explained to me, "Without them, I would not know what to do!" His shortcomings were his gift to his people. All benefited from the wisdom of his leadership. I had found the most perfect social expression of true democracy that I was ever to know, a democracy free of self-righteousness and personal bias. At the Pow Wow honoring his death, thousands of people danced in gratitude and honor for the gift of his being.

REFERENCES

1. Brown, Joseph E. Teaching Spirits. Oxford University Press. 2001

2. Clinton, Hillary R. It takes a Village. Simon and Schuster. 1996

3. Gill, Sam D. Native American Religions, 2nd Ed. Wadsworth Co-engage, Learning, Belmont, CA 1983

4. Mead, George H. Mind, Self and Society: The Definitive Edition.

5. Charles W. Morris, Ed. University of Chicago Press. 1934-2015

6. Simmel, Georg. "The Stranger", an essay. On Individuality and Social, Ed. University of Chicago Press, 1908-1971

7. Tonnies, Ferdinand. Community and Civil Society. Jose Harris, Ed. University Press, Cambridge. 1887-2001

HUMANISM IN CHILD NEUROLOGY (FROM A BUDDHIST AND SPIRITUAL PERSPECTIVE)

Thananchai Tejapañño Sugsai, B.A.
Phrakru Dhammarata, The Ecclesiastical Honorific Rank
Teacher, Wat Nyanavesakavan, Bachelor of Communication
Arts, Bangkok University
Graduate Diploma of Tripitaka Studies, Mahachulalongkorn-
rajavidyalaya University
Dhamma Scholar, Advanced Level, Pali Scholar, Level 3

Thasanporn Toemthong, DDS.
Rajanukul Institute, Department of Mental Health, Ministry
of Public Health, Thailand

HUMANS ARE PART OF NATURE AND FOLLOW THE LAWS OF NATURE.

Buddhism aims to uncover the truth that all things in the universe – human beings, animals, trees, rocks, mountains, rivers, and so on – are part of nature and proceed according to causes and conditions. When looking from the perspective of a human being, we can refer to this truth as a set of natural laws. In Pali, 'natural laws' are called "niyāma," which means 'fixed order' or 'absolute process.' When specific causes and conditions exist, they invariably lead to certain outcomes. It is possible to separate these laws into five categories [1].

1. Laws of nature relating to physical phenomena and the external environment, specifically temperature, weather, and the seasons (utu-niyāma)

2. Laws of nature relating to reproduction, genetics, and so forth (bīja-niyāma)

3. Laws of nature relating to the workings of the mind (citta-niyāma)

4. Laws of nature relating to human behavior, in particular the process of intentional action and its results (kamma-niyāma)

5. Laws of nature relating to the interrelationship of phenomena and the general process of cause and effect (dhamma-niyāma)

Actually, the first four laws can be subsumed within the fifth law, that is, the term 'dhamma-niyāma' incorporates all five laws. However, when looking from a human perspective, kamma-niyāma is the most important because it is directly related to human existence. Karma – volitional action – shapes the trajectory of our lives, beginning with conception in the womb.

The value of being human comes from our actions and behavior.

Because the law of karma is directly related to human affairs, shaping the course of individual people's lives and the direction of society, Buddhism gives it great importance. As the Buddha said: kammunā vattatī loko, meaning: 'The world turns by way of karma' [2]. In any case, the law of karma (kamma-niyāma) is only one of many laws of nature.

Because of that, when a person is born sound or impaired, either physically or mentally, and experiences happiness or suffering, we should not blame all these circumstances on karma. The differences apparent in each individual person accord with natural causes and conditions, or laws of nature, which apply equally to all people. This equality is a basic attribute of all humankind.

The teachings on karma focus on intentional actions by way of body, speech and mind, corresponding to the Buddhist passage: 'Cetanāhaṃ bhikkhave kammaṃ vadāmi,' meaning, 'It is intention, bhikkhus, that I call kamma.' With intention, people then act by way of body, speech, and mind [3]. Buddhism thus deems that human beings are equally at freedom to develop and improve themselves, even surpassing the grandeur of devas and Brahmas. People's virtue, skills, and conduct are the criteria for determining their degree of excellence or inferiority, not caste, social class, race, etc. Self-development is not dependent on luck or fortune or on prayer and supplication, for example by petitioning external forces. Desired results and goals are achieved by way of effort and active engagement requiring self-reliance and perseverance. As the Buddhist texts say: 'Na jaccā vasalo hoti na jaccā hoti brāh-. maṇo kammunā vasalo hoti kammunā hoti brāhmaṇo' – 'One is not a Brahman by birth, nor by birth an outcaste. By action (kamma) is one a brahman, by action is one an outcaste' [4]; 'Danto seṭṭho manussesu' – 'Amongst human beings, those well-trained are the most noble' [5]; 'Vijjācaraṇasampanno so seṭṭho devamānuse' – 'One fully accomplished in knowledge and conduct is best among devas and humans' [6].

HUMANS MUST PRACTICE TO BE NOBLE, WITH A VIRTUOUS FRIEND OPENING THEIR EYES TO VARIOUS FACTORS OF ACCOMPLISHMENT.

When people clearly discern their own basic disposition in the present, and improve and develop themselves correctly in line with the law of karma, even such conditions as illness, or physical, emotional or cognitive shortcomings, won't be seen as a hindrance to improving their quality of life. In any case, success or failure is linked to various factors that either support or obstruct the bearing of fruit of particular actions. In Buddhism, the term 'sampatti' refers to a fulfilment of associated factors promoting intended positive results, and the term 'vipatti' refers to a deficiency of such factors thus undermining positive results. The four factors favorable to the ripening of good karma are: residence (gati), physical health (upadhi), time (kāla), and undertaking (payoga) [7].

When you are aware of these factors, even if you are deficient in any of them you should not be upset or discouraged, but you should rather strive to develop other virtuous qualities. Knowing what qualities need to be strengthened and increased, you will hasten to act based on an understanding of the law of karma.

Such informed engagement is beneficial even for children and adolescents with neurological, cognitive, or developmental disabilities. The starting point of this process, however, requires a virtuous and supportive friend who has firm confidence in the potential of children in respect to the universal human condition of being able to develop and also requiring some form of training.

NO MATTER HOW BAD LIFE MAY BE, ONE MUST STILL CULTIVATE THE THREEFOLD TRAINING AND THE FOURFOLD DEVELOPMENT.

It has already been stated that human beings are a part of nature and are subject to natural laws, in particular the law of karma. Moreover, every individual is fully entitled to engage in training and cultivation despite being born with neurological, cognitive, or developmental disabilities. In Buddhism, however, improving one's quality of life must accord with the Threefold Training (sikkhā) and be validated by the four kinds of development (bhāvanā). This improvement is holistic. The Threefold Training involves promoting physical and verbal actions favorable to oneself, society, and the natural environment (sīla-sikkhā), cultivating the mind by making it bright and joyous and imbuing it with virtuous qualities like kindness, fortitude, patience, stability, and readiness for work (citta-sikkhā), and growing in wisdom which discerns the conditioned nature of things and understands all things according to reality (paññā-sikkhā) [8].

Assessing people's quality of life in accord with the four kinds of development begins with an examination of whether their use of the five senses is beneficial to their lives or not (kāya-bhāvanā). This is followed by an examination into how harmonious their relationships are with fellow human beings and other living creatures (sīla-bhāvanā),into the level of their mental aptitude, proficiency, and health (citta-bhāvanā), and to what extent their understanding of human life and the world conforms to reality (paññā-bhāvanā) [9]. Improving the quality of life for children with neurological, cognitive, or developmental disabilities requires care and a determined effort to provide wholesome causes and conditions. Caretakers must know the natural disposition of each and every one of the children along with the aforementioned factors that either support or obstruct healthy development. We must not forget that caretakers, whether this be parents, relatives, or medical personnel, are an essential factor for the children's development. Moreover, behaviour consistent with one's understanding of relevant causes and conditions ensures that one's work will be successful.

FOR CHILDREN TO DEVELOP WELL, THEIR MENTORS MUST CULTIVATE THE SUBLIME STATES OF MIND.

In terms of improving quality of life, we should recognize and respect that an individual's existence is tied up with other people ever since they are in the womb. When a child is born, they depend on other people's love, care, support and instruction at almost every stage of growing up, until they can live and survive by themselves. Buddhism gives these relationships great importance as they are seen as harbingers of improving quality of life.

Self-awareness, which is the starting point of self-development, relies on external factors, namely, supportive people who enable progress and maturity. In particular, those individuals with disabilities and developmental impediments require kindness and support from virtuous companions including parents, relatives, medical personnel and other members of society. These virtuous companions should maintain an attitude of goodwill based on an understanding of truth and an appreciation of human interrelationship, and they should be able to foster conditions suitable to children's development.

Technically speaking, there are four basic qualities a virtuous friend should be endowed with, known as the four sublime states of mind (brahmavihāra): 1) Loving-kindness; the wish for all beings to abide in peace and well-being (mettā); 2) Compassion; a wholehearted willingness to help others escape from suffering (karuṇā); empathetic joy; 3) Rejoicing and offering encouragement when others prosper and meet with success (muditā); and 4) Equanimity; knowing the right time to support and teach others (upekkhā) [10]. When one is endowed with these qualities then one's actions are naturally in line with the four bases of social solidarity (saṅgaha-vat-thu), namely:

1) Generosity; renunciation; sharing material possessions, knowledge, and teachings (dāna); 2) Kindly speech; pleasing, reconciliatory and respectful forms of communication; beneficial and reasonable words inducing others to do good (piyavācā); 3) Acts of service; providing assistance both to individuals and to the public; promoting ethical conduct (atthacariyā); and 4) Even and equal treatment of others; offering constant friendship; behaving appropriately in relation to other people's social standing and to various circumstances by considering the common good (samānattatā) [11]. This fourth factor is dependent on equanimity, which goes hand-in-hand with wisdom and leads the way in fostering conditions that improve people's quality of life.

The inner qualities of a virtuous friend, as well as their ability to effectively help others, are generated by practicing the Threefold Training: by refining conduct by way of body, and speech and enhancing the relationship to the natural environment; by cultivating the mind; and by understanding the truths of nature. The Threefold Training is a means for improving the quality of human life in harmony with natural laws, in particular the law of karma, in order to live a virtuous life conducive to assisting others.

UNDERSTANDING DHARMA AND REFINING KARMA: GENERATING GOODNESS FOR ONESELF AND SOCIETY.

Buddhism – also known as 'Buddha-Dhamma' – has a unique perspective on human existence. It urges us to understand the interrelationship of all things and to apply this understanding in order to benefit society, the environment, and ourselves. The Buddhist path involves training and development until one realizes the supreme goal: an escape from all bonds and a freedom from all suffering. The result is a life of true peace and well-being.

We must also acknowledge that human knowledge is limited. For this reason we should aim to understand those truths that can be applied to improving the quality of our lives. In this manner, each individual can draw upon their own degree of intelligence to fulfil their aspirations.

Although people's quality of life will vary due to their own personal factors of development, this diversity does not exclude any human being from self-improvement or realizing the supreme goal. Moreover, the Buddhist teachings emphasize that if one is not yet able to reach the ultimate goal, one should put forth constant effort to do so, as confirmed by these proverbs: 'Vāyametheva puriso yāva atthassa nippadā' – 'Make unremitting effort until the goal is attained' [12]; 'Anibbindiyakārissa sammadattho vipaccati' – 'Carry on undauntedly; the desired goal will be fulfilled' [13]. These quotes indicate the importance of making diligent effort and abstaining from vague and dubious expectations. These principles accord with the law of karma – the natural order of actions and results –, which has a direct bearing on human beings. As mentioned above, intentional actions shape the course of individual people's lives and the direction of society. Indeed, making diligent effort can be equated with the Pali term 'puñña-kusala' which refers to wholesome and skilful actions that benefit both oneself and others.

Improving the quality of life of children with neurological, cognitive, or developmental disabilities should follow the same principles, both in terms of the children themselves and of their carers. Initially, people should establish a correct understanding of natural truths including the fact that human beings require education and training and that everyone possesses the ability to develop according to their own unique circumstances.

This process requires the assistance of virtuous friends and mentors. Within this relationship both parties – the children and their careers – should view this as an opportunity to learn and grow in line with the Buddha's teachings, to make diligent effort based on wisdom until they reach the highest goal.

REFERENCES

1. Dighanikaya Atthakatha (Sumaṃgalavilasinī) No.2 Page 34

2. Majjhimanikaya Majjhimapaṇṇāsaka Vol.13 No.707

3. Anguttaranikaya chakkanipāta Vol.22 No. 334

4. Majjhimanikaya Majjhimapaṇṇāsaka Vol.13 No.707

5. Khuddakanikaya Suttanipata Vol.25 No.306

6. Khuddakanikaya Suttanipata Vol.25 No.33

7. Dighanikaya Pātikavagga Vol.11 No.72

8. Abhidhammapiṭaka Vibhanga Vol.35 No.840

9. Dighanikaya Pātikavagga Vol.11 No.228

10. Anguttaranikaya Pañcakanipāta Vol.22 No.79

11. Anguttaranikaya Pañcakanipāta Vol.22 No.129

12. Dighanikaya Pātikavagga Vol.11 No.140

13. Samyuttanikaya Sagāthavagga Vol.15 No.891

FURTHER RESOURCES

1. Khuddakanikaya Jataka (including its Atthakatha) Vol.27 No.2444 Numbers 2-13 referenced from the Pāli Canon or Buddhist Canon (the Official Siamese version or Syāmaraṭṭhassa Pāli Tepiṭakaṃ) Available from: Trapitaka v1-45 2470-1-22-2018pdf (chula.ac.th)

2. Buddhadhamma : the laws of nature and their benefits to life Somdet Phra Buddhaghosacariya (P. A. Payutto) (Thai Version)

3. Buddhadhamma : the laws of nature and their benefits to life Bhikkhu P. A. Payutto (Somdet Phra Buddhaghosacariya) ; Translated into English by Robin Philip Moore. (English Version)

4. The Nectar of Truth: A Selection of Buddhist Aphorisms Somdet Phra Buddhaghosacariya (P. A. Payutto) Translated into English by Professor Dr. Somseen Chanawangsa (Pāli-Thai-English Version)

HUMANISM FROM A BUDDHIST PERSPECTIVE IN CHILD NEUROLOGY

Venerable Mae Chee Sansanee Sthirasuta
Founder of Sathira-Dhammasathan, Bangkok, Thailand
Founder of Bodhisattva Valley (Sathira-Dhammasathan2),
Phetchaburi, Thailand
Co-Chair of Global Peace Initiative of Women

As a spiritual leader in the Buddhist tradition, we give importance to the present moment, because we cannot change the past nor know the future. The only time that we can act is here and now, so the present moment is a precious moment. Acting in the present creates the cause and the result is the future. We usually say we are reborn every day, meaning we can start doing good things every day. Once we create a good cause, there is no doubt of the good result.

We might guide the special child or child neurologist to realize that the here and now is the first priority, even if the child has a genetic disorder. We have to act on a belief that they are similar to others. Please do not compare them with other children. If you compare them, special children will feel inferior, and then will receive fewer opportunities. I have been working with special children for 33 years. I have been telling doctors, nurses, and their parents that the present moment is what is most important to their children.

The here and now of reality is composed of the harmonization of bodily action, verbal action, and mental action. The present is the most powerful tool to help lift the spirits of special children so that they can discover their own value. We cannot change their genetics nor their birth, since that is all in the past. If we treat them in the present with respect and love them unconditionally, it will help them understand and accept themselves. Happiness will start appearing in their hearts. Unconditional love means to love them the way they are, not based on our own desires. In this way, we can truly help draw out their inner strength. We have to learn to accept them, no matter the outcome.

When we respond to them in the present with our pure hearts in our speech and actions, we also teach them to be in the present where there is no past or future, no comparison, no competition, and no winner or loser. Then they will not be considered unfortunate children but be able to shine and be proud of good little things that they find in themselves. Happiness will grow. They will experience the inner development of their happiness. With this strength, they will be able to move on with their lives in a normal way. We have to respect their own normal way of being. Certainly, when one acts with a totally pure heart, mind, and speech, the results are always good, without any doubt.

Let's work in the present with a pure heart to uplift their souls, help them to feel secure, and to be happy every day they live in this world.

CHRISTIAN HUMANISM TO TREAT PATIENTS WITH NEUROLOGICAL DISORDERS

WHAT IS MAN?

Felipe Roman Larrea
Doctor in Spiritual Theology (2021), Pontifica University of the Holy Cross
Rome, Italy

The Bible tells two stories of creation; they are symbolic stories that convey profound truths about man. In Gen 1: 26-27, we read:

And God said, 'Let us make man in our image, according to Our likeness; and let them have dominion over the fish of the sea, and over the birds of the air, and over all the wild animals of the earth, and over every creeping thing that creeps upon the earth.' And God created the man in his own image, in the image of God he created him; male and female he created them [1].

The second narration is found in chapter two of Genesis. When God speaks of the creation of man, he says:

Then the Lord God formed a man from the dust of the ground and breathed into his nostrils the breath of life and man became a living being [2].

From the two narrations, we see that man is a special creature within all creation because he is made in the likeness of God. When he says in the second narration that God blew on his nose and breathed life into him, he is explaining to us that God gives man a spiritual soul that is what properly resembles God, who is a spirit. That is why humans have such a special dignity, because being creatures who enjoy spirituality, we are destined for eternity. We know that our life does not end with death, but with death begins Eternal Life, which is the destiny to which all men are called.

To what this first book of the Bible says, we must add the teachings of Jesus, who is the same God who became a man to save us and to teach us the way to eternal life. Jesus our Lord, the one who created himself, knows in depth what man is. Pope John Paul II said: "Christ manifests man to man himself" [3], since no one but Him fully knows human nature. It must be added that God, by taking our nature, elevates human dignity to levels no one ever imagined. Since we share the same nature as God, in some way we have become deified. Throughout his life, Jesus constantly worried about the sick and the poor and taught his followers always to be aware of them. When he talks about what the final judgment will be like at the end of time, he says the following words:

"When the Son of Man comes in his glory, and all the angels with him, he will sit on his glorious throne. ll the nations will be gathered before him, and he will separate the people one from another as a shepherd separates the sheep from the goats. He will put the sheep on his right and the goats on his left. "Then the King will say to those on his right, 'Come, you who are blessed by my Father; take your inheritance, the kingdom prepared for you since the creation of the world. For I was hungry, and you gave me something to eat, I was thirsty, and you gave me something to drink, I was a stranger and you invited me in,36 I needed clothes and you clothed me, I was sick and you looked after me, I was in prison and you came to visit me.' "Then the

righteous will answer him, 'Lord, when did we see you hungry and feed you, or thirsty and give you something to drink? When did we see you a stranger and invite you in or needing clothes and clothe you? When did we see you sick or in prison and go to visit you?' "The King will reply, 'Truly I tell you, whatever you did for one of the least of these brothers and sisters of mine, you did for me.' "Then he will say to those on his left, 'Depart from me, you who are cursed, into the eternal fire prepared for the devil and his angels. For I was hungry, and you gave me nothing to eat, I was thirsty and you gave me nothing to drink, I was a stranger and you did not invite me in, I needed clothes and you did not clothe me, I was sick and in prison and you did not look after me.' "They also will answer, 'Lord, when did we see you hungry or thirsty or a stranger or needing clothes or sick or in prison, and did not help you?' "He will reply, 'Truly I tell you, whatever you did not do for one of the least of these, you did not do for me.' "Then they will go away to eternal punishment, but the righteous to eternal life" [4].

With these words, the Lord makes us see that behind each man or each sick child with neurological problems, we have to see Him, that is to say, he again emphasizes with renewed strength that each man is the same image of God.

Therefore, each child with autism, cerebral palsy, or intellectual disability has a value in themselves, regardless of their race, sex, age, economic position, beliefs, health condition, and in any other way that people can be segregated. A child is more than a number or a statistic. Everyone is a unique person and loved by God as a son, because that is what God our creator wanted. Men from the moment of their conception until their natural death, have an absolute dignity for being the reflection of the same God.

Another fundamental teaching that Jesus brings us is the sense of pain. Before Jesus came, he had the idea that pain was absolute evil.

Jesus shows us that pain accepted with resignation and offered for love is one of the best ways to achieve Christian and therefore, human perfection. This concept may be difficult for a child to understand, but not for the parents in the context of deeply held Christian thought. Since Jesus died on the cross, even though he had not committed any sin, it became clear to Christians that by way of the cross we could achieve true happiness in this life and also that it is the way to reach heaven.All Christians who have come to understand the positive meaning of pain have discovered "the secret of happiness." Saint Josemaría, a saint of the 20th century, said: "Authentic love brings joy: a joy that has its roots in the shape of a cross [5]. "The man who learns to offer his pain and lovingly unites this pain with the pain of Jesus on the cross becomes immune to sadness; nothing in this life can take away his joy. Therefore, the criterion for pain in disease in this case of a neurological nature is this: if it can be removed or decreased it is done; if it cannot be done, the pain is offered to God.

How should we behave with every man?

Having laid the foundations of the dignity of man, let us see what Church documents say about the treatment to be had with men. Let us begin with a few words from the last great Council that the Church had, the Apostolicam Actuositatem. The decree says:

For this exercise of charity to be truly extraordinary and appear as such, it is necessary to see in the neighbor the image of God according to which he has been created, and Christ the Lord to whom in reality what is given is given to the needy; the freedom and dignity of the person receiving the aid are considered as the maximum delicacy; let the purity of intention not be tainted with any self-interest or desire to dominate; above all, the demands of justice are satisfied, and what is already due as a title of justice is not offered as an offering of charity; the causes of the ills are removed, not just the defects, and aid is ordered so that those who receive it gradually release themselves from external dependence and suffice for themselves [6].

From these words that shine by themselves, I would like to highlight that of not acting for their own use, it seems to me that, something that enhances the doctor (the pediatric neurologist, in this case), is that in his professional performance, do not forget that he is not doing only a job, but is dealing with a person.

Therefore, the material use of the doctor goes to a second place, being the human treatment of you to you that must be given between doctor and patient. A doctor's job changes when he is aware of his vocation of humanitarian service. The doctor is not only a professional; he is in his task a dispenser not only of physical health, of preserving brain functions, but of integral well-being. The doctor, aware of his own dignity and the personal dignity of his small patient affected by neurological problems, establishes a "human" bond in which the mere doctor-patient bond is transcended and it is understood that in this relationship the benefit is mutual.In other words, not only does the patient win, but the doctor also can enrich himself in that relationship if he is truly human. When we learn from children with hemiparesis, for example, is that instead of giving up, they fight with great spiritual strength to recover and over time make their deficits imperceptible.

At the Conference of Latin American Bishops meeting in 2010, the Manual of Theology and Pastoral Health was created and from this, I extract the following advice that it seems to me every pediatric neurologist who wants to provide Christian treatment to his patients should know:

The suffering person is cause for concern and concern in the missionary action of the Church. Suffering and pain affect the person not only in their physical appearance but also affect their integrity and their family and social environment; they are inseparable companions of humanity. To alleviate pain, medicines and painkillers are needed. To alleviate suffering, we need to find answers about the meaning and significance of human life [7].

Although we are talking about the mission of the Church here, it can be applied to every doctor who wants to reach the integrity of the person, who will be concerned not only with physical health, treating the patient as any living organism. It should help the patient see a deep meaning behind their pain, so that they understand that this pain can help clean the stain that sin has left in their life, can help to strengthen their character, and can help as a prayer offered to God, since God, when he sees the suffering man, is when he has the most mercy on him. God is a loving father and like any father, he is closest to his sick and suffering children.

Later the same Manual tells us:

Health is a harmonic process of physical, psychological, social, and spiritual well-being ("well-being") and not only the absence of disease, which enables the human being to fulfill the mission that God has assigned him, according to the stage and condition of life in which it is. Health is a "biographical" experience: it encompasses the different dimensions of the human person and is closely related to the person's experience of his own embodiment, of his place in the world and the values on which he builds his existence. In short, we could say that health is harmony between body and spirit, harmony between person and environment, harmony between personality and responsibility [8].

We cannot forget that the man is a social being and that therefore he is integrated into a family and a culture. If the doctor wants to provide truly humane treatment, they have to work together with the family, or with the human group that surrounds the patient, since the authentic well-being of the individual can only be achieved if the entire nucleus is treated. This point is key, especially when the doctor has to treat long healing processes, as is often the case in pediatric neurology. In these cases, the relationship with the patient is not enough. The patient's recovery process must be linked to their intimate community, which in most cases will be their parents (in the case of young people), or their spouse and children (in the case of older people).

On the other hand, putting the disease in contact with a supernatural perspective is essential, since it will give the patient and their parents a global vision of their situation. Remembering that this life is not everything and that after this life there is eternal life, is something that gives a new perspective to disease. We have not been created just for this world, but we have been created to live in love for all eternity. This life is only a space of time that man has to learn to love. Illness and pain are key in the process of learning love since he truly loves the one who learns to think of others more than himself. Love's greatest enemy is not hatred, but selfishness. Like all men (from Original Sin), we have a natural tendency to selfishness, we only learn truly to love when we go through pain, and we learn that the Ego diminishes. Great loves are always forged amid difficulties and the disease process offers us enormous possibilities. How many times do people think they love another person when they really love themselves?

To convert the act of caring for a child affected by neurological problems, the specialist strips off all selfish perspectives and tries to understand his patient from his perspective, with the eyes of the other, as true love would. That is why love is tested in contradiction; it is there where a man comes to light where his hopes are placed.

Neurological problems are sometimes chronic and unfortunately, occasionally regressive or degenerative. Families suffer many pains together: economic problems, the education of their children amid many hardships, and complicated family relationships.

To be successful and last in adversity, families have to know how to forgive, and they have to learn to yield to one another. This is true love, because it is not based on their own satisfaction, but on the search for the good of the other. Illness and pain give man the possibility of achieving pure love, teach a man not to focus on himself, and to think of others. For this reason, it is critical that the whole family is involved in healing since everyone can take advantage of the pain that one of their members is suffering.

Finally, I want to speak to pediatricians who are Christian and, in particular, Catholic pediatric neurologists. If the person treating a disease is a Catholic, the good of his acts and their repercussion depend to a great extent on the union the doctor has with Christ. In the parable of the Vine and the Branches, Jesus said: "Without me, you can do nothing," obviously referring to the fact that we cannot do anything of real value. Concerning the subject we are dealing with, the union of the doctor "to the Vine" (that is to say, to Christ), gives a new perspective to his treatment of the patient, because he is no longer just a doctor who is treating a patient. That doctor becomes a representative of God.

The Holy Mass is for the Christian the Mystery of the Salvation of men since the Mass is the celebration of the same Passion, death, and Resurrection of Christ that are made present in a mysterious way at every moment of history. I copy what the Catechism of the Catholic Church says verbatim when it speaks about the Mass:

In the Liturgy of the Church, Christ primarily signifies and realizes his paschal mystery. During his earthly life, Jesus announced with his teaching and anticipated his acts the paschal mystery. When his Hour arrived, he lived the only event in history that does not happen: Jesus dies, is buried, rises from the dead and sits at the right hand of the Father "once for all." It is a real event, happened in our history, but absolutely unique: all other events happen once, and then happen and are absorbed by the past. The paschal mystery of Christ, on the contrary, cannot remain only in the past, because by his death he destroyed death, and everything that Christ is and everything that he did and suffered for men, participates in the divine eternity and thus he dominates all times and remains permanently present in them. The event of the Cross and of the Resurrection remains and draws everything towards Life [9].

Whether the doctor or the patient is Catholic, understanding what the Holy Mass means is vitally important, since everything we do can be united to the Passion of Christ through the Holy Mass. In this way, the pain and setbacks that a person suffers become part of this Savior. The doctor who links his work to that Sacrifice of Christ makes his work part of the history of Salvation. In this way, the doctor-patient relationship is not only a human relationship, but it becomes something divine because it participates in the transcendence of Christ who is fully united by communion with God, who makes His own Blood boil through His Mystical Body, which is the Church. Thus, work becomes something holy and divine, which not only improves this world in which we live but also prepares us to achieve eternal life.

What a great opportunity doctors have to improve this world if they care not only for the bodies of their patients but also for their souls. How much good can they do if they remember that their work is not only a professional task but also a fully human activity in which they can teach many people to love? The only thing that can genuinely improve this world is love. If the doctor loves his patients, if he does his work for the love of God and neighbor, if he teaches how to love to those who have to heal and elevates the patient's gaze to the supernatural realm, he is building a new world, the world that God wants to live; he is building the Kingdom of God in the middle of the world.

REFERENCES

1. Bible Reina-Valera, Gn. 1, 26-2

2. Bible Reina-Valera, Gn. 2,7

3. Gaudium et Spes, no 22

4. Bible Reina-Valera 1960m Nt. 31-46

5. Saint Josemaria Escriva de Balaguer, Forja, pt. 28

6. Vatican Council II, Apostolicam Acuositatem, pt

7. Missionary Disciples in the World of Heath, Guide for Heath Ministry in Latin America and the Caribbean, Department of Justice and Solidarity CELAM Pastoral health, Guatemala 2010, pt.

8. Missionary Disciples in the World of Heath, Guide for Heath Ministry in Latin America and the Caribbean, Department of Justice and Solidarity CELAM Pastoral health, Guatemala 2010, pt. 8

9. Catechism of the Catholic Church, pt 1085

HUMANITY IN ISLAM FOR CHILD NEUROLOGY PROVIDERS

Yasmine Elhefnawy, MD
Pediatric Neurologist at Boston Medical Center
Boston University School of Medicine
Boston, Massachusetts

INTRODUCTION

Islam is one of the monotheistic religions; meaning that it calls for believing in one God who is Allah, Almighty (ﷻ). The word Islam means "submission," and it refers to "submission to God's will." Islam started in 610 CE when prophet Muhammed, peace be upon him (ﷺ), was sent a message from Allah ﷻ and he became the messenger for Islam. Mohammed ﷺ is the last of a long chain of prophets and messengers starting with Adam and including Abraham, Moses, Jesus, and many others. The words of Allah ﷻ were revealed to prophet Muhammed ﷺ which was then written in one book named "Quran". This book is considered the holy book of Muslims. The rules and directions for Islam are derived from the holy book "Quran" and the sayings of prophet Muhammed ﷺ which is called the "Sunna". The third reference is what is called "Ijtihad" which is deductive logic laws about aspects not mentioned in the two former primary sources. Those aspects are increasing every day with the recent advances in modern life, especially in the medical field. Islamic scholars are the responsible ones for those deductive laws where they use the general essence of the similar issues mentioned in the Glorious Qur'an and Sunna to produce "Fatwa" or advisory opinion. It is not uncommon to have two contrast opinions about the same issue from two different Islam scholars. In such cases, the individual is free to choose what he thinks is the best judgment [1]. Most of the references for this chapter are obtained from the Glorious Qur'an and Sunna.

It is important to be aware of the background of the Muslim patient's beliefs. Dealing with a Muslim patient holds the same grounds of professionalism that are well known for medical personnel. Cultural and religious sensitivity is one important core value of professionalism. Child neurology providers see a wide range of patients in all ages and get involved in a lot of poor prognostic conditions and brain death cases. This chapter will go through some values and differences that are worth to be aware of while dealing with a Muslim patient.

Medicine and Islam

Medicine was always valued since the Islamic old culture. When Europe had mainly the priests providing medical care in sanatoriums and annexes to temples, the Islamic world had hospitals with a structure similar to the present, with wards, medical records, and pharmacy [2]. Multiple prominent Islamic figures were known to have changed the history of medicine. A lot of examples are well known in history in different parts of the old Islamic world. Ibn-Alnafis lived in the 13th century described the pulmonary circulation 300 years before William Harvey [2,3]. Abu Al-Qasim Al-Zahrawi was a surgeon and pathologist in the 10th century who described hydrocephalus along with other congenital diseases. He described a procedure for evacuation of superficial intracranial fluid in hydrocephalic children [4]. Ishaq ibn Ali al-Ruhawi lived in the 9th century and was the first one to write a book about medical ethics in the Islamic world [5]. Ibn Sina (or Avicenna as known in the western world) is known as the Prince of physicians in the west. He had a lot of contributions in clinical and pharmacological science but most importantly he was the founder of what we call today Holistic Medicine which is treatment using herbs and diet in combination with addressing the physical and psychological factors [2].

DEMOGRAPHICS OF MUSLIM IN USA

There are 3.45 million Muslims of all ages living in the U.S. which makes up about 1.1% of the total U.S. population based on a study in 2017 made by Pew Research Center. It is estimated that US Muslims increase by a rate of 100,000 per year mainly due to migration. By 2050, the number of American Muslims was projected to be twice the size of the 2017 Muslim population. More than a third of the Muslim American adults were born in the United States. Foreign-born Muslims originate from 77 different countries mostly from the Middle East, North Africa, and South Asia countries [6].

INSIGHT FOR BEING DISEASED

Muslims believe that Allah ﷻ is the creator of all living beings on earth including humankind. The fates of individuals are written and controlled by Allah ﷻ especially what is related to birth, disease, and death. They believe that Allah ﷻ grants health and wealth and is also capable to inflict diseases, poverty, and death [7,8]. The Muslim's perception for this affliction is either a test or a consequence for their wrong deeds from Allah ﷻ. The religion of Islam encourages patience and tolerance to affliction awaiting salvation from Allah ﷻ [9]. As the prophet ﷺ has mentioned that Allah ﷻ is the one who created illness and he is the one who guides human beings to the treatment [10]. There a lot of Muslims find a lot of comfort in retrieving their faith and reciting the Holy Quran during hard times. Sometimes also they find that helping their pains and suffering in a way that mindfulness and meditation work to alleviate physical symptoms. In the end, Allah ﷻ promises who accept illness and afflictions in general with patience, satisfaction, and submission the best reward during life and on the day of judgment.

The Muslim perceives his life as a long test where he is expected to obey and follow the laws of Islam. His eventual goal is to win the blessings of Allah ﷻ and gain access to heaven and avoid being punished through the hell on the judgment day. The Muslim believes that the day that he dies is predestined since he was born. They believe in the doomsday "Yawm Al-Qeyama" that after the death of all human beings on earth, Allah ﷻ is going to revive all, tell each one about how he/she did through life [11].

The Muslim believer's standard is to conduct himself/herself in the best manner possible at all times and places. He/She is encouraged to take good care of his/her physical state like cleanliness and health [12,13].This is also simply evidenced by the fact that Muslims are obliged to wash their faces, mouths, hands, and feet as mandatory steps before their daily prayers. Prophet Muhammed ﷺ even had a lot of sayings encouraging Muslims to brush their teeth using "Siwak," the old days' toothbrush [14].

EXPECTATIONS FROM PHYSICIANS

Patients all over the world expect not only to treat and cure their diseases but expectations extend to heal and care for them sincerely. The expectations of Muslim patient, in general, is not so different from the broad frame of medical ethics that get taught in medical schools.

The physician in the old Islamic world in the middle east used to be called "al-hakim" which means the wise one and the one who possesses ethics. The virtues that a good Muslim believes in do represent the moral qualifications that he/she seeks when dealing with his physician. For example, honesty, trustworthiness, compassion, respect and to be humble and to not abuse his/her status or power. Those are few yet important character traits that are honored in Islam [15].

A good Muslim has the will to abide by all of those morals even if nobody is watching. This is related to the strong belief that Allah 🕮 can see and hear all that we do and say and even what we think of [16]. Appreciation of beliefs, concepts, and perspectives of the Muslim patient is crucial in building a good rapport with him/her.

Muslims in the US originated from different countries and various cultures and backgrounds as mentioned before. What all Muslims learn about Islam is the same, as the references for Islam are the same across the boards. However, one should be careful and conscious about the baseline educational level and awareness of healthy lifestyle standards as well as the cultural background to provide an appropriate counseling plan for the patient.

SENSITIVITIES DURING THE MEDICAL INTERVIEW AND PHYSICAL EXAMINATION

Holding a culturally sensitive medical interview is very important to gain the trust of the patient. It is also important to provide appropriate counseling that is relevant to the patient. It is important to be aware of the basic obligations and taboos for the Muslim patient so the provider won't get surprised by certain practices or ask inappropriate questions.

It starts with the apparel, where the classic clothing for Muslim women is covering all their body except hands and face. This is usually known as "Hijab," which is an Arabic word meaning veil or barrier. This is encouraged in Islam for identification, protection, and chastity. Some Muslim women moreover cover their faces and hands and they keep only a slit in their clothes for their eyes to see around. It is not appropriate to ask a veiled Muslim female to uncover herself except if medically necessary. A lot of Muslim females prefer female physicians for that purpose [17]. A lot of men in Islam also follow some regulations in their clothing like avoiding shorts above the knee as well as tall pants that cover the heels or drags on the floor. It is not surprising to have a Muslim patient with a little unusually short pants [18].

It is well known in Islam that intimate relationships and sexual intercourse are forbidden outside of marriage frame. It is not acceptable for the Muslim patient to do hugs or kisses for salutes and some are even sensitive to handshakes from the opposite sex. Handshaking is an important aspect of professionalism when introducing to a patient, however, the provider must not be discouraged or feel rejected if a Muslim patient refrains to shake hands [19].

One other well-known Islam law is avoiding eating pork or its derivatives. Muslim patients needs to be given alternatives if it comes to any medicine or treatment that is derived from pigs. It is always appreciated to be prepared to answer the question of the ingredients or constituents of recommended treatments and if they contain any pigs' derivatives.

Heavy alcohol drinking is known for its long-term neurological sequelae. Alcohol drinking is forbidden in Islam with many references from both the Quran and Sunnah. This fact may play an augmentative role while counseling an adolescent about alcohol drinking and anything that hurts his body as mentioned before.

DILEMMAS

A lot of commonly encountered issues in the medical field are still points of debate among Islamic scholars. Some of those issues are already settled with established judgment agreed among different scholars and some are still in conflict. A lot of those issues are commonly encountered in the medical field and it may be interesting for some to know Islam's laws about those.

There is a general framework that guides the decisions. This includes maintaining human life and intellect, the right to know one's pedigree, preservation of honor and integrity, protection of an individual's freedom of belief, and protection of property [20].

End-of-life decisions are hard to deal with among all human beings. It is an instinct to wish to maintain life for oneself and his beloved individuals. However, when that wish faces the facts regarding specific disease prognosis and quality of life following a certain diagnosis, different harsh decisions come to the surface. In that case, health care providers go over this tough conversation of goals of care with the family. This conversation is generally difficult with religious individuals who think that a disease or an injury is a divine entity and that miracles can happen. This conversation is even more challenging with the Muslim family as withdrawal of care violates the law of maintaining human life. Also, Islam encourages not to be desperate from Allah's ﷻ mercy. However Islamic jurists and scholars have agreed on certain indications for withdrawal of medical care. Those are futility of continued therapy, the depressed neurological status of the patient or brain death in other words, and compounding harms from continued clinical care. While life support measures may be withheld, ancillary measures like hydration, nutrition, and pain control should continue. There are a lot of yet unclear distinctions that aren't settled in regards to specific situations, especially that the above-mentioned indications are so broad and depend mainly on physicians' expertise and trustworthiness which carries the possibility of being wrong or corrupt. Hence, there is a consensus in most Muslim countries to seek the opinion of three expert physicians before deciding that one of the indications for withdrawal of health care is fulfilled. Similarly, the decision for DNR/DNI can only be taken if three expert physicians agree that the patient has a terminal disease, facing inevitable death, irreversible brain damage causing coma or chronic cardiac and pulmonary failure that is impossible to reverse [21].

It was explained formerly that Muslims believe that Allah ﷻ is the creator of human bodies and is their ultimate owner. Those bodies are combined with the souls for the period of a lifetime and then eventually both return to their creator when the individual dies. Allah ﷻ ordered to keep those granted bodies healthy. The bodies are considered to be trusts that need to be rendered safe and sound back to its creator; Allah ﷻ. It is also preferred and encouraged to bury the dead body as soon as possible following death. Hence, organ donation is another sensitive issue that is material for debate among Muslim scholars. After long years of arguments, the laws of organ donations were passed in most Islamic countries regarding living organ donation like kidney and bone marrow transplant. Non-living organ donation in the case of brain death is still a matter of debate until today. Health care providers should expect a lot of hesitation from Muslim families in that regard [22].

Genetic research is proliferating at a vast pace. Stem cell transplantation is the future for conquering a lot of diseases. However, care should be taken not to violate any of the Islamic laws, so only somatic cells can be used to avoid any changes in the individual hereditary characteristics [20].

Adoption is frowned in Islam because of the usual process of transfer of parental rights where the child carries the last name of the adopted parents. This poses a lot of conflicts in the lineage, asset inheritance, and future marriage of the adopted child. On the other side, fostering is accepted and actually highly encouraged where the fostered child retains his father's name [23].

Donor breast milk usage for premature babies if the mother is unable to produce enough breast milk has been a great advance in Neonatology. In Islam, regulations, as stated in the Glorious Qur'an, entails that breastfeeding from the same mother generates kinship between unrelated children. This makes marriage in the future between the "breast milk brother and sister" prohibited. With the current system in the United States regarding pooling and banking the donor breast milk, it is impossible to know the origin of the donated breast milk. This fact makes the donor breast milk not accepted in Islam [24].

CONCLUSION

Muslims represent a growing population in the western world. They have different beliefs and insights that are derived from their religions. A lot of the usual circumstances and decisions that we go through every day during our practice in Child Neurology may be handled differently with the Muslim patient to ensure the best outcomes, patient satisfaction, and trust. Hence, knowing the basic background of Islam is necessary. When in doubt, as we connect with patient's therapists and teachers when needed, as Child Neurology providers, we should also be open to connecting with the Mosque Imam (leader) to facilitate the best health care for our patients in a religiously sensitive fashion. That makes patients more comfortable accepting given medical advice without possibly violating any of the Islam laws, and at the same time making sure that the correct medical information is relayed accurately to the Imam to give a valid opinion.

REFERENCES

1. "Wabisah bin Ma'bad (May Allah be pleased with him) reported: I went to Messenger of Allah (ﷺ) and he asked me, "Have you come to inquire about piety?" I replied in the affirmative. Then he said, "Ask your heart regarding

it. Piety is that which contents the soul and comforts the heart, and sin is that which causes doubts and perturbs the heart, even if people pronounce it lawful and give you verdicts on such matters again and again." Riyad as-Salihin, Book 1, Hadith 591, sunnah.com.

2. Majeed A. How Islam changed medicine. BMJ. 2005;331(7531):1486-1487. doi:10.1136/bmj.331.7531.1486

3. Akmal M, Zulkifle M, Ansari A. Ibn nafis - a forgotten genius in the discovery of pulmonary blood circulation. Heart Views. 2010;11(1):26-30.

4. Aschoff A, Kremer P, Hashemi B, Kunze S. The scientific history of hydrocephalus and its treatment. Neurosurg Rev. 1999;22(2-3):67-95. doi:10.1007/s101430050035

5. Aksoy S. The religious tradition of Ishaq ibn Ali al-Ruhawi: the author of the first medical ethics book in Islamic medicine. Journal of the International Society for the History of Islamic Medicine. 2004;3:9–11.

6. https://www.pewforum.org/2017/07/26/demographic-portrait-of-muslim-americans/

7. "[He] who created death and life to test you [as to] which of you is best in deed-and He is Exalted in Might, the Forgiving", The Glorious Qur'an, Chapter 67, Verse 2.

8. "And We will surely test you with something of fear and hunger and a loss of wealth and lives and fruits, but give good tidings to the patient(155) Who when disaster strikes them, say, indeed we belong to Allah, and indeed to Him we will return(156) Those are the ones upon whom are blessings from their Lord and mercy. And it is those who are the [rightly] guided. (157)", The Glorious Qur'an, Chapter 1, Verses 155-157.

9. "And when I am ill, it is He who cures me", The Glorious Qur'an, Chapter 26, Verse 80

10. The Prophet (ﷺ) said, "There is no disease that Allah has created, except that He also has created its treatment." Narrated Abu Huraira, Sahih al-Bukhari 5678, sunnah.com.

11. "On the Day when Allah will resurrect them all and inform them of what they did. Allah had enumerated it, while they forgot it; and Allah is over all things, Witness." Glorious Qur'an, Chapter 58, Verse 6.

12. "And spend in the way of Allah and do not throw [yourselves] with your [own] hands into destruction [by refraining]. And do good; indeed, Allah loves the doers of good." The Glorious Qur'an, Chapter 1, Verse 195.

13. "Indeed, Allah loves those who are constantly repentant and loves who purify themselves". The Glorious Qur'an, Chapter 1, Verse 222.

14. "If it were not that it would be difficult on my nation, then I would have ordered them to use the Siwak for each prayer." narrated by Abu Hurairah, Jami` at-Tirmidhi 22, sunnah.com.

15. Arawi TA. The muslim physician and the ethics of medicine. J IMA. 2010;42(3):111-116. doi:10.5915/42-3-5403

16. "Undoubtedly Allah knows what they conceal. And what they reveal. Verily He loves not the arrogant." The Glorious Qur'an, Chapter 16, Verse 23.

17. "O Prophet, tell your wives and your daughters and the women of the believers to bring down over themselves [part] of their outer garments. That is more suitable that they will be known and not be abused. And ever is Allah Forgiving and Merciful", Glorious Qur'an, Chapter 33, Verse 59.

18. Abu Hurairah (May Allah be pleased with him) reported: The Prophet (ﷺ) said, "What is below the ankles of a lower garment is condemned to the Fire (Hell)." Sahih al-Bukhari 5678, sunnah.com.

19. It was narrated that Ma'qil ibn Yassaar said: the Messenger of Allaah (peace and blessings of Allaah be upon him) said: "For one of you to be stabbed in the head with an iron needle is better for him than that he should touch a woman who is not permissible for him." Narrated by al-Tabaraani in al-Kabeer, 486. Shaykh al-Albaani said in Saheeh al-Jaami', 5045

20. Gatrad AR, Sheikh A, Medical ethics and Islam: principles and practice Archives of Disease in Childhood 2001;84:72-75.

21. Mohiuddin A, Suleman M, Rasheed S, Padela AI. When can Muslims withdraw or withhold life support? A narrative review of Islamic juridical rulings. Glob Bioeth. 2020;31(1):29-46. Published 2020 Mar 22. doi:10.1080/11287462.2020.1736243

22. Ali, A, Ahmed, T, Ayub, A, et al. Organ donation and transplant: The Islamic perspective. Clin Transplant.2020; 34:e13832. https://doi-org.ezproxy.bu.edu/10.1111/ctr.13832

23. "And He has not made your adopted sons your [true] sons"The Glorious Qur'an,Chapter 33,Verse4

24. "Prohibited to you [for marriage] are your mothers, your daughters, your sisters, your brother's daughters, your sister daughters, your [milk] mother's who nursed you, your sisters through nursing...", Glorious Qur'an, Chapter 4, Verse 23

JUDAISM IN PEDIATRIC NEUROLOGY

Rabbi Sharon Clevenger
The Rashi School
Dedham, Massachusetts

Rinat Jonas, MD
Assistant Professor of Pediatric and Neurology
Director, Child Neurology Residency Program
Director, Pediatric EEG
Boston Medical Center
Boston, Massachusetts

INTRODUCTION

Pediatric neurological conditions account for a significant proportion of serious pediatric illnesses, whether acute or chronic, and represent a major cause of impairment and disability. As Pediatric Neurologists, we not only diagnose and treat neurological conditions but as important, we build long-term relationship with our patients and their families, to guide and help them through challenging and difficult health struggles. In such times, many of our patients seek additional advice and support from religion, tradition and spirituality. In the current healthcare system, where we focus on modern, scientific, and time efficient treatments, it is essential not to forget the importance of humanistic, culturally competent medical care as an important aspect of quality patient care. A humanistic physician demonstrates respect and is sensitive to the patient's cultural and ethnic background, values, social and religious needs and provides skilled compassionate and empathetic care. In this article, we will touch on a few religious, cultural, and historical factors that may help pediatric neurologists better understand Judaism and its attitude towards medical care.

Judaism is the world's oldest monotheistic religion, dating back nearly 4,000 years to biblical times. Today there are around 15 million Jews in the world, of which 45% live in Israel and 45% in the United States. Except for Israel, where the Jews are considered the majority, in the rest of the world they are a religious and cultural minority.

The central idea of the Jewish faith is that there are one God and that people must follow Gods laws, which govern daily life.

The foundation of Jewish laws and ethical thinking is the Bible-Torah, often referred to as the Five Books of Moses. In the roughly 3,300 years since the Torah was given to Moses by God in Mount Sinai, Rabbis have interpreted and adapted those written as well as oral laws to apply to life in each new place and time. These are summarized in 3 important collections- Talmud from Babylonian times and Later the Mishna and Shulchan Aruch. A collection of laws or Mitzvot-Commands total of 613 which addresses every aspect of Jewish life, is called Halacha, which means, 'the way we go."

As with other religions, there is no single representative of "the Jewish people." They can be divided into 3 main groups based on their difference in understanding or interpreting of the Torah. Some Jews would identify themselves as secular (they don't believe in God but follow many Jewish traditions as a culture) and others as religious but liberal (because they follow some Halacha and many Jewish traditions but adapt it to the current modern life). An important minority in the Jewish community is Orthodox, meaning they are strictly observant with the laws of Halacha. Within the Orthodox Community, there are different divisions: the modern Orthodox and the ultraorthodox.

Medical professionals are most likely to face most of the cultural or religious challenges such as complex code of religious observance, delicate balance between patient autonomy and rabbinic authority and fear of stigma associated with illnesses, when treating the Ultra-Orthodox, or most traditional group of Jews. And yet, even many secular Jews will seek guidance and comfort from tradition and faith when grappling with impossible, life and death decisions.

Jewish tradition has reflected on the treatment of patients with neurological disorders since Biblical times as demonstrated in the story of the Shunamite woman. Her only young son, which she conceived after years of infertility as a gratitude for her hospitality to the healer Elisha, dies after a presumable rupture of a brain AV malformation. Tragically, the first episode recorded of the boy's life begins when, he cries out, "Oh, my head, my head," at which point he is brought, to his mother: "And the child sat on her lap until noon; and he died."

Elisha the prophet and healer was brought in. First, he prayed to God. "Then he bent over the child and put his mouth on its mouth, his eyes on its eyes, and his hands on its hands... and the body of the child became warm. Thereupon the boy sneezed seven times and opened his eyes." Elisha said, 'Pick up your son.' She came and fell to his feet and bowed low to the ground; then she picked up her son and left." The Shunamite women as a woman of faith, does not submit to death, but works to sustain her son's life and demands that Elisha, the prophet and healer, revives him.

This ancient story of a sick child, a desperate parent and a healer who needs to show compassion to parents and child, one who will try anything in order to heal the patient, must feel familiar to any pediatrician and especially child neurologists who often deal with chronic often devastating and incurable disorders. It also serves as a wonderful launching point to understand Jewish attitudes about the value of life, body, God, and importance of medical care.

Genesis 1:27 states: "And God created man in his image, in the image of God he created him, male and female he created them." That fundamental connection between people and God sits at the foundation of Jewish beliefs about life and death, illness and healing. Judaism very clearly includes people with differences such as physical or developmental disabilities, whether from birth or due to illness or accident, in the category of being created in God's image. This accepted truth also informs the tremendous value that Jews place on medicine and medical professionals, and significantly informs the ethos of most of the faithful Jews who will be patients in your offices. To save a life is to save the very likeness of God.

JUDAISM, HEALING AND THE PHYSICIAN'S ROLE

What does Jewish tradition seek to teach about illness and healing? Human life has infinite value and improvement of the patient's quality of life is a constant commitment. The Torah states: "Heal, you must heal" from which the Rabbis derive that a doctor has to heal and that the practice of medicine is in accordance with the will of God." The Jewish code of law states: "we have to use all available knowledge to heal the ill, and 'when one delays in doing so, it is as if he has shed blood." It is important to acknowledge that illness is not a punishment from God and the person does not have to suffer; on the contrary, the patient is commanded to seek healing from the physician and to prevent illness if possible.

The work of healing and the role of the physician is so vital that, "Whoever destroys a life... it is as if he destroyed an entire world. And whoever saves a life... it is as if he saved an entire world." Lifesaving is so valuable that while doing so the person may violate almost any other laws of the Halacha, such as observing the Sabbath.

Rabbis from Talmudic times (Third through Seventh Centuries CE), compared the work of physicians to the work of farmers. God created the human body just as God created the earth, both need the care in order to thrive: "A tree, if it is not composted, weeded... will not grow... So, too, the human body is a tree, a healing potion is the compost, and a physician is the tiller of the soil." Jews have a long and proud tradition of serving as medical professionals. The great Maimonides, a 12th Century Torah scholar, supported himself as a physician, and even treated the Sultan of Cairo. The tradition of Jews in medicine continues today, even inspiring the joke about the first Jewish president being sworn into office. His mother nudges the person next to her and says, "See that man with his hand on the Bible? His sister is a doctor."

The Jewish tradition emphasizes that healing does not only happen through medical intervention. The simple act of being present for the suffering patient, getting close enough, showing compassion and respect holds a significant power and importance (see Elisha's obvious concern for the Shunamite woman, and his willingness to get very close to the ill boy).

In medicine, the ultimate goal is, of course, cure, but in many cases, especially in Pediatric Neurology that is impossible. In such cases, the goal must be to try and do the most to improve the patient's quality of life and make suffering manageable. How do Jews understand suffering? To repeat, Jewish tradition does not see suffering as a sign of God's punishment, nor is it something to be borne stoically. Suffering is not welcome to people, and it is not seen as having some ultimate reward. Instead, suffering can be seen as an opportunity for reflection: 'How can I live my most meaningful life while living with my suffering?'

THE ROLE OF THE RABBI

This is where the intersection of the physician's role and the rabbi's role become very important. As the physician is responsible for healing the body, the Rabbi cares about the suffering and the soul of the congregant. The Rabbi holds a significant place in the personal lives of the family and is viewed not only as a spiritual leader who is knowledgeable about traditions and the Jewish law but also as a counselor and educator. In the most observant communities, the Rabbi serves as the "ruler/decisor" in controversial matters of the Jewish law (Halacha) that portray to every aspect of the Jewish life including medical decisions.

It is important to understand that Orthodox Judaism does not have a single central authority. Many decisions related to modern medical treatment and Jewish law require interpretation and extrapolation from ancient sources. As a result, Rabbis with different approaches to interpreting rabbinic texts may come to different, but equally valid, rulings about a course of action. This is part of the reason there is variability in some aspects of religious practice within the ultra-Orthodox community. Health care professionals should not be surprised if two Orthodox Jewish patients with similar medical situations receive different guidance from their respective Rabbis.

In the US, the ultra-Orthodox Jews are mainly the ones to involve Rabbis in healthcare and medical decisions making in order to ensure that their actions are in accordance with Jewish law and hence God's will. However, a study from Israel showed that not only religious and ultra-Orthodox Jews consult Rabbis but also a considerable number of secular and traditional Jews consult Rabbis when facing serious medical issues. They do so for emotional support, guidance in making difficult medical decisions and to receive blessings for success or a miracle for cure.

JUDAISM AND END OF LIFE EUTHANASIA

When healing or even management proves impossible, where do Jews stand on end of life issues? Though individual Jews may have varied opinions, the religious movements of Judaism all directly oppose active euthanasia and consider it murder even if the patient wishes to die. "The value of human life is infinite and beyond measure, so that any part of life - even if only an hour or a second - is of precisely the same worth as seventy years of it. Just as any fraction of infinity, being indivisible, remains infinite." The Rabbis of the Talmud put it quite succinctly: "One who closes the eyes of a dying person while the soul is departing sheds blood." Today, Jewish leaders, especially from the Orthodox and Conservative movements, oppose active euthanasia.

Passive euthanasia is less clear. Jewish law says that doctors (and patients) have a duty to preserve life, and a doctor must do everything they can to save a patient's life - But there is a fine line for doctors and patients in cases where a patient is terminally ill. Although a doctor cannot do anything that hastens death, in Shulchan Aruch, the author states: "If there is anything which hinders the departure of the soul, such as a knocking noise, or wood chopping, near the patient's house" a doctor can remove whatever is preventing the dying person's soul from departing, as there is no act involved in this other than the removal of the impediment." Modern Jewish medical ethicists use this text as a basis for turning off respirators or removing feeding tubes on patients who have no hope for recovery. For example, if a child with Tay Sachs is nearing the end of its life and the parents request that the child not be put on a ventilator or stop ventilatory support when it is clear that the child would die if not for the ventilator, Jewish law allows for the removal of the support. Another example is when a dying patient suffers great pain, he should not be kept alive by artificial means if the treatment does not cure the illness but only prolongs his life temporarily.

The trauma of the Holocaust, which is beyond this paper, also contributes to how Jews view euthanasia and any deliberate taking of human life.

DETERMINATION OF BRAIN DEATH

The determination of brain death is important in Jewish laws for many reasons but especially for medical needs such as termination of medical interventions and organ transplantation. In previous generations, before the advances in medical technology such as cardiac respiratory support, the moment of death happened with the cessation of both breathing and cardiac activity. During the late 1960's most countries accepted the term "Brain death/death by neurologic criteria" as the legal definition of death in adults and children over 5 years and later in the 80's also for younger children. Brain death is defined as irreversible and permanent cessation of all brain function, unresponsive coma with loss of capacity for consciousness, brainstem reflexes, and the ability to breathe independently all while cardiac function and blood circulation could remain intact. Currently most authorities agree that it is not necessary to perform ancillary testing such as EEG or brain scans.

The Jewish view on how to determine brain death originates from two different interpretations of one story in the Talmud. The story is about a man that was buried under a pile of rocks on the Sabbath and the debate whether bystanders were allowed to clear the rubble that buried him on Sabbath, as only lifesaving work is allowed on this sacred day. The decision was to clear the rubble to uncover the person's nose and check for breathing. If he was breathing, then it was allowed to continue and clear the rest of the rubble to save his life. However, if he was not breathing, they had to wait until the end of Shabbat to clear the rest of rubble as he was already dead and it was not a lifesaving action. Some Rabbis interpreted this as allowing to determine death when a person stopped breathing. However, other Rabbis concluded that if breathing was not detected, then the bystander had to continue and dig further to uncover the heart and check for lack of pulsation before determining death and stopping the lifesaving action.

In modern times most Jewish movements including the Israeli chief rabbinate agree with the concept of Brain death/death by neurologic criteria. However, this opinion is not accepted by many ultra-Orthodox Rabbis in Israel, Europe and the US, who require cessation of breathing and heartbeat before determining death. In some states such as NY and NJ there is legislative recognition of religious exceptions to death determination that takes into consideration the patient's religious beliefs and wishes and allows to declare death on the basis of cardiorespiratory criteria. In Israel, due to objections of the ultra-Orthodox community to the neurological criteria of brain death, it is recommended to add an extra ancillary test, like EEG or doppler, before determining brain death by neurological criteria

GENETICS AND JUDAISM

One of the most important mitzvot (commandments of the Torah) for Jews is to procreate. "God blessed them and said to them, 'Be fruitful and multiply and fill the earth...'" Rabbinic authorities already recognized in ancient times the increased risk for genetic inheritable disorders in the Jewish population and tried to minimize them. It was prohibited in Halacha "to marry a woman from a family of epileptics or lepers" as the illness may be genetically transmitted to future generations.

Because of the common heritage that Jews share, recessive disease-causing mutations appear in Jewish populations more than in the general population. In fact, one in every 3-4

Ashkenazi Jews (descendants of central and eastern Europe) is likely a carrier of a mutation for a recessive neurological disorder, especially neurodegenerative and neuromuscular disorders. The most common Ashkenazi treatable genetic disease is Gaucher disease type 1, carriers status of 1:12. The most common neurological disorder is Tay Sachs with carrier status of 1:26. Tay Sachs is a progressive, not curable, lysosomal sphingolipid storage disorder caused by deficient hexosaminidase A. Infants who were born normal start to regress around 6 months of age, have refractory epilepsy, lose vision, motor and communication skills and progressively become dependent on G tube feeds and ventilators and die by age 3-5 years. Other common disorders include familial dysautonomia (1:32), Canavan disease (1:40),) Maple Syrup Urine disease (1:80), Nieman Pick type A (1:90), Glycogen storage disease type 1 (1:70), Jubert type2, Mucolipidosis IV, Nemaline myopathy, Walker Warburg and Torsion dystonia.

It is important to recognize that carrier state of recessive mutations is not only present in Ashkenazi Jews but also in Sephardic Jews (descendant of Mediterranean and Arab countries). For instance, the carrier frequency for Spinal Muscular Atrophy is 1 in 10 for Egyptian Jews and only 1 in 41 for Ashkenazi Jews.

In face of fulfilling the mitzvah to reproduce, while limiting the chance of producing a child who surely will die shortly or is destined to suffer, all Jewish denominations encourage screening for these genetic mutations. However, they may differ in the approach to timing of the genetic screening and what to do with the results. In most denominations the screening is performed after marriage before conception and the results of the carrier status are known.

In the ultra-Orthodox communities, marriages are arranged through a matchmaker. Being a carrier of a genetic disorder or having a relative with a presumably genetic disorder poses a stigma and grief to the carrier and the entire family and make the unmarried members of the family not desirable for a match.

The community recognized the need for genetic screening to avoid an increase in inheritable recessive genetic disorders, especially as abortions are prohibited except for when the mother's life is in danger. At the same time, they tried to minimize the stigma of being a carrier. The solution was to recommend genetic screening already pre-dating/marriage and keep the carrier status anonymous. This is currently done through different services such as Dor Yeshorim (Upright or Righteous Generation). In the last year of high school, Ashkenazi boys and girls are screened for carrier status for common genetic disorders, but they or their families never receive the carrier status. Instead they are given an ID number and their Rabbi or matchmaker can check whether the couple is genetically compatible before suggesting or disapproving dating and marriage. The couple and their family will not know who carries what gene mutation. Since the introduction of carrier testing, the incidence of Tay Sachs has decreased by 90%.

Jewish law- Halacha- allows and even encourages use of modern technology such as use of gene therapy and other applications of genetic engineering to cure or prevent genetic disorders. These are considered legitimate implementation of the biblical mandate to heal. Jews are also allowed and encouraged to participate in clinical trials, as they are allowed to take some risks to preserve life and have the religious obligation to help others.

JUDAISM AND PEOPLE WITH DISABILITIES

Children with neurological conditions often have a typical development such as autism or intellectual disabilities. There is detailed Jewish material about children with physical and intellectual disabilities and whether they can live a fully meaningful Jewish life. Jews believe that "God made us all in his image" and therefore all humans are of equal, infinite and ultimate value, even if they vary considerably in their physical or intellectual abilities or personalities. Life is a gift for all and nothing could be more valuable, and no one is less valuable.

It is a Jewish obligation for individuals, family and society to help children and people with disabilities lead as full and productive a life as possible.

A lesson by an Orthodox Rabbi talks about providing Jewish education: "The "child who cannot ask questions" (Intellectually disabled) cannot be neglected. Even though this child appears unable to talk and is apparently without intelligence, we are not to assume that the child has no potential. With proper patience, love and perseverance, one is apt to open his mouth. The child's maximum potential is to be reinforced and galvanized. This will require dedication and labor, but those who devote themselves to this endeavor will become partners with God by infusing life and joy into the stagnant existence of these children. There is no nobler cause than dedication to the ushering of joy and meaning into the lives of intellectually disabled people.

Children and adults with disabilities are encouraged to embrace all aspects of Jewish life, including being able to become bar mitzvah (the legal status afforded to Jewish boys at age 13 and girls at age 12). Communities may think creatively about ways for Jews with disabilities to fulfill the commandments (such as deaf people using sign language for prayer or people with intellectual disabilities getting similar exposure to Jewish teaching, even if they are able to learn less material than their neurotypical peers). When possible the community and family must work to their utmost to help people with disabilities avoid institutional care. It is most important for physicians to know that families hope that their children with neurological disorders will still live rich and meaningful Jewish lives.

CARE OF SEVERELY HANDICAPPED NEWBORNS

Until a newborn reaches 30 days of life he is not considered to be a person whose life is confirmed. Therefore, if a newborn is born with severe disabilities that threaten their lives, it is OK not to apply heroic measures for treatments. While it is not allowed to do anything actively to hasten the newborn's death, we may, according to Halacha, do less to sustain its life, except, of course, if the intervention holds out significant promise of curing the infant of the disease or condition. Most rabbinic authorities would not require surgery or medications beyond those necessary to relieve the newborn's pain.

Tips for the pediatric neurologist taking care of Jewish patients

When treating a Jewish patient, not always can the physician guess, just by their appearance, whether they are from a liberal or stricter observant Jewish denomination. It is important to ask the patient what cultural, religious, spiritual, or lifestyle beliefs may impact the kind of health care they want to receive. It is important to document these preferences in the patient's chart so other providers can honor them. Continuity of cultural appropriateness within the care team is essential.

Orthodox Jews avoid unnecessary physical contact between men and women. This does not apply to doctors treating patients, however some may prefer and feel more comfortable with a same gender provider, or may ask to leave the office door a crack open during exams. Outside of the context of treatment, or when meeting with family members of the patient who are not the same gender as the physician, physical contact may be unwelcome. Parents of a patient, or patients who have reached the age of adulthood (13 for boys, 12 for girls) may prefer not to shake the hand of a provider of the opposite gender. It is best to wait for the family to set the tone if they want to shake hands or not or just simply ask about their preference.

The Sabbath: Medical providers should know that the Sabbath (called Sabbath or Shabbos), which begins at sundown on Friday and concludes an hour after sundown on Saturday, is the most sacred day of the week. Shabbat is a day for rest and reflection and during that time Orthodox Jews will not engage with technology (use of phones, TV, computers, elevators, etc.), nor will they cook food, drive or write. All of the prohibitions of the Sabbath are suspended in the case of danger to life and Orthodox Jews would not decline lifesaving medical treatment. There is a traditional Jewish teaching that "preservation of life" (pikuah nefesh) precedes all rabbinic and biblical prohibitions, even strict observance of the Sabbath.

However, for any non-life saving care the Orthodox Jews will prefer to postpone treatment until Saturday night (for instance, dealing with severe migraine at home rather than seeking help in the emergency room). When a physician takes care of Orthodox Jewish patients it is important to weigh the urgency of the medical needs against the mandate to keep the Sabbath. We as Child Neurologists should incorporate into a seizure action plan specific instructions for seizure management on Shabbat, which may be different than everyday management. The patient will appreciate guidance on when it is acceptable to observe the child safely at home and when it is a "lifesaving" situation that required violating the Sabbath and coming to the emergency room.

It is important that the physician understand that their professional opinion actually carries a great deal of weight in Halacha and they are considered the final authority concerning the necessity of suspending the laws of the Sabbath. The Halacha recognizes the possibility that conditions that are currently not life threatening such as short self-resolving focal seizures in Dravet syndrome, may escalate rapidly into life-threatening status epilepticus when the child is febrile. In such a scenario when the clinical situation may evolve into a life-threatening situation, it is allowed to violate the Sabbath. However, if conditions are not life threatening and are not likely to become life threatening, the physician should err on the side of allowing the Jewish patient to maintain their observance of the Sabbath at home.

When a Jewish patient is hospitalized on Sabbath, they may prefer to avoid use of any electric devices, such as an IV pump, and would prefer to give verbal rather than written consent for necessary procedures. The patient is not allowed to perform simple daily tasks like turning of the lights in the room or asking someone to do it for them. However, it is permissible to indirectly hint to a non-Jewish person, "The lights are on..." The healthcare provider should be able to understand that it is a cue to turn off the light.

Many Jews, especially Orthodox and Conservative, observe kashrut, laws about eating certain foods and avoiding others (not eating pork or shellfish or dairy and meat products together). You may receive questions about the kosher status of certain medications or treatments or about taking certain medications during Passover, the Jewish festival of unleavened bread, if they are not deemed kosher for Passover (contain wheat products). A patient may consult the Rabbi with these questions, but know that Jewish tradition is clear that preservation of health is more important than following the laws of kashrut (for example, Jews can receive a pig's heart valve if they need a valve replacement, even though pigs are not kosher). When a patient is hospitalized, the hospital should make every effort to provide kosher food.

There are a few fasting days in Jewish traditions, most notably Yom Kippur. Jewish adults (over age 12 for girls and 13 for boys) are obligated to refrain from eating and drinking for a full 25 hours. While most observant Jews will take medications that are life preserving, they may choose to refrain from other medications, only doing the minimum necessary to maintain health. Physicians should speak with their patients about a clear plan for successfully and healthfully navigating a fast day.

As pediatric neurologists, we are occasionally involved in end of life decisions and determination of brain death. Especially in children, it is always tragic and highly emotional to both physicians and families. We must be sensitive to the beliefs of some Jewish denominations that do not accept the current brain death by neurological criteria and regard it a murder, to withdraw ventilatory support when the heart is still beating. As mentioned before in some states such as NY and NJ, there are legal considerations that allow for keeping a child in the ICU on ventilatory support even if legally brain dead, until the heart stops beating. Insurance companies in such states cannot deny ICU payments; however, in most other states or countries it is at the discretion of the attending physicians to respect the cultural and religious beliefs of the family. The physician should not issue a brain death certificate before allowing the medical teams and the family to consult their Rabbinical authority and reaching a compromise regarding level of care to allow asystole to occur as soon as possible. Studies show that asystole usually occurs within a few days of brain stem death even if limited supportive care is continued.

The physician-patient and Rabbi: As Mentioned above, the Rabbi plays a central role not only in providing spiritual and emotional support but in some Jewish denominations also in guiding the patient to make medical decisions that are aligned with the Jewish Law of Halacha.

It is important for physicians to respect the patient's decision to consult a Rabbi, as faith in religion and Rabbis does not reflect lack of faith in conventional medicine. The physician has the medical and scientific knowledge and has a duty to put it fully at the disposal the patient. The patient has a duty to take care of himself and obtain all the necessary medical information and match it with his own understanding of his own needs. And the Rabbi gives halachic guidance and pastoral support to the patient and physician in their critical decision-making process, while observing the values of the Jewish tradition. In most complex cases, none of the three has the absolute decision-making power. The physician with the patient's permission should offer to speak directly with the Rabbi to provide clinical information and a chance to ask questions. The physician should be open minded and listen without judgment while discussing openly all the ramifications of the decision-making process. The physician should understand the importance of reaching a solution that is at the same time medically, ethically and halachically proper.

The Rabbis usually supports and encourages the patient to follow the conventional medical treatment offered by the physicians and usually leans to recommend more care rather than less care ("If you saved one person as if you saved the word")

Prayers are an important part of the Jewish religion and every adult man is obligated to pray 3 times a day. During illness and distress, these activities will likely intensify and it is common to see family members at the bedside reciting palms and being involved in religious study. Jews believe that physicians are God's partners in the ongoing act of healing but that ultimately life and death, sickness and health are in God's hands. During prayers for a critically ill child, especially at the time of death, the family may desire the presence of a prayer quorum, or minyan, of at least 10 men so that specific prayers can be recited as the patient dies. In an acute care setting, this request can be challenging to meet. However, recognizing the spiritual significance to the patient and family at this critical time can help clinicians be as flexible as possible in their efforts to accommodate.

CONCLUSION

Judaism is a religion of law, dating back almost 4000 years. The traditional, observant Jew incorporates the laws into their everyday life, including decisions regarding health care.

Just as importantly, Judaism is a religion of life and all biblical laws are temporarily waived in order to save a human life, even the strict laws of observing Shabbat.

In Judaism, physicians are obligated to heal patients, decrease suffering and cure disease whenever possible. Similarly, patients are obligated to lead healthy lifestyles, to consult physicians when they are sick and to be compliant with the physician's therapeutic recommendations.

Judaism also recognizes that life is not infinite and so, when faced with death, Jews, like all people, seek to die with dignity and surrounded by family.

It is important that we as physicians approach our patients with sense of humility and real curiosity about their lives and encourage our patients from diverse religious and cultural backgrounds to feel comfortable expressing their cultural health beliefs and practices. It is our duty to be familiar with and respectful of various traditional healing systems and beliefs and where appropriate, integrate these into treatment plans. We should actively self-reflect whether the way we are treating our patients is how we ourselves wish to be treated. When healthcare professionals give humanistic care, patients are more likely to adhere to their medical orders, which results in better health outcomes.

RESOURCES

1. Biblical citations: II Kings chapter 4. Exodus 21:19

2. Babylonian Talmud Sanhedrin 37a, Babylonian Talmud Shabbat 151b

3. Shulchan Aruch, Yorei De'ah 336:1

4. Orech Chayim339:1

5. G Goldstein et al. Bioethics for clinicians: Jewish bioethics Can Med assoc J. 2001;164(2):219-22

6. Victor Frankl. Man's searching for meaning. 1964

7. Y Keshet et al. Coping with Illness and Threat: Why Non-religious Jews Choose to Consult Rabbis on Healthcare Issues. J Relig Health (2014) 53:1146–1160

8. JD Hoffman et al. The Ashkenazi Jewish carrier screening panel: evolution, status quo, and disparities. Prenat Diagn. 2014 Dec; 34(12):1161-7.

9. HJ Schwartz et al. Management of the Asthmatic, Sabbath-observant Jewish Patient. Some Guidelines in the Light of Jewish Law. Chest, 1983 Dec;84(6):762-5.T Bressler et al. Ethical Challenges When Caring for Orthodox Jewish Patients at the End of Life. J Hosp Palliat Nurs. February 2018 Volume 29 (1):36 – 44

10. H Zukier. The Soul in Medicine: Rabbinic and Scientific Controversies. J Relig Health (2016) 55:2174–2188

11. BN Dorff . The Jewish Tradition: Religious beliefs and health care decisions. Handbook series published by the Park Ridge Center for the Study of Health, Faith, and Ethics. 2002.

12. E, Gabbay et al. The Care of the Ultra-Orthodox Jewish Patient. J Relig Health (2017) 56:545–560

13. F Rosner. The Jewish Patient in a Non-Jewish Hospital. J of Relig and Health. 1986 Vol. 25: 316-324

14. M Koch. Judaism and Disability. BA, Yale University, 2002

15. E Gabbay et al Go in Peace: Brain Death, Reasonable Accommodation and Jewish Mourning Rituals. J Relig Health. 2019 Oct;58(5):1672-1686

RELIGIOUS PERSPECTIVES AND HUMANISM IN CHILD NEUROLOGY—A VEDANTIC PERSPECTIVE

Jaskaran Singh Lamba
Undergraduate student
Frederick S Pardee School of Global Studies
Boston University
Boston, MassachusettS

Mandeep Rana, MD
Assistant Professor Pediatrics
Boston University School of Medicine
Boston Medical Center
Boston, Massachusetts

The American Humanist Association describes humanism as "a progressive philosophy of life that, without theism or other supernatural beliefs, affirms our ability and responsibility to lead ethical lives of personal fulfillment that aspire to the greater good." It is a system of thought that emphasizes the importance of the human over the divine. It may be described as an outlook that focuses on the essential goodness of the human being. Religion, on the other hand, is the worship and belief in the control of a superhuman power, such as a god or gods, who are above the individual. The 30,000 feet view is that both share similar goals: engagement in the phenomenon within the self, awareness of oneness, union with oneness, and acceptance of the self and the divine/force/energy within us and in all things around us. Both are steps on a spiritual journey.

Child neurology deals with the physical manifestation of this force or energy and involves the examination and treatment of disorders of the brain and spinal cord, peripheral nerves, and muscles. These disorders include cerebral palsy, migraine, epilepsy, and neurodevelopmental diseases, such as autism, and metabolic, genetic, and degenerative disorders [1]. Caring for children with complex medical and neurologic issues requires not only a medical approach but also a humanistic approach, that is, understanding the religious and cultural practices of our patients and their families and respecting the personal integrity and uniqueness of each patient and family.

INFLUENCES OF INDIAN CULTURE ON HEALTH

India is a multicultural, multiethnic, pluralistic society with enormous socioeconomic and educational disparities and beliefs. The term Hinduism has been used as a common geographical, cultural, and religious identifier for people living on the Indian subcontinent and has come to encompass Hindus, Sikhs, Muslims, Christians, and Buddhists, among others. The majority of Asian religions are united by common cultural and religious practices. They offer a unique perspective on God and the material world, particularly with regard to understanding illness. Religious beliefs can exert positive influences on health by acting as a source of inspiration or release, as well as negative influences when linked with guilt, punishment associated with karma, and societal stigma. Some Asian religions also engender a sense of fatalism, a belief that someone other than the individual or something else is in control. The identification of an external locus of control can have an impact on health behavior [2]. When caring for families from these regions, it important to keep in mind that religious and traditional therapies are likely to play a role either in isolation or as an adjunct to conventional medical therapy. The mind is often given the highest tribute owing to its potential influence on conscious and creative energy, and its association with the soul in the physical body [3] commonly used in Asian communities.

MAJOR HINDU RELIGIOUS TEXTS

The Vedas are ancient religious texts that define truth for Hindus. They contain fundamental knowledge relating to underlying cause and function of and one's personal response to existence. Life is considered sacred, eternal, and of enormous value. One of the Mahavakyas or "The Great Sayings" of the Upanishads is Aham Brahmasmi: I am Brahman or I am Divine, I am Absolute Reality, in other words, I am a complete being. The purpose of human life is to recognize one's higher self (the Atman, Brahman) and perform whatever dharma (duty) one has been given with proper karma (action) in order to free one's self from the cycle of rebirth and death. When an individual finally breaks the bonds associated with dharma and karma, Oneness with the Creator is achieved.

BHAGAVAD GITA

The Bhagavad Gita (Song of the Lord) is one of the most popular Hindu texts, a smriti text or remembered tradition. The Bhagavad Gita is a book of wisdom offering advice on how to live a righteous life. It describes the struggle between what we know is right and good and difficult and what we know is often not right, not good, but definitely easier. It guides us in making choices in this life. We can choose what to eat and wear, but when it comes to moral choices, Krishna, who lives in all of us, provides the voice of our conscience, telling us what we should be doing and guiding us on the way. We can choose to hear and heed, and we can choose to ignore.

GURU GRANTH SAHIB

The Guru Granth Sahib is the religious text of the Sikhs. It is based on the concept of Oneness: Ek Ongkar, there is only oneness, only one God that exists in each and every heart. That Oneness/God permeates the whole of creation. God is not far away. God is within you. The goal is to find that Oneness, that state of permanent truth, the state that dissolves the duality between man and God. The answer can be found in the text, Hukam Razai Chalna, Nanak Likhya Naal (Walk in the will of His order, flow with the universe). Challenging the flow of the Universe would be like trying to swim in the opposite direction of the flow of the river. When you walk with the will of God, every moment has the possibility of being sweet: Tera kiya meetha lage. Most holy texts attempt to walk us to a common destination: self-realization/inner strength/state of being, self-love and love for each other—a philosophy shared with humanism.

THE PHYSICIAN'S ROLE IN HUMANISM

Approaching the patient from a humanistic perspective can help physicians demonstrate respect for their patients' cultural and religious beliefs. Doing so promotes a conscious cognitive process to understand an individual's values and beliefs, and raises awareness to higher standards. The goal becomes the common good, for both patient and physician— doing your best for the patient lifts the doer (dharma) and releases you from debt (karma). It helps set the stage for providing medical care at a holistic level for the ultimate good of the patient. Whether caring for a child on the autism spectrum disorder or a child with cerebral palsy or an intellectual disability, the physician will see the child as more than just an interesting patient or statistic, but as a human being with immense potential, regardless of their race, beliefs, or socioeconomic status.

Seeing patients through the window of their beliefs also em-powers and supports them. Ismail and colleagues observed that in an adult patient with epilepsy, "... everything comes from up there; everything's from Allah and the one who fixes it is Allah as well. You see, that's our Muslim belief, what do you think? You see, the doctors gives you your medication, but the cure comes from Allah" [2].

The reality is that we do not choose neurologic conditions and associated mental disorders. Yet many parents and families view it as karma of parents or the child. This mindset carries with it a tremendous amount of guilt. Neurologic disorders, such as epilepsy and intellectual disabilities are seen as un-natural phenomena carrying stigma at a familial, social, and structural level. At the individual level, it manifests in the form of diminished self-esteem, self-confidence, and isolation [4].

It is interesting to note that some neurologic disorders have been described in ancient texts. In one such instance, Klein-Levin syndrome, a rare disorder among adolescents, associat-ed with periodic episodes of hypersomnolence, hyperphagia, hypersexuality, and other behavioral and cognitive difficul-ties, was described in the character Kumbhakarna in the ma-jor Sanskrit legend of the events of Ramayana, another major Sanskrit epic of Hindus [5].

CASE STUDY #1

This reminds me of a patient I saw during my internship. A 15-year-old child from rural Rajasthan was diagnosed with juvenile myoclonic epilepsy. Her parents, who were school-teachers, were overwhelmed by the fact that this type of epilepsy entailed life-long seizures. After much counselling regarding this disorder, its treatment and the importance of medical compliance, the family became worried that no one would be inclined to marry this girl child. Furthermore, what would happen if their community found out about this? Thus, they took her to a traditional healer and suffered with the guilt that this illness was a punishment for sins committed in a past life. One morning after studying for most of the night for a high school final exam, the child had a seizure. She fell and fractured her maxilla and had several other injuries to her face. My attending child neurologist and I met with the family on several occasions for further education not just about the epilepsy but their role as parents in their daughter's life. My attending quoted from the Bhagavad Gita:

karmaṇy-evādhikāras te mā phaleṣhu kadāchana

mā karma-phala-hetur bhūr mā te saṅgo 'stvakarmaṇi

(You have the right to perform your prescribed duties, but you are not entitled to the fruits of your actions. Never consider yourself to be the cause of the results of your activities, nor be attached to inaction.) Fortunately, this reminder resonated with the family and they agreed to medical therapy, but also used traditional therapies as an adjunct rather than as a substitute.

CASE STUDY #2

Another case involved a young aspiring physician couple who moved to United States to pursue further medical training with their 6-month-old daughter. A few months after their arrival, they noted abnormal movements in their child's hands and the lack of eye contact. The neurologist also recognized that the child's head circumference was trending down. A clinical diagnosis of possible Rett syndrome was later confirmed by genetic testing. The family was heartbroken and grieved deeply. At every visit, both parents were in tears and their eyes always questioned, "Why us; why my child"? After much thinking, the mother decided to leave her residency training and devote all her life to taking care of her child. They met with their priest who discussed the lack of power and control we have as human beings in deciding what we get in this life.

We do not choose our own existence, let alone what comes with it. This was incredibly touching for the family. The mother felt strengthened and resolved to return to her residency and take care of her daughter as well.

This reminded me of two quotes from Japji Sahib from the Guru Granth:

1. Hukmae andar sabh ko baahar hukam na koye, nanak hukmai jay bujhai ta ha-umai kahai na koay. (We are all with in the fold of order, none is outside (His) order. If one realizes the order, he will not fall prey to ego.)

2. Aakhan jor, chupai nah jor, jor na mangan, dayn na jor, jor na jeevan maran nah jor, jor na raaj mal man sor... (Neither speech nor silence in with in one's power,neither begging nor giving is within in one's power, nether life nor death is with on one's power. Only "He" wields the power and nobody is good or bad. We can work hard to remain connected with magic and wholeness of this life and continue to move forward.)

Supporting families in the decisions they make on religious grounds is humanism, while recognizing that parenting is an "ultimate spiritual journey, the equivalent of deep awakening of the isolated monk, the pilgrimage to Mecca or Jerusalem, or the climb up Mount Everest" [6].

CASE STUDY #3

I was amazed and struck by a family in which the mother had been in a car accident toward the end of her third trimester, resulting in placental abruption. The newborn suffered severe hypoxic ischemic injury to the brain stem, as confirmed by brain MRI. He had to be on a ventilator for respiratory support, and nasogastric tube for feeding. Following several family meetings, the family was able to come to terms with the dismal and poor prognosis of the child. The family was given the option to continue life support or withdraw care. They went home, read the Bhagavad Gita, and decided to let the spirit free and not have it suffer. It was amazing to see the confidence in this family's eyes and the peace they derived from their decision. They believed he would always be with them, even though not physically. Mother noted, "We all have to focus on doing our duty and let the universe take care of the consequences." This family found great comfort in their beliefs.

This experience reminded me of a passage from the Bhagavad Gita:

na tv evaham jatu nasam

na tvam neme janadhipah

na caiva na bhavisyamah

sarve vayam atah param

(Never was there a time when I did not exist, nor you, nor all these kings before you and neither will we cease to be in the future.)

A Model for Humanism in Medical Practice

The pediatric neurologist often sees children when parents or caregivers seek care for nervous system disorders. This often involves long term care for chronic and some neurodegenerative disorders. Thus, trust must be built from the onset.

In addition to reviewing the issue that required referral by their primary care provider or hospital admittance, it will be important to explain carefully the tests the child will be undergoing and why. In some cases, the child can be engaged in the process, using photos of equipment and describing who will be with them during the process, how long it might take, and where they will be transferred.

When treating patients and meeting families, it will be important to approach them as individuals who might be leaning on a set of particular beliefs regarding their child's condition. Explore their beliefs, examine their understanding and that of other family members, and attempt to allay any unwarranted fears. Seek understanding, if you are unfamiliar with their religious texts, such as the Guru Granth or the Bhagavad Gita. The Internet is a wonderful tool. Although it can lead you to the correct sites, it will not necessarily give you a complete understanding of the information you might find. Allow the family to guide you. While you provide medical expertise and information, permit the family to express their understanding of their religious texts and individual beliefs. Ask questions and show that you respect their culture and seek to understand it.

Above all, as you practice medicine, put the humanistic approach into practice:

1. Take time to discuss with family members the psychosocial aspects, misconceptions, and misunderstandings they might have about the neurologic disorder affecting their child;

2. Correct false notions families might have and provide accurate information;

3. Familiarize yourself with and attempt to understand and recommend meditative techniques derived from Indian philosophies for families who subscribe to Hindu practices, such as tantra and yoga, and how they can bring changes about in the structure and function of the nervous system as adjunctive treatment to various diseases [7,8];

4. Recognize the importance of parents and families in the fight against stigmas associated with neurologic disorders;

5. Help parents overcome stress and the stigma associated with disorders, such as epilepsy;

6. Encourage families and their children to transcend the physical and step into a higher dimension;

7. Emphasize the treatability of neurologic disorders rather than their link to the supernatural;

8. Help create awareness among lay persons through health camps and informative brochures [1];

9. Identify the life goals of patients with long-term neurologic disabilities;

10. Raise awareness, change attitudes, and offer information, counseling, and personality development workshops, yoga, and support groups as recommended by the Indian Epilepsy Association.

REFERENCES

1. Singh S, Mishra VN, Rai A. Myths and superstition about epilepsy: a study from North India. J Neurosci Rural Pract. 2018;9(3):359-362.

2. Ismail H, Wright H, Rhodes P.Religious beliefs about causes and treatment of epilepsy. Br J Gen Pract. 2005;55(510)26-31.

3. Shamasundar C. Relevance of ancient Indian Wisdom to modern mental health- A few examples. Indian J Psychiatry 2008 ;50 (2): 138-143. [FURTHERUIRED]

4. Sanjeeve . Confronting the stigma in epilepsy. Ann Indian Acad Neurol. 2011;14(3):158-163.

5. Lakhani OJ, Lakhani JD. Kumbhakarna: Did he suffer from the disorder of the hypothalamus? Indian J Endocrinol Metab. 2015;19(3):433-434.

6. Miller L. "The Spiritual Child: The New Science on Parenting for Health and Lifelong Thriving." Picador. New York, NY.

7. Venkatraman A, Nandy R, Rao SS, Mehta DH, Viswanathan A. Tantra and modern neurosciences: is there any correlation? NeuroIndia. 2019;67(5):1188-1193.

8. Mooventhan A, Nivethitha L. Evidence based effects of yoga in neurological disorders. J Clin Neurosci. 2017;43:61-67.

ETHICS, MORALITY, RELIGION, AND MEDICINE – THE IMPLEMENTATION OF HUMAN VALUES IN MEDICAL PRACTICE

Jorge Vidaurre, MD, FACNS, FAES
Director, Pediatric Clinical Neurophysiology Program
Director EEG laboratory
Associate Professor, Pediatric Neurology
Nationwide Children's Hospital – The Ohio State University

Hector Jose Castaneda, MD
Director Instituto de Neurociencias, El Salvador
Medical Director, Hospital Diagnostico, San Salvador, El Salvador
Medical Director, Free Sai Clinic, San Salvador, El Salvador

Hari Conjeevaram, MD, MSc, FACP, FACG
Program Director, GI Fellowship Program
Medical Director, Student Run Free Clinic
Professor of Medicine
Division of Gastroenterology and Hepatology
University of Michigan
Ann Arbor, Michigan

The world health organization (WHO) defines health as a state of complete physical, mental and social well-being and not merely the absence of disease or infirmity. In order to promote this "mental and social wellbeing," physicians need to take a more holistic approach when treating patients with specific health conditions. In fact, 'ideal medical care' should be provided each and every time when caring for patients in an atmosphere of compassion, tolerance and respect for human dignity, as stated by the American Medical Association.

The core moral principles for the practice of medicine are embedded in the "Hippocratic oath" written in the fourth century BC [1]. The oath establishes the principles of beneficence ("Whatever houses I may visit, I will come for the benefit of the sick"), non-maleficence and justice ("I will keep them from harm and injustice"). The main principles established in the oath are still valid in modern medical practice, as they are based in long-lasting moral values. These principles protect the best interests of the patients and define the basis for the doctor-patient relationship [2].

Many of the values described in the original Oath are taught in medical schools. These include respect for one's colleagues and the practice of humility, but the adoption of these values into daily practice need to be fostered by intentional behaviors, mindfulness and role modeling [3].

Nowadays, the practice of moral behavior in the medical field encounters multiple obstacles, including emphasis in observable behaviors, such as tasks directed to patient care, academic performance or specific milestones and competencies [4]. Such an environment may stimulate competition between students, trainees and medical staff and risk not practicing ideal medical care and also lead to burnout and reduced wellness among healthcare givers.

This overemphasis on science and academic productivity may have its origins in the early 20th century. In 1910, the medical education system in America experienced a radical transformation, with the institution of the biomedical model and removal of proprietary schools, as a consequence of the

Flexner report [5]. Flexner was commissioned by the Carnegie foundation to evaluate US and Canadian medical schools. His previous experience with German education and admiration for their system influenced the report [6]. This hyper rational approach was very successful to create excellence in science, which was, however, not balanced with enhancing excellence in clinical care [5].

Prominent physicians, including William Osler, emphasized the importance of the study of humanism in medicine, to avoid nurturing the formation of "Doctors- Technicians" [6,7]. Since then, medical schools have incorporated courses of medical ethics. Ethics use facts, logic and values to decide the best course of action in specific circumstances and can offer flexible solutions. Ethics provides physicians with tools to deal with problems encountered in daily medical practice. These problems can be simple and straightforward or very complex. Ethicists use basic values, including autonomy, justice, beneficence and non-maleficence. Different ethicists can have different point of views when analyzing the same problem, so ethics do not provide a unique answer or solution about the right action during specific circumstances.

Morality is an essential part of human activities and it is based on beliefs, which are centered on personal point of views or religious beliefs. Actually, data suggests that religion appears to be an important element in the practice of medicine, but science and religion share a complex, and at times controversial history [8]. Despite this, it is important to be open-minded and accepting when caring for patients, who view religion as an integral part of their own healing.

In a study of 1000 adult participants in the US who were polled, 79% of those who responded believed that spiritual faith helps in the healing process. 63% thought doctors should discuss spiritual faith with patients [8,9]. A survey of doctors showed that most believed religious beliefs are part of the healing process [8,10] and in fact, a growing number of US medical schools are incorporating religion and spirituality in their curricula [8,11,12]. This could contribute to a more humanistic approach to medical practice or at least promote tolerance to religious 'beliefs'. It is also important to recognize that faith can infuse strength and hope in patients through the healing process.

In 1983 at the World Health Assembly, 22 countries with different religious beliefs prepared a draft with the objective to incorporate the spiritual dimension into the WHO definition of health. This was proposed at the 101st session by the WHO regional office for the Eastern Mediterranean. In 1998, the executive board adopted the resolution EB101.R2 recommending the change to the general assembly. The change proposed was as follows: 'Health is a dynamic state of complete physical, mental, spiritual, and social well-being and not merely the absence of disease or infirmity.' Nevertheless, the proposal was not discussed in the general assembly held in 1999, due to differences of opinions and arguments between delegates, with the notion that "health" belongs to the domain of nature-natural science and spirituality to the domain of culture [13-15].

Adding of a spiritual dimension to the actual definition means recognizing that each individual is a spiritual being and not just a biological organism. This will likely create some central changes related to health care delivery and medical education and therefore to the whole medical educational system.

The integration of courses of ethics, religion and human values into the academic curricula of multiple medical schools reflects an effort to bring this holistic view into clinical practice.

Physicians still face multiple challenges to implementing these values into their daily practices. This is not an easy task when doctors are already dealing with fatigue, stress, frustration and burnout symptoms [16]. Medicine has also become more fragmented and sub-specialized. There is overemphasis in academic and curriculum development or productivity goals, adding pressure to medical professionals and stimulating competition. Medical institutions need to develop plans to incorporate these moral principles into daily practice, creating an evaluation system where the practice of these values is encouraged.

Morality actually comes from the Latin word "moralitas," meaning character or manner. Morality is involved in the differentiation between right and wrong. A number of factors, including biological, socio-cultural and religious, determines an individual's moral values [17].

The practice of human values is necessary for the proper functioning of society. and their universal applicability has been thought since ancient times. One of the oldest bodies of philosophy is the Vedanta or vedantic philosophy (constituted by different scriptures). Vedanta provides the instructions to discriminate, choose and perform moral and righteous actions, even in difficult situations [17,18]. The universal values in this philosophy are love (prema), peace (shanti), righteousness (dharma), truth (satya) and non-violence (ahimsa).

In this philosophy, 'love' is considered one of the most important values. The philosophy teaches to express love towards all beings, instructing that the same divine energy is the unifying current in all. Love is expressed as compassion, kindness, selflessness and sacrifice [17,19]. It emphasizes that true education should foster compassion instead of focusing solely on knowledge [19]. This type of education instructs that no harm, pain, or grief should be inflicted on another and stimulates the practice of selfless – service [20]. Practicing 'truth' fosters honesty, inquiry, self-knowledge, integrity, and equality. 'Peace' promotes calmness, humility, contentment, endurance and happiness. 'Righteousness' inculcates a sense of duty, good-ethical behavior, respect and responsibility. 'Non-violence' implies appreciation and tolerance to different cultures, castes or creeds and involves consideration, cooperation, respect, social justice and avoidance of harm.

The practice of these principles may benefit not only the patients but also the physician practicing them, serving as antidote for depersonalization and humanizing the doctor-patient relationship. It is important to not only listen to our patients, but also to practice inclusiveness, as we participate in decision-making. We should shape our policies on how best to provide medical care to maintain high ethical standards. In this regard, constant peer review with a thoughtful assessment of the required benchmarks and of performance in overall patient care is very important.

We tend to focus on making our medical students 'ideal doctors' and instill human values, but these values are already intrinsic in them. It is the responsibility of all involved in medical training to serve as a good role model and provide the right environment for students to reflect their intrinsic values.

Physicians can transform the culture of the workplace by the practice of human values. Fostering an attitude of respect, caring and service, not only towards patients, but also colleagues and learners is necessary in doing so. When medicine is practiced with the attitude of service as the primary goal, we may be able to provide better medical care and improve our sense of self-satisfaction. Physicians will then become an important aspect of the healing process with a truly holistic attitude, rather than only scientists with a very concrete approach.

REFERENCES

1. Edelstein L. The Hippocratic Oath: Text, Translation and Interpretation. Baltimore: Johns Hopkins Press, 1943.

2. Askitopoulou H, Vgontzas AN. The relevance of the Hippocratic Oath to the ethical and moral values of contemporary medicine. Part II: interpretation of the Hippocratic Oath-today's perspective. Eur Spine J 2018;27(7):1491-1500.

3. Gruppen LD. Humility and respect: core values in medical education. Med Educ 2014;48(1):53-58.

4. Irby DM, Hamstra SJ. Parting the Clouds: Three Professionalism Frameworks in Medical Education. Acad Med 2016;91(12):1606-1611.

5. Duffy TP. The Flexner Report—100 years later. Yale J Biol Med 2011;84(3):269–276.

6. Weisberg DF. Science in the service of patients: lessons from the past in the moral battle for the future of medical education. Yale J Biol Med 2014;87(1):79-89.

7. Nuland SB. The uncertain art: Thoughts on a life in medicine. New York: Random House, 2008.

8. Sloan RP, Bagiella E, Powell T. Religion, spirituality, and medicine. Lancet 1999;353(9153):664-667.

9. McNichol . The new faith in medicine USA Today, 1996. Available at:

10. Benson H. Timeless Healing: The Power and Biology of Belief. Fireside, New York, 1996.

11. Levin JS, Larson DB, Puchalski CM. Religion and spirituality in medicine: research and education. JAMA 1997;278(9):792-793.

12. Puchalski CM. Spirituality and medicine: curricula in medical education. J Cancer Educ 2006;21(1):14-18.

13. Chirico F. Spiritual well-being in the 21st century: it's time to review the current WHO's health definition. J Health and Soc Sci. 1. 11-16. 10.19204/2016/sprt2.

14. Nagase M. Does a Multi-Dimensional Concept of Health Include Spirituality? Analysis of Japan Health Science Council's Discussionson WHO's 'Definition of Health' (1998). Intl J Applied Sociol 2012;2(6),71–77.

15. Ministry of Health, Labour and Welfare, Press release data on what follows after the proposal to revise the 'definition of health' in the WHO Charter—Results of 52nd WHO General Meeting. Available at: http://www1.mhlw.go.jp/houdou/1110/h1026-1_6.html

16. Patel RS, Bachu R, Adikey A, Malik M, Shah M. Factors Related to Physician Burnout and Its Consequences: A Review. Behav Sci (Basel) 2018;8(11):98.

17. Srivastava C, Dhingra V, Bhardwaj A, Srivastava A. Morality and moral development: Traditional Hindu concepts. Indian J Psychiatry 2013;55(Suppl 2):S283-S287.

18. Brodd J. World Religions. Winona, MN: Saint Mary's Press; 2003.

19. Summer showers in Brindavan 2000 discourses of bhagavan sri sathya sai baba sri sathya sai books & publications trust prasanthi nilayam, anantapur district andhra pradesh - 515 134.

20. Summer showers in Brindavan 1972 discourses by bhagavan sri sathya sai baba delivered during the summer course held for college students at whitefield, bangalore, india page ii © sri sathya sai books and publications trust prashanthi nilayam, anantapur district andhra pradesh - 515 134.

PART 3

HUMANISM IN CLINICAL PRACTICE

HIPPOCRATIC OATH

Alcy R. Torres, MD, FAAP
Associate Professor of Pediatrics and Neurology
Assistant Dean of Diversity and Inclusion
Director of the Pediatric Traumatic Injury, International and Bilingual Programs
Boston University School of Medicine
Boston Medical Center
Boston, MA, USA

Relfa Proano Ponce, MD
Boston Medical Center
Boston University School of Medicine
Boston-MA, USA

The Hippocratic Oath is an oath of ethics historically taken by physicians. It is one of the oldest and most well-known Greek medical texts. It is attributed to Hippocrates, a Greek physician who was born on the island of Cos, and is usually credited as one of the first people who took a new approach to medicine by making it centered more towards rational science than holistic views. In its original form, it requires a new upcoming physician to swear, by several healing gods, to uphold specific ethical standards [1,5,6]. It tries to get the individual to practice medicine with their whole abilities and correct judgment and to defend medicine and trained doctors when it's seen as necessary. The oath is the earliest expression of medical ethics in the Western world, establishing several principles of medical ethics that remain of paramount significance today. These include the principles of medical confidentiality and non-maleficence. As the seminal articulation of certain principles that continue to guide and inform medical practice, the ancient text is of more than historic and symbolic value. Swearing a modified form of the Oath remains a rite of passage for medical graduates in many countries [1].

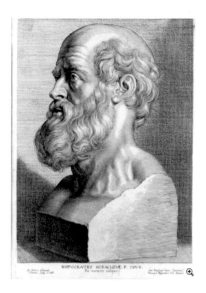

Hippocrates is considered the father of medicine [1,4,9]

Hippocrates was a philosopher and physician who lived from 460 to 377 BC. He is known as the "father of modern medicine". He is one of the first people to be credited as believing that diseases were caused naturally either by something environmental, the diet of the person affected or their living habits and standards and not by the anger of any deity, separating medicine from religion. He and his followers were the first that kept a record of many diseases and medical conditions, and provided the first description of clubbing in the fingers, for this reason, this condition is sometimes referred to as "Hippocratic fingers". He also is one of the first documented chest surgeons; his teachings remain important for today's medicine. Not much is known of his life, but his works included the Hippocratic Oath which described the basic ethics of medical practice and laid down a moral code of conduct for medical professionals. This was part of his manuscript "Hippocratic Collection".

The father of modern medicine was the creator of a great number of documents that include 72 books and 59 treaties.

Together they are known as the Hippocratic Collection, which was organized by Ptolomeo in the Library of Alexandria. Here, he built a cultural center with the idea of assembling the human insight; The Hippocratic Collection includes anatomy, physiology, psychiatric diseases, surgical procedures, diagnostic, prognosis, and treatment concept relevant to ethics.

The fundamental aspects of the document are:

a) the respect for the teachers, classmates and disciples.

b) The treatment of the patient with the intent of total recovery.

c) The absence of all evil or damage: Do not administer mortal medicines, even if requested, do not provoke abortions or practice surgeries.

d) if incapable or underqualified; transfer the patient to someone who is capable [3]

The practice of the art in a healthy and pure way, maintaining the professional secret of human intimacy. Do not seduce women or children, and swear to perform all these precepts positively, without falseness.

The classical Hippocratic Oath has been translated and interpreted over time, and it has been handed down to new generations of doctors who have changed it into various versions [1,4,7].

THE ORIGINAL VERSION, WRITTEN BY HIPPOCRATES, READS:

"I swear by Apollo Physician, by Asclepius, by Hygieia, by Panacea, and all the gods and goddesses, that, according to my ability and judgment, I will keep this Oath and this stipulation:

to reckon him who taught me this art equally dear to me as my parents, to share my substance with him, and relieve his necessities if required; to look upon his offspring in the same footing as my brothers, and to teach them this art, if they shall wish to learn it, without fee or stipulation; and that by precept, lecture, and every other mode of instruction, I will impart a knowledge of the Art to my sons, and those of my teachers, and to disciples bound by a stipulation and oath according to the law of medicine, but to none others.

I will follow that system of regimen which, according to my ability and judgment, I consider for the benefit of my patients, and abstain from whatever is deleterious and mischievous.

I will give no deadly medicine to any one if asked, nor suggest any such counsel, and in like manner I will not give to a woman a pessary to produce abortion. With purity and with holiness I will pass my life and practice my Art.

I will not cut persons laboring under the stone but will leave this to be done by men who are practitioners of this work. Into whatever houses I enter, I will go into them for the benefit of the sick and will abstain from every voluntary act of mischief and corruption; and, further, from the seduction of females or males, of freemen and slaves.

Whatever, in connection with my professional service, or not in connection with it, I see or hear, in the life of men, which ought not to be spoken of abroad, I will not divulge, as reckoning that all such should be kept secret.

While I continue to keep this Oath unviolated, may it be granted to me to enjoy life and the practice of the art, respected by all men, at all times. But should I trespass and violate this Oath, may the reverse be my lot."

Some common criticisms of the classical Hippocratic Oath include its dedication to the ancient Greek gods, as well as its prohibitions against euthanasia, abortion, and any form of surgery [1].

The classical version also instructs doctors that they should teach aspiring physicians for free, which is impractical today [1,6,7].

THE CLASSICAL HIPPOCRATIC OATH HAS BEEN SUMMARIZED AS:

Of solidarity with teachers and other physicians.

Of beneficence (to do good or avoid evil) and non-maleficence (from the Latin 'primum non-nocere', or 'do no harm') towards patients.

Not to assist suicide or abortion.

To leave surgery to surgeons.

Not to harm, especially not to seduce patients.

To maintain confidentiality and never to gossip.

Contrary to what is commonly believed, the first Hippocratic oath was vastly different from the version doctors use today. For example, in the original version it never states that a physician should "do no harm" [6]. It was phrased in a broader way by having a promise to, "abstain from whatever deadly medicine to anyone if asked" and also "abstain from every voluntary act of mischief and corruption". And, yes, "First not harm" was a motto used various times by Hippocrates, but it was used in other texts rather than in the Hippocratic oath. The original also calls for the "use of the knife" even for small procedures, which is impossible for how modern medicine conduct's itself.

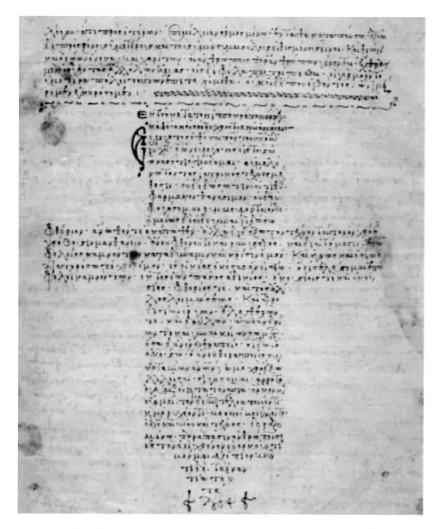

A section of the oath on Papyrus Oxyrhyncus 2547 [1,3,9]

There were no findings of any written direct punishment for breaking the Hippocratic Oath. There are various accounts of physicians from that time who assisted with the suicide of their terminal patients, a practice otherwise known today as euthanasia [3]. Therefore, one might think that not all doctors at the time swore or were faithful to the oath. Today's equivalent of breaking the oath could be interpreted as medical malpractice. The punishment for this varies depending on the gravity of the physician offense, but it could end up with losing their license and their right or privilege to practice medicine.

Modern versions have been proposed, using many of the basic principles of the original. The original version couldn't take into consideration contemporary issues such as the ethics of experimentation, team care, and the physician's legal responsibilities and how those affect the patient and the treatment because there were no such things at the time [3,4,7]. However, for the time when it was created, its writings were considered modern and innovative for medicine. The document was not translated into English until somewhere in the 1700s, it was then when scholars started taking notice of it and began to use it regularly [1,2].

Many people think that doctors still swear the Hippocratic Oath. It is not compulsory but many medical schools now hold a ceremony where graduating doctors do swear an updated version. The British Medical Association (BMA) drafted a new Hippocratic Oath for consideration by the World Medical Association in 1997 but it was not accepted and there is still no one single modern accepted version [3,6]. In some medical schools, the Declaration of Geneva physician's oath is used [1,3]. In others, an oath individualized by the institution is used. Doctors are supposed to be kind and compassionate. Doctors are supposed to respect the beliefs and values of their patients. Doctors are not supposed to cause patients to suffer. Doctors are not supposed to kill their patients. Although it is true that certain expectations of physicians, such as the ones stated above, are understood without being stated, many rules do need to be explicitly written for the sake of maintaining a uniformly practiced code of ethics within the constantly evolving field of medicine. Woodbury states that a "physician may view 'medicine' as a means to help the sick, an institution, a lifetime of personal relationships, a profitable business, an organic expression of human empathy, a rigorous application of scientific innovation, or a disciplined body of knowledge" or a multitude of other definitions. This ever-expanding collection of interpretations of the word 'medicine' further necessitates the implementation of a single code/set of guidelines to serve as a foundation and source of reference for the ethical constraints of medical practitioners. Many agree that the Hippocratic Oath can no longer serve as this code of ethics due to its complete modern irrelevance and lack of philosophical grounding and, as a result, the world has seen the creation of numerous "modern Hippocratic Oaths" to replace the original document. However, this creation of multiple codes has led to inconsistency and unreliability in terms of having a uniform set of guidelines for practitioners to follow [2].

Out of the total percentage of Oaths sworn upon at graduation ceremonies of medical students, "only 14% of these oaths prohibit euthanasia, 11% reference a deity, 8% forbid abortion, and 3% prohibit sexual relationships with patients; 50% of them do not reference accountability at all" [3,4]. The solution to this problem is for the medical community to agree upon a single document that is assertive and all-inclusive of the previously mentioned subjects. This document should be Edmund Pellegrino's Precepts, which was founded on the "patient-physician relationship as the central unique bedrock of medicine," and contains parallels to modern society that the Hippocratic Oath so desperately lacks. Pellegrino's Precepts would make a more relevant, reliable medical code of ethics that would better support physicians in their endeavors to approach the new challenges of modern-day medicine in an ethical and socially just manner [5].

This is not a matter that just affects those studying medicine. It is a subject that applies to anyone who has ever visited or plans on visiting a doctor of any kind to get better and expecting to be treated properly. Society might eventually move towards adapting a new, modern Oath.

Nowadays the White Coat Ceremony is a ritual for the medical students. The Arnold P. Gold Foundation instituted it in 1993 at Columbia University's College of Physicians and Surgeons. During this ceremony, a white coat is placed on each student's and the Hippocratic Oath is rehearsed, signifying their entrance into the medical occupation, currently implemented at most medical schools in the United States, medical schools in 19 other countries, 360 schools of nursing and in numerous physician assistant programs [3]. It provided to greet students to healthcare society and increase the value of humanism as the center of healthcare. It provides a strong significance on compassion in combination with scientific quality. Individual schools decide what their commemoration will look like. But all ceremonies include an oath, orators and some way to celebrate the occasion, whether it be with the introduction of a white coat to each apprentice or some other icon, such as the stethoscope.

The newest version is still used in some of the US medical schools today [3,7,8]:

"I swear to fulfill, to the best of my ability and judgment, this covenant.

I will respect the hard-won scientific gains of those physicians in whose steps I walk, and gladly share such knowledge as is mine with those who are to follow.

I will apply, for the benefit of the sick, all measures [that] are required, avoiding those twin traps of overtreatment and therapeutic nihilism.

I will remember that there is art to medicine as well as science, and that warmth, sympathy, and understanding may outweigh the surgeon's knife or the chemist's drug.

I will not be ashamed to say "I know not," nor will I fail to call in my colleagues when the skills of another are needed for a patient's recovery.

I will respect the privacy of my patients, for their problems are not disclosed to me that the world may know. Most especially must I tread with care in matters of life and death. If it is given me to save a life, all thanks. But it may also be within my power to take a life; this awesome responsibility must be faced with great humbleness and awareness of my own frailty. Above all, I must not play at God.

I will remember that I do not treat a fever chart, a cancerous growth, but a sick human being, whose illness may affect the person's family and economic stability. My responsibility includes these related problems, if I am to care adequately for the sick.

I will prevent disease whenever I can, for prevention is preferable to cure.

I will remember that I remain a member of society, with special obligations to all my fellow human beings, those sound of mind and body as well as the infirm.

If I do not violate this oath, may I enjoy life and art, respected while I live and remembered with affection thereafter. May I always act so as to preserve the finest traditions of my calling and may I long experience the joy of healing those who seek my help."

It seems as if there were more versions of the Hippocratic oath than one can count. In addition, even though the Hippocratic Oath is not used anymore in its original form and it does not apply anymore for the form of modern medicine we adhere to now, the oath's message is still important for the people who work in the medical field nowadays. The idea that the purpose of medical science is to care for the ill and that the patient should be the physician's top priority is still an important theme to take into note. Even if medical professionals have evolved from what they were before and medicine is a more difficult and diverse science, the principles remain.

Today's oath is not as binding as the Hippocratic oath. It is seen as ideal for modern medicine, it is a meaningful tradition that doctors, nurses, and all of the medical staff and practitioners use in the long tradition of taking care of ill patients.

REFERENCES

1. Edelstein, Ludwig (1943). The Hippocratic Oath: Text, Translation, and Interpretation. p. 56. ISBN 978-0-8018-0184-6.

2. Norman, Jeremy. "Perhaps the Earliest Surviving Text of the Hippocratic Oath". HistoryofInformation.com. Retrieved April 26, 2018.

3. Markel, Howard. "I Swear by Apollo" — On Taking the Hippocratic Oath" (PDF). Massachusetts Medical Society. Retrieved 1 March 2017.

4. Raphael Hulkower The History of the Hippocratic Oath: Outdated, Inauthentic, and Yet Still Relevant (PDF)ojs.library.einstein.yu.edu/index.php/EJBM/article/view/42.

5. EricW.Weisstein19962007HippocratesofCos(-460ca370BC)https://scienceworld.wolfram.com/biography/HippocratesofCos

6. Laura McPherson. The History of the Hippocratic Oath. June 03,2015

7. Peter Tyson. The Hippocratic Oath Today. March26.2001.

8. Sritharan, Kaji; Georgina Russell; Zoe Fritz; Davina Wong; Matthew Rollin; Jake Dunning; Bruce Wayne; Philip Mor-

gan; Catherine Sheehan (December 2000). "Medical oaths and declarations". BMJ. 323 (7327):14401. doi:10.1136/ bmj.323.7327.1440. PMC 1121898. PMID 11751345.

All pictures in this article have been obtained from the public domain

HUMANISM IN CHILD NEUROLOGY

Alcy R. Torres, MD, FAAP
Associate Professor of Pediatrics and Neurology
Assistant Dean of Diversity and Inclusion
Director of the Pediatric Traumatic Injury, International and Bilingual Programs
Boston University School of Medicine
Boston Medical Center
Boston, MA, USA

This essay will offer an introduction to "Humanism" applied to Child Neurology. I will attempt to offer a neutral view and my objectives are to:

- Define humanism and demonstrate that it is a core construct in the education and everyday practice of child neurologists

- Differentiate between humanism and professionalism

- Demonstrate educational techniques to foster and encourage humanism

Humanism is a philosophical stance that emphasizes the value and agency of human beings, individually and collectively. Pediatric neurology or child neurology is the science and practice of establishing the diagnosis, prognosis, treatment, and prevention of disease in children who have problems with their nervous system during the neonatal period, infancy, early childhood, and adolescence. A child neurologist is a physician who is trained to provide the highest standard of care while at the same time offering compassion and empathy to the patient and their families, mostly their parents. Like other pediatric specialties, however, it has many challenges that require, for example, the ability to work with patients who may have limited or nonexistent verbal skills, who might not be able to understand or follow commands, and whose level of interactions with others could be severely impaired. Providing humanistic care to this group of patients and stressed parents can be challenging and overwhelming to the child neurologist and a real test for even the most equipped among us.

When we ask aspiring medical students why they want to study medicine, they invariably will answer that they would like to help other people. While sometimes this could sound like a cliché phrase, we still need to ask. With time, however, child neurologists with deep "vocation" feel this as an instinct, almost a reflex, yet when we reflect on a much deeper level, taking care of children with neurological disorders gives us a sense of purpose and meaning to our lives and that is the connection between medicine, child neurology and humanism.

Our professional organizations recognize the contributions of our members in different areas: scientific, lifetime achievement, research, and the "Humanism Award" to recognize those physicians that accomplish both skilled and humanistic care. This is not an easy task, because many child neurologists worldwide have outstanding accomplishments and their humility is such that they would prefer not to be recognized. Reaching that level of humanism, however, might be challenging at times due to financial limitations, administrative demands, and systemic organization failures.

On occasion, I heard about poor interactions between patients and their physicians. Sometimes it can be the result of a bad moment, a circumstance, an unfortunate sequence of events, or unpredictable events. Still, when you hear that time after time, I can't avoid asking myself the questions I asked myself before entering medical school: Aren't we supposed to be kind, compassionate, interested, prepared, with excellent bed manners, and to be good to our young patients and their families and by extension to our communities? Isn't this the reason we study medicine and become doctors? Everybody has the right to a decent life, but there is a difference when the priorities place profit over people.

It is true we child neurologists are different in many ways, but there is not a lot of room for variation when it comes to being interested in helping others. You must be committed to what you are doing and feel the need to serve and help others; then, you are loyal to yourself and will enjoy what you do. Trying to understand what moves our minds to develop these behaviors, I became interested in humanism, the values that can help us understand what it is, and how to apply this knowledge in every interaction. Humanism helps us try to understand our patients, including those with neurological problems like chronic refractory headaches, severe behavioral problems, profound neurodevelopmental disabilities, neurodegenerative disorders, complex pain syndromes, or our patients with poor recovery from neurovascular disorders, brain tumors or traumatic brain injuries.

Humanistic movements worldwide have emphasized a non-religious posture but other groups approach humanistic values inspired by their own traditions and beliefs. I think that whatever your motivation, it does not and should not influence the way you practice medicine. Humanism refers, regardless of the source or sense of purpose, to a respectful and compassionate relationship with the patient and their families, and other team members. It reflects attitudes and behaviors sensitive to the values and the cultural and ethnic backgrounds of others.

Three elements are important when considering the humanism approach to our medical practice in the care of young children with severe neurological damage or neurodegenerative disorders: Reality, Morality, and Meaning.

1. Reality: As humans became more complex, they started asking questions to understand our nature and our habitat. In many ways, the answers to these questions were influenced by beliefs, cultures, and traditions of that group of humans at that point in time as either spiritual, humanistic, or mixed.

2. Morality: Morality is the differentiation of intentions, decisions and actions between those that are distinguished as proper and those that are improper. Some of these behaviors and instincts build the foundation of what we as conscious animals today call morality. It is about seeing yourself in the face of the other person and respecting them for the same reasons you respect yourself, but with a twist of the Golden Rule, which is to treat others, the way they would like to be treated. Reason, empathy and thinking about the best way to live are the consequences of this view of morality, according to Andrew Copson.

3. Meaning: The view that is associated with a humanistic attitude is that meaning is not something up there waiting to be discovered, but something that we create, that we give to create a sense of purpose in our own lives, that we are the ones who ascribe meaning to the experiences that we are having.

In combination, these ideas are found everywhere that there have been human communities writing down their thoughts. You can find these ideas as far back as 2.5 thousand years ago in India, China and Europe. The theologian Friedrich Niethammer coined the term at the beginning of the 19th century to refer to a system of education based on the study of classical literature ("classical humanism"). Of course, they are all over the world today and we call this approach to life, Humanism.

We are all familiar with the Hippocratic Oath, which many medical schools require graduating medical students to take.

Hippocrates established some basis to practice humanism in medicine, when he said it is the physician's duty to benefit the sick and keep them from harm and injustice.

The same way as Hippocrates, William Osler, a Canadian doctor who was one of the co-founders of Johns Hopkins Hospital and one of the most quoted physicians of all times, said, "It is much more important to know what sort of person has a disease than to know what sort of disease a person has." The professional organizations that regulate the practice of medicine have noted the importance of developing physicians with the highest humanistic values. The American Board of Pediatrics lists six professional sub-competencies or milestones a pediatric resident should acquire. Five are related to humanism and only one to medicine. The Liaison Committee on Medical Education (LCME) is an accrediting body for educational programs at schools of allopathic medicine in the United States and Canada. They have mandated that medical schools must ensure that the learning environment for medical students promotes the development of humanistic values.

We see ourselves instead quite properly as being on one far edge of the spectrum of those sorts of humanistic-like behaviors. The conscious attribution of meaning to experience and the time spent trying to explore the questions to explain our own nature is indeed a very human endeavor.

Humanists have talked about how we should live well in the one life we have, and that sort of talk is guided obviously by humanist convictions. Acceptance of the human person's finite nature in time has consequences for the question of how we should live and what meaning we might give to our lives. Spiritual thinkers see this more as a path to something bigger, but regardless of what you think or what your honest motivation is, these behaviors are still quite similar when it comes to how we treat our patients with neurodevelopmental disabilities.

This life is not just an episode in our existence, and so the development of the whole person and the search for the answer to the question of how best to live has added a sense of urgency; consequently, it tends to shift our thinking away from the meaning of life to talk instead of the good life. What is the good life, and how should we live it? We should not look for a purpose outside ourselves, but within our experience, in the existence that we have.

A phrase like living a good life immediately faces objections; people will say it is good to talk about the good life, but a good life is impossible for many people. Human life is simply not just the pursuit of nice things and interest in personal development and fulfillment; a considerable amount of human life is full of tragedy. There are people today who have painful lives, and that is how they were born and unfortunately, also how they will die. The most graphic embodiment of that is probably, I think, something that we all accept, which is the global inequality that exists in the world today.

Acknowledgment in a sense of our universal human tragedy for humanists provides the functional basis for compassion. The humanist's answer to the question of whether we can speak of human experience in a universal way faced with this inequality is something that, according to Norman, we not only can but must meet.

We are talking about the good life and the way to live now. In a sense, again and again in the lapse of a thousand years, the idea that has persisted and reasoned repeatedly is that life's purpose should be to pursue happiness; this is the overarching aim in an individual human being's existence.

Equally, however, to the point Epicurus is making is that pleasure comes from creativity, from our relationships with others, from internal endeavor, and a plethora of other sources.

The pursuit of happiness is not just the pursuit of pure sensation, but it is also the pursuit of personal development.

Sometimes we encounter several walls that challenge our humanistic character. Stress, fatigue, and the chaos of modern medical organizations are hurdles we need to face. Physicians might respond with irritability and by being short; patients became the problem instead of the reason we are here. All of this leads to a lack of self-care, loss of empathy, feelings of burning out, early retirement, or even suicide.

Disruptive behaviors occur among us physicians in up to 95% of colleagues. Respondents to a survey were aware of potential adverse events that may have occurred because of disruptive behavior in up to 60%. Nurses, physicians and administrators have witnessed unprofessional physician behavior and, in fact, some get trained to deal with these abusive behaviors. Finally, up to 30% of providers knew a nurse who left their organization because of a physician's behavior.

But is there a recompense if you wish to be humanistic? Numerous studies support the notion that humanistic behavior will impact patient care, better patient outcomes, improve adherence to therapy, and increase patient and physician satisfaction.

The Arnold P. Gold Foundation has a mnemonic (IECARES) that includes the major characteristics of a humanistic child neurologist. IECARES stands for: Integrity, Excellence, Compassion and Collaboration, Altruism, Respect and Resilience, Empathy, and Service. Or a good way to accomplish this it is with the method of the 5 T's: time, talk, tact, touch, and trust.

Let us review some of the reflections of several physicians who have been distinguished because of their humanistic traits by their colleagues and patients. The patient-centered model is considered a very humanistic approach. To accomplish this, you might need to remember the Golden Rule with the twist:

treat others as they would like to be treated. Our patients are not numbers or a collection of symptoms and signs; everyone wants to be recognized as an individual.

It is worth remembering that underneath every person, there is a world to be discovered. Keep in mind that people you are dealing with are suffering, and you still need to find common ground despite the obstacles: "We are in this together," "We are all human beings," "We all get sick," "We all have problems," and "We are all mortal." You should become an advocate and a problem solver. We should actively work to show empathy and acknowledge the emotions of our patients and their families for effective communication. Remember, everybody needs that extra touch of humanity; it is not just science. This little extra step sometimes goes the distance.

Remember, humans need to connect. We matter to each other, and so we should nurture our relationships and respect them. This is hard to teach and it is better to model them; to be successful, we need mindfulness and to be aware. Make appropriate eye contact and avoid distractions, such as sending messages. Typing, editing and looking at the electronic medical record excessively might prevent you from having good communication with a patient. Smile to children; ask an adolescent what interests them. Look at the whole person, not just the disease process. Even worse, don't label a child with the name of their disease; for example, "the sickle's," instead of Jack, Joe, or Chloe. If you see something that is not right, ask yourself, Why not? Is it because of bad people or a bad situation? Consider what you would do if you were in the same situation.

Reach out to the human being in front of you with dignity and value the moment, even if it includes giving bad news. Make progress from patient to patient because these skills take some time to develop. Once you are satisfied with yourself is when humanistic moments are likely to keep happening. Sometimes we do not know what we have until we lose it. Sometimes we need to say good-bye and only then we realize how much we have built together. Some of the most incredible shows of emotions happen when patients whom we have followed in our practices for years need to leave, and then we know we got it right! Even when an outcome is not good, sharing and helping might be meaningful to our patients and families. It is better not to assume, and a real effort to get to know the people we take care of is a powerful humanistic trait. This is a process, however, and it takes time. We need to be realistic. There is a balance between best intentions and constraints. If it seems you have forgotten, remember why you came to medicine, to care for others but then to change their reality. Your talent needs to consider going beyond the medical office with your impact.

You cannot prescribe medications and be indifferent – indifference is a negative trait. We must build a rapport, a relationship and establish a therapeutic bond, which is dictated not by schedule but by the needs of our patients and their families. To grow these skills, we must have patience and dedication with our patients, colleagues, coworkers and even people with whom we do not find many things in common. It is important to understand that what altruism means for you might not be the same for others. Humanism in medicine requires love, kindness, humility, and a genuine curiosity to learn.

Can we measure how humanistic we are? How do you measure a privilege? Yes, because being a doctor is a privilege, being able to be part of the lives of children and their families. This is an art, however, and we should do this without harming ourselves. You are not useful to anyone if you are not good to yourself and your family. Take time for yourself, to be at your best. Physicians deal with difficult situations and cannot provide the best advice if we do not have a balance. In one sentence, we should appreciate that we are human beings ourselves; you cannot go home feeling how every patient feels. We should use our time effectively and reflect on what is this person feeling, and how can I help?

There has been an evolution of humanistic models in medicine and consequently in child neurology from a paternalistic model to a patient-centered model and, depending on how active patients are, to a collaborative model for effective care. The result is a combination of time, trust, and autonomy to get an effective care plan.

There are many child neurologists that are inspiring and certainly could be mentioned here but that might be unfair to some of you, so instead I am going to concentrate on Dr. Gold of Columbia University, who started the Foundation that carries his name. The Arnold P. Gold Foundation promotes humanism in the US and abroad. For Dr. Gold, these are the most important traits and yes, I agree that those of you who can give the worst news in the most loving way, are already at another level.

Quite reasonably, scholars of humanism, like Jeaneane Fowler, have characterized humanist views about meaning in life as optimistic. You are what you make yourselves. You will need courage, tenacity, motivation and a good sense of humor on the route. Quality of character, happiness, and the fulfillment of potential and human needs can be improved through changed values, and through redirection of individuals through personal change and personal evolution. There is no journey ever successful if you begin expecting the worse and, in fact, you make success much more likely if you set out with a positive determination. Humanists cannot really see what is wrong with optimism in that sense.

Let us consider the faces of the patients we see, and then reflect that behind every face there is a heart and a soul; there are many stories, some unique that I am sure will make you feel as the great human being you are in the broad sense of the word.

CONCLUSIONS

The practice of medicine and any specialty, including child neurology, requires not only knowledge but also strong humanistic traits. Physicians want to be the best they can be, but life challenges might prevent the practice of humanism to the fullest extent, with subsequent impact on patient care. Child neurologists and their professional organizations should make an effort to educate, practice, and advocate for humanism in child neurology.

RESOURCES

1. Nicolas Walter's Humanism – What's in the Word (London: Rationalist Press Association, 1997 ISBN 0-301-97001-7)

2. Gaufberg E. Mapping the Landscape, Journeying Together: The Gold Foundation's Model for Research-Based Advocacy in Humanism in Medicine. Acad Med. 2017 Dec;92(12):1671-1673. Doi: 10.1097/ACM.0000000000001987. PMID: 29019801.

3. Giglio AD. Medicine and humanism. Rev Assoc Med Bras (1992). 2016 Sep-Oct;62(5):387-8. Doi: 10.1590/1806-9282.62.05.387. PMID: 27656845.

4. Marcum JA. Professing clinical medicine in an evolving health care network. Theor Med Bioeth. 2019 Jun;40(3):197-215. Doi: 10.1007/s11017-019-09492-x. PMID: 31377897.

5. Niño Amieva A. Psychiatry and humanism in Argentina. Int Rev Psychiatry. 2016 Apr;28(2):133-53. Doi:

10.3109/09540261.2016.1158702. Epub 2016 Apr 22. PMID: 27102381.

6. Schiffman F. Treating the Patient, Not the Disease: Fred Schiffman on Humanism in Medicine. Oncology (Williston Park). 2017 Apr 15;31(4):246-7. PMID: 28412774.

7. Of Science, Humanism, and Medicine. JAMA. 2015 Aug 18;314(7):734. Doi: 10.1001/jama.2014.11930. PMID: 26284733.

8. Agnew LR. Humanism in medicine. Lancet. 1977 Sep 17;2(8038):596-8. Doi: 10.1016/s0140-6736(77)91440-4. PMID: 71409.

9. Bonaldi A, Vernero S. Slow Medicine: un nuovo paradig-ma in medicina [Italy's Slow Medicine: a new paradigm in medicine]. Recenti Prog Med. 2015 Feb;106(2):85-91. Italian. Doi: 10.1701/1790.19492. PMID: 25734598.

10. Heusser P. Integrative medicine and the quest for humanism in medicine. Forsch Komplementmed. 2011;18(4):172-3. Doi: 10.1159/000330650. Epub 2011 Jul 25. PMID: 21934315.

11. Pérez Tamayo R. Humanismo y medicina [Humanism and medicine]. Gac Med Mex. 2013 May-Jun;149(3):349-53. Spanish. PMID: 23807338.

12. Miles A. Science, humanism, judgement, ethics: person-cen-tered medicine as an emergent model of modern clinical practice. Folia Med (Plovdiv). 2013 Jan-Mar;55(1):5-24. Doi: 10.2478/folmed-2013-0001. PMID: 23905483.

13. Kvesić A, Galić K, Vukojević M. Humanism influencing the organization of the health care system and the ethics of medical relations in the society of Bosnia-Herzegovina. Philos Ethics Humanit Med. 2019 Sep 14;14(1):12. Doi:

10.1186/s13010-019-0082-7. PMID: 31521184; PMCID: PMC6744621.

14. Craxì L, Giardina S, Spagnolo AG. A return to humane medicine: Osler's legacy. Infez Med. 2017 Sep 1;25(3):292-297. PMID: 28956551

15. Lang JH. The philosophy and humanism of medicine. Chin Med J (Engl). 2011 Jan;124(2):318-20. PMID: 21362388.

16. Richard Norman – Emeritus Professor of Moral Philosophy, founder-member of the Humanist Philosophers' Group, and a Vice-President of Humanists UK humanism.org.uk/about/our-people/patrons/professor-richard-norman. Humanism UK2020.

17. Dr. Christos Yapijakis,- ,Epicurus.The Philosophy of Epicurus: Humanism and Science Aiming for Happiness societyofepicurus.com/the-philosophy-of-epicurus-humanism-and-science-aiming-for-happiness 2020 Feb.

18. Copson Andrew, What is Humanism? https://humanists.international/what-is-humanism/ UK2015.

19. Jeaneane Fowler, Humanism: Beliefs and Practices (The Sussex Library of Religious Beliefs and Practices) Epub 1999 Sep 9. ISBN 1898723702.

HUMANISM IN THE INTENSIVE CARE UNIT

David L. Coulter MD.
Associate Professor of Neurology at Harvard Medical School.
Senior Associate at Boston Children's Hospital.
Boston Children's Hospital.
Boston, Massachusetts

For 25 years (1975-2000) I provided neurologic consultations to the Neonatal Intensive Care Unit (NICU) and the Pediatric Intensive Care Unit (PICU) first at the University of Michigan Medical Center, then at the University of Texas Medical Branch in Galveston, and then at Boston City Hospital. I not only saw the patients in the ICU and read all of their EEGs, I also followed them in clinic after discharge. These are their stories.

Poor Brad. He was such a sweet teenage boy. It took me a while to realize that he had Kearns-Sayre Syndrome. But then his mitochondrial disorder swept him away, and he spent three months in the PICU on a ventilator in what was basically a vegetative state. It was 1977. His parents and I were together at his bedside when he died. I felt totally helpless.

Joey was another nice teenage boy who started having myoclonus in 1978. He had had measles years ago. The EEG suggested he had SSPE. Joey asked me, "Doc, please tell me what is wrong with me so I can know what it is." We sent the tests which took 6 weeks to come back and eventually confirmed the diagnosis of SSPE. But by that time, Joey could no longer understand anything I said to him.

Some years ago I was called to see a patient in the NICU at Boston City Hospital. The boy had been born prematurely at 32 weeks of gestation but had done well otherwise. The routine head ultrasound showed that he had cystic periventricular leukomalacia. His examination was unremarkable, but I had to tell his parents that I thought he would probably develop spastic diplegic cerebral palsy, which he did. James is now 25 years old. He is seated in a wheelchair but enjoys spending time with his father (a retired Post Office letter carrier) working in their garden together. He had bad epilepsy a long time ago but now is doing well. His quality of life is just fine.

I was called to see another patient in the NICU at Boston City Hospital who had been born at full term but had suffered severe perinatal hypoxic-ischemic encephalopathy. She was not doing well. I told her mother that I thought she would never walk or talk and would be profoundly disabled. Ayana is now 28 years old. She is able to walk (with a hemiparesis) and talk and is the joy of her mother's life. She had some behavioral issues in the past related to her intellectual disability but those have largely subsided. She is on no medications.

I cared for a boy who had had a normal birth but then suffered an anoxic event at 10 days of life and was in our PICU on a ventilator. He stabilized but had profound brain damage I told his parents that I thought we should put in a tracheostomy tube and a gastrostomy tube and send him to a pediatric rehabilitation facility. They said, "Are there any other options?" Their parish priest was very supportive and came to visit the boy and his parents frequently. He finally told them that it was okay for them to withdraw life support and let the boy go to Heaven. After the boy died, his 4 year old sister wrote a letter addressed, "Dear God, please take good care of my little brother."

Many years ago I was doing medico-legal consultations to supplement my marginal academic income. The lawyers asked me to see a patient whose mother had filed a malpractice claim. The lawyers provided me with all of the obstetrical, birth and neonatal records, which I reviewed. The boy's mother was a poor Black woman who had given birth to him in the hallway of a crowded public hospital. The baby had no heart-beat and was not breathing. After 20 minutes of resuscitation, his heartbeat was 30 but he was still not breathing. He was placed in a corner of the nursery so that he could die peaceful-ly. The attending obstetrician wrote in the chart, "Prepare the body for an autopsy." 12 hours after birth the baby was still alive so they transferred him to the NICU at a local children's hospital. He was having continuous seizures so they did a lumbar puncture and discovered that his cerebrospinal glu-cose level was zero. He survived and went home. His mother said she never went back for follow - up because the doctors all said he was a "vegetable." I saw him when he was 12 years old. I reviewed the psychological tests that showed he had an IQ of about 70. I examined him in detail and concluded that he had a completely normal neurological examination. Let me be clear, I saw all of the records and examined the boy myself. I have told his story many times to remind us all to be humble about our predictions for babies who had a troubled birth.

Another time I was called to the NICU to evaluate a baby who had been born with hydrocephalus. The CT scan showed that he had Dandy-Walker Syndrome. His unmarried teenage par-ents were told that he would have profound disabilities, so they declined permission for a life-saving shunt. The NICU nurses told me, "They can't do that, right?" I agreed and called the hospital lawyer, who then got a judge to come to the NICU, take custody and order the shunt. He was eventually dis-charged into foster care and adopted. At age 7, he had normal intelligence and a normal neurological examination (except for a big head). I asked him what his favorite hobby was and he said he liked to play chess. He survived a severe shunt mal-function at age 12, overcame a drug dependency as a teenager, became a peer advocate for other young people dealing with drugs, and then died tragically from another shunt failure at age 23.

I was called to the PICU once to evaluate an 18 year old college freshman with diabetes who had tried to kill himself with an overdose of insulin. He was in coma and soon transitioned to a vegetative state. Because of his age, they had consulted an adult neurologist who had said, "Send him to a nursing home, he will never recover." His parents wanted a second opinion so they called me. The boy was still within the 3 month window for potential recovery from a vegetative state, so I said they should send him to a rehabilitation facility instead. One month later I visited him at the rehabilitation facility. He got up and walked with me around the unit and talked to me about what he was feeling and how he was doing. He never returned to college but he has thrived in the community ever since.

I saw another unfortunate patient in the PICU at Boston City Hospital. He was a teenage boy who had done all of the wrong things to upset his parents and make them think he was worthless, so he hanged himself and hoped to die. But he lived and ended up in a vegetative state instead. His father came to see him one last time in the PICU and said, "I always thought you would kill yourself, but I never expected that you would end up like this." I do not know whatever happened to him.

I helped care for a couple of twin premature babies in the NICU at Boston City Hospital. Their mother was a poor immigrant from China. Both babies had severe brain damage. We of course wanted them to go to a rehabilitation facility and expected that they would eventually develop profound cerebral palsy and intellectual disability. Their mother said, "In China, we would let them die. We would honor them as part of our family forever and reunite them with our ancestors. They will soon have new brothers and sisters."

I was the attending on the neurology service one Sunday morning when we got a transfer from the NICU. It was a 2 month old boy who had been admitted with seizures. I noticed that his CSF glucose was less than 30. The NICU had not noticed or reacted to this. I called Dr. DeVito's lab in New York early that Sunday morning and told them, "I think this baby may have GLUT-1 deficiency." We sent the tests which confirmed the diagnosis. He has been on a ketogenic diet ever since and is now a totally normal teenager.

Child neurologists who consult in the NICU and the PICU have a special obligation to try to see the present and the future for our patients. The stories do not always turn out well, but sometimes they turn out better than we expected. Experienced child neurologists approach these encounters with their professional skills, experience, humility and love. And, as the stories suggest, we also need to respect the cultural expectations of the families. In the end, we are all pilgrims traveling on the same road together.

BIBLIOGRAPHY

Coulter DL, Allen RJ: Abrupt neurological deterioration in children with Kearns-Sayre syndrome. Archives of Neurology 1981; 38:247-250

COMMUNICATING WITH FAMILIES ABOUT BRAIN DEATH

Nina A. Fainberg, MD
Fellow Physician, Pediatric Critical Care Medicine
Department of Anesthesiology and Critical Care Medicine
Children's Hospital of Philadelphia

Wynne Morrison, MD MBE
Associate Professor, Department of Anesthesiology and Critical Care Medicine
Perelman School of Medicine at the University of Pennsylvania
Attending Physician, Pediatric Critical Care Medicine and Palliative Care Medicine
Justin Michael Ingerman Endowed Chair in Palliative Care Medicine
Children's Hospital of Philadelphia

Matthew P. Kirschen, MD PhD
Assistant Professor, Departments of Anesthesiology and Critical Care Medicine, Neurology, and Pediatrics
Associate Director, Pediatric Neurocritical Care
Perelman School of Medicine at the University of Pennsylvania
Attending Physician, Pediatric Critical Care Medicine
Children's Hospital of Philadelphia

Introduction

Historical Perspective & Definitions

Public Perception

INTRODUCTION

Christopher was a previously healthy 6-year-old boy who fell out of a tree and sustained a severe traumatic brain injury. He is receiving aggressive medical management for increased intracranial pressure. He underwent a decompressive craniectomy and remains on a ventilator. In spite of these therapies, he fails to demonstrate evidence of neurologic recovery. You feel it is clinically indicated to evaluate him to see if he meets criteria for brain death. You meet with Christopher's family and share your concerns about a dismal prognosis and your plan to evaluate him for brain death. The next day, two separate neurologic evaluations confirm that he has met criteria based on your institutional protocol for brain death. He is declared dead. You must now communicate this diagnosis to his family. How do you approach this conversation? What key pieces of information do you seek to convey, and in what way?

The concept of brain death was introduced in the late 1960s and for decades has been recognized clinically and legally throughout the world. First termed irreversible coma, brain death was further described in the late 1970s and was defined as irreversible cessation of all functions of the entire brain, including the brainstem [1]. The diagnostic criteria later put forth by the American Academy of Neurology included coma or unresponsiveness, absence of brainstem reflexes, and apnea [2]. Pediatric-specific guidelines were first introduced in 1987 after initial hesitation to diagnose brain death in young children. They were most recently revised in 2011 with specifications regarding the timing of the examinations, who and how many providers should perform the examinations, how the apnea test should be conducted, and how ancillary testing should be utilized [3].

Though a diagnosis of brain death is a legal declaration of death, its meaning remains nebulous to many individuals. Families of patients declared brain dead frequently equate brain death with coma and believe there may be some chance of recovery [4]. Moreover, mistrust of the medical community regarding brain death, fueled by the media's depiction of highly publicized cases, presents unique challenges in communicating this diagnosis. It is therefore essential to be intentional in one's approach to communicating this diagnosis with families. How such conversations are approached may have far-reaching consequences, including trust in the medical team and the decision to donate organs [4,5].

This chapter will examine nuances of communicating the diagnosis of brain death to families, and will offer a framework with which to discuss this complex topic.

HISTORICAL PERSPECTIVE & DEFINITIONS

The concept of brain death was first introduced in the middle of the 20th century following the invention of positive pressure ventilation, cardiopulmonary bypass, and intensive care units, all of which led to a new ability to support organ function in patients with devastating neurologic injury [6]. These technological advances presented a new set of clinical, ethical and legal dilemmas as the boundary between life and death became blurred. Previously, cessation of function of the heart and lungs indicated death; this belief had been deeply rooted in medicine, culture and society across the globe for millennia. Now this sole definition was challenged. While some patients who had experienced neurologic injury and were supported on a ventilator would recover partial or full neurologic function, others remained in what appeared to be an unconscious state indefinitely, with no brainstem reflexes, no drive to breath, and no activity on electroencephalogram. These observations forced clinicians to re-examine the concept of death more generally. Whereas some considered such patients to be dead, others were hesitant to equate this state with death and instead proposed the term beyond coma [1]. Further complicating the determination of death was the new ability to resuscitate individuals from death following the first successful defibrillation of a human heart by Claude Beck in 1947 [7].

In 1968, an ad-hoc committee at Harvard was convened to address ethical questions brought on by what was deemed the "hopelessly unconscious patient" [8]. There, the first clinical definition of an "irreversible coma" was put forth along with a diagnostic framework for its determination. It was suggested that patients could be pronounced dead as a result of neurologic injury prior to the occurrence of cardiopulmonary arrest. This spurred state legislatures and courts to legally recognize this new standard of determining death, but there was variability in these definitions. The desire for increased standardization culminated in the Uniform Determination of Death Act (UDDA) released in 1981, which proposed that death could be defined as "irreversible cessation of circulatory and respiratory functions" or "irreversible cessation of all functions of the entire brain, including the brainstem" [9]. The report put forth the notion that brain death was equivalent to cardiac death because the brain confers integrative unity onto the body, transforming a disparate collection of organs and tissues into the whole organism [10].

The UDDA was approved by both the American Medical Association and American Bar association, and served as a piece of model legislation intended to guide individual states in establishing their own brain death laws. It did not, however, establish a standard set of criteria that should be used to reach the diagnosis of brain death. Instead, it left this to the discretion of the medical community, and included a statement allowing for changes in interpretation or diagnostic tools over time, stipulating that "...a determination of death is made with acceptable medical standards" [1]. In the 1990s, the American Academy of Neurology (AAN) sought to standardize the means by which adult patients should be declared brain dead. Their published document advocated that the three clinical findings in brain dead patients were coma, apnea, and loss of brainstem reflexes, and specified practice parameters and protocols for diagnosing brain death. The process includes identifying a mechanism of brain injury expected to produce brain death, such as trauma or spontaneous intracranial hemorrhage; excluding conditions that may confound examination results, such as hypotension, hypothermia, and electrolyte derangements; performing a complete neurologic examination, including assessment of brainstem reflexes; and conducting the apnea test [11]. Since then its recommendations have been revised, with updated criteria for adults published by the AAN in 2010.

There was initial reticence to apply adult recommendations to pediatric patients because of the belief that children's brains have a higher propensity for recovery from catastrophic injury. Initially, guidelines were applied only to children over 5 years of age [12]. Later, in 1987, a specialized task force published recommendations to be applied to all pediatric patients. Guidelines for children and adults are largely similar but do have important differences, a key one being that two examinations and apnea tests are currently required in children to exclude the potential for recovery [3,9].

Since it was introduced over 50 years ago, the concept of brain death has become widely accepted but there remains considerable inconsistency among states and institutions in protocols for establishing its diagnosis in both children and adults [13,14]. The AAN has advocated for uniformity in the declaration of brain death and believes this is essential for providers in gaining the trust of the public [15,16]. The following section will examine public attitudes toward brain death, which is key in informing physicians in their approach to disclosing this diagnosis to loved ones.

Public Perception

It is unsurprising that a topic rife with philosophical, ethical and legal implications has remained a subject of controversy in the eyes of the public. Though many have accepted the concept of brain death over the years, there are individuals who believe brain death is a legal fiction created for the purpose of organ transplantation policy. While organ transplantation and brain death have been historically intertwined, this is a simplistic reduction. Nonetheless, beliefs about this relationship have no doubt influenced public opinion about both brain death and organ transplantation.

In addition to mistrust and skepticism about brain death, there is confusion amongst the public about what brain death means in actuality. A widely-cited survey of 1,351 Ohio citizens in 2004 found that while 98% of respondents had heard of brain death, only one-third believed that a diagnosis of brain death meant that a patient was legally dead [5]. Many equated the term brain death with coma or vegetative state and/or believed there was a chance of recovery, and 28% believed individuals declared brain dead could hear. Less than half stated that they believed brain dead patients were "as good as dead." A national survey released the same year produced similar results [17].

Popular media may contribute significantly to misperceptions about brain death. One recent study evaluated public perception of brain death by analyzing the most commonly accessed resources on the Internet. The findings suggested widespread lack of knowledge about the subject, negative emotions toward brain death and the medical community, and a significant amount of misinformation available. The majority of websites mentioned organ donation in conjunction with brain death and this association was universally discussed in a negative light [18]. Another study examined articles about brain death in newspapers in the United States and Canada. Less than 3% of articles examined presented a definition of brain death, and there were numerous examples in which death was stated in specific cases to have occurred twice: once by neurologic criteria, and again after organ procurement [19]. Highly publicized cases around brain injury and brain death, such as those of Terry Schiavo and more recently of Jahi McMath, have contributed to the confusion and controversy about brain death as well as more general public mistrust of the medical system [20].

In summary, it is apparent that there is considerable cynicism and confusion surrounding the meaning of brain death. There is often mistrust of the medical community, which may result from the media and other information-sharing platforms and also from historical inequities in health care. The general public's uncertainty and trepidation about the subject makes it all the more imperative that providers take great care in disclosing and explaining brain death of a loved one.

Family Experiences & Cognitive Dissonance

What do we know of family members' perceptions of and experiences with receiving a brain death diagnosis? As it turns out, similar to the general public, family members of patients declared brain dead exhibit confusion about what this diagnosis means, even when they decide in favor of organ donation. One analysis of interviews of families found that only 28% were able to provide a completely correct definition of brain death; just 15% linked brain death with death and one-fifth believed their loved one may recover [21]. Another study demonstrated that an astonishing number did not realize their brain dead loved one was dead at the time of organ procurement [4].

Potentiating this misunderstanding is the fact that brain dead patients who are potential organ donors may not appear to be dead; they will remain on ventilator support, have frequent lab draws, and be given therapies to normalize their physiology. They will have good color, are warm to touch, have a beating heart and a chest that rises and falls with each breath. The cognitive dissonance that results from having a brain dead loved one who appears "alive" is challenging to comprehend [22,23]. Family members of patients declared brain dead who have later been interviewed often express this difficulty: "She was breathing. Her heart was going...they're telling you she's dead but she's still there" [4]. Thus, via visual and sensory cues, families receive the paradoxical message that their loved one appears alive, in contrast to the message that they are dead.

There are other aspects of the hospital experience that contribute to families' lack of knowledge regarding the brain death diagnosis. Communication in the ICU surrounding brain death is often inconsistent [23]. For example, usage of the term coma or brain damaged is frequently employed in conjunction with brain death; this provides a mixed message to families. Providers will sometimes state that patients declared brain dead "will not survive" or will even go so far to say, "they will not live off the ventilator" rather than emphasize that they are already deceased [24]. These and similar ambiguous messages are counterproductive and may fuel families' cognitive and emotional difficulties in accepting this diagnosis.

CULTURE, RELIGION & BRAIN DEATH

Different religious and cultures have beliefs about life, death, and the mind-body interface that will affect perceptions of brain death in ways that must be acknowledged. The diagnosis of brain death can be challenging when such beliefs are not aligned with the concept of integrative unity in which personal identity resides in the brain. In general, Western philosophies are more accepting of brain death as the mind and body are viewed as separate entities, whereas in Eastern cultures, the body and mind are more often perceived as integrated [25]. In Japanese culture, for instance, Kokoro describes the unity of heart, mind and spirit, with its center located in the chest. Similarly, in Buddhist teaching, one's collective identity does not exclusively reside in the brain and hence death of the brain does not confer death of the individual [26].

Traditional beliefs about life and death have influenced global practices related to both brain death and organ transplantation, and there is considerable variance worldwide [27,28]. In 1968, when one of earliest heart transplantations in the world was performed in Japan, the surgeon who completed the operation was accused of illegal experimentation. National objections to brain death were pervasive and influenced the passing of legislation related to organ transplantation; the second heart transplant in Japan was performed over 30 years later in 1999 [26,29].

In addition to spiritual beliefs, rituals and legal code will affect perceptions of brain death. In Judaism, for instance, Halachah is a prescribed set of laws that govern day-to-day life. Rabbinic leaders' perceptions of brain death according to Halachah is variable. There is considerable heterogeneity in both knowledge and beliefs about brain death among Rabbis across Jewish denominations; those who object to brain death seem to hold more influence among Orthodox Jews in the United States [30,31]. In Judaism and Islam, the declaration of brain death can delay the prescribed sequence of end-of-life observances that begin immediately after death, such as purification of the body and funeral preparation. In these situations, the temporary maintenance of somatic support following brain death determination may delay performance of these rituals [31,32].

Challenges can arise when religious and cultural beliefs result in rejection of the concept of brain death. It is important for institutions to have policies and procedures in place regarding how to address such objections both prior to and after brain death declaration, and for the care team to acknowledge these beliefs when framing conversations about the status of the patient and to provide compassionate end-of-life care. Collaboration with clergy and other religious leaders can be helpful in these scenarios.

Effective Communication in the Intensive Care Unit

Prior to discussing communication strategies about brain death, it is useful to discuss communication in the ICU more generally. The benefits of successful communication in the ICU may seem intuitive but have been found to have widespread positive effects. Patients and families have identified good communication with their providers as equally important to their hospital experience as the team members' clinical skills [25]. Good communication has been associated with improved health outcomes and is correlated with decreased length of ICU stay [26,27]. Traumatic stress disorder in parents of children admitted to the ICU is correlated with their perception of the severity of illness, which does not correlate with actual illness severity – a discrepancy modifiable by clear and consistent messaging by providers [28].

In spite of its importance, communicating effectively with families in the intensive care unit can be quite challenging. There is an overwhelming amount of data that families must grapple with to interpret the status of their loved one and they hence become increasingly dependent on the care team for information. Meanwhile, the pace, acuity and unpredictability of the ICU can make interactions with families hurried and ineffective. Rapid clinical changes can create extraordinary circumstances, in which the provider may have no prior rapport with family members and thus no context with which to inform their communication of events. Moreover, the multidisciplinary nature of modern healthcare can contribute to a "too many cooks in the kitchen" problem, in which communication failures, misunderstandings and/or disagreements between care team members leads to inconsistent messaging to families [29]. When discussing a topic that can be difficult to grapple with, such as brain death, this can be increasingly problematic.

To address these challenges, it is helpful to think of communication as a procedure. Like other procedures, it requires preparation, can be learned and taught, and improves with practice. Many authors have developed tools to aid in the effective delivery of difficult news; several popular and well-cited examples are the SEGUE and SPIKES frameworks developed in the early 2000s, which have been since been studied and validated [30,31]. Common elements include preparation; gathering information from the patient or family; transmitting the medical information; providing support and expressing empathy; and eliciting collaboration in identifying next steps. These will be discussed in the context of brain death in the following section.

DISCLOSING A DIAGNOSIS OF BRAIN DEATH

Sharing the diagnosis of brain death can be daunting and provoke discomfort as it presents a unique set of challenges. Because there may be confusion amongst family members about what brain death means, it is critical for providers to be thoughtful in their approach to breaking this bad news. We provide commentary below about communicating the diagnosis of brain death in the context of Christopher's case.

Preparation

Before breaking difficult news to Christopher's parents, it is critical to prepare in advance. Think about what you wish to communicate and ensure you have accurate information – take time to review Christopher's chart and speak with consultants to ensure there is a shared mental model about his status and clinical trajectory. Be knowledgeable about your state's and hospital's brain death policies. Decide which individuals will be present during the discussion. This includes establishing which care team members will participate and who the family would like present for support. Ensure an interpreter is present if his family is non-English speaking if possible. Avoid using family members as interpreters as this places undue burden onto them, may affect family dynamics and may alter the message the team seeks to deliver [32]. Reserve an appropriate space for the conversation. Ideally this will be a private area with seating available to allow for eye-level communication. Identify which provider will be the primary communicator and deliverer of the difficult news. If it is an option, providers present should request that colleagues hold phones and/or pagers to minimize interruptions. Finally, especially if a large group is present, begin the meeting with introductions and by clearly articulating the purpose of the conversation.

Eliciting Information

Following preparation and prior to disclosing the difficult news, it is useful first to solicit from the family what they understand about their child's diagnosis. Use open-ended questions, such as "What have you been told about your child's medical situation?" or "What is your understanding of how Christopher is doing?" This allows providers to tailor the conversation in a way that the family will understand and may also provide insight into their emotional state and values. It also will reassure the family that the care team seeks to listen and engage them in a conversation rather than deliver a monologue.

Sharing Information

The initial shock of bad news can leave families with little retention of the details of the discussion. To lessen the blow as well as facilitate information processing, some advocate beginning the disclosure with a "warning shot," such as "I am afraid I have some difficult news to share" [33]. This introduction followed by a pause can allow the family to brace themselves and prepare to hear the news. Deliver information in digestible pieces and allow sufficient time for emotional processing and discussion after each bit of news is shared. Avoid phrases such as "there is nothing more we can do" as this contradicts the notion that family members may have other care goals for their loved one besides a cure [34]. Often visual aids are helpful if appropriate. For instance, showing Christopher's family the CT scan of his brain and pointing out the blood may set the stage for anticipated bad news. Take care in the words used to communicate with the family during the early stages following his traumatic brain injury; if the term "brain death" is used too early, it may create confusion if he is later not declared as such. On the other hand, if there is a high risk of progression to brain death, it might be of value to mention this possibility early on to prepare the family for what is to come, emphasizing that it is a diagnosis that takes time and special examinations to determine.

Once the diagnosis of brain death is suspected, decide along with other care team members whether you wish to invite the family to be present during the brain death examination. While it is often not practice to do so, some research suggests it may aid in their understanding and acceptance of the diagnosis [32-33]. If Palliative Care is available at your hospital, consider whether there would be added benefit to involving another team for their expertise in end-of-life care and comprehensive family support.

After brain death is declared, do not be ambiguous. Christopher's parents must be told unequivocally that Christopher is dead. Provide his family with a clear, straightforward and jargon-free headline statement and avoid beating around the bush: "We performed the exam we discussed to look for any evidence of brain function in Christopher. I am so sorry to say that we did not find evidence of any brain function. This means that Christopher is dead." It is important to be transparent about this, because the transition from being "alive" to brain dead may seem arbitrary to Christopher's family; after extensive testing is carried out, without any other clinical change, Christopher, who was considered alive just prior, is now dead. Do not deliver mixed messages, such as "Christopher is in a coma" or "it is unlikely that Christopher will recover" as this creates confusion about the potential for improvement.

Should Christopher's family experience cognitive dissonance in seeing signs of life – a warm body and beating heart – it is important to empathize with them and gently remind them that his organs are being maintained, but that he is dead. That being said, the above can (and should) be delivered in a tender and empathetic manner; examples of language to use (and not to use) are summarized in the section below and in Tables 1 and 2. There should be ample time devoted to allowing his parents to process this devastating news and the provider should take care in responding to their emotions. A reasonable amount of time should be given for the family to come to terms with this diagnosis and for loved ones to say goodbye if desired before removing ventilatory and other organ support.

Responding to Emotion

There is a spectrum of emotional reactions exhibited by families upon receiving devastating news – anger, frustration, tears, silence, shock. Identifying these emotions and helping the family process what they are feeling is vital. The previously published NURSE mnemonic is an example of a framework to guide the provider in responding to emotion when delivering difficult news (naming, understanding, respecting, supporting, exploring) [37]. For example, the family member may become tearful and say, "I can't believe this. This is what we were afraid of," to which the provider may respond, "I know this isn't the news we hoped for; I wish things were different." During the conversation, pause often and be comfortable with silence; following a statement with a pause increases the likelihood that family members will share their concerns, values or hopes [38]. Table 1 below summarizes examples of NURSE statements that can be used to respond to family members' emotions.

Consider how Christopher's siblings should be supported during the evolution of his clinical status. Older children often cope better with illness and death if informed honestly about the situation in an age-appropriate matter. Members of the care team and Child Life services if available can provide sibling support and guidance [39].

Determining Next Steps

Following the conversation, the meeting should be summarized and the providers should discuss next steps with Christopher's family. Decisions regarding organ donation, funeral plans and other logistics may be temporarily deferred to a separate meeting depending on the family's need to process the news they have just received. If this is the case, be clear that you will be speaking with them again soon and give them a sense of the timeline in which a future meeting will occur. Allow time for questions and ensure they know whom to contact before the next meeting should new questions or concerns arise. Removal of the ventilator and other organ support should not be presented to the family as something they have to make a decision about – the timing of ventilator removal will be discussed, but not whether to remove it.

Because Christopher is brain dead, he is considered eligible for organ donation; institution-specific policies exist for approaching this with families. The decision to donate can be a highly emotional one and is affected by a multitude of religious, socioeconomic, educational, cultural and spiritual factors. Representatives of the regional Organ Procurement Organization or a specially trained staff member will generally initiate the discussion regarding organ donation. The discussion will involve communicating with Christopher's family about the process of organ donation, what they can expect during each step, and how the decision may benefit recipients of his organs and tissues. When discussing organ donation with his family, it should be made clear that Christopher's organs will be procured after he has died; the moment of death does not coincide with removing ventilator support or with the removal of his organs, but rather it has already occurred. When the diagnosis of brain death is suspected, consider reaching out to your local Organ Procurement Organization early and be aware of your hospital's particular protocols for doing so.

Navigating Doubt

In talking with Christopher's family, anticipate that feelings of doubt may arise weeks, or even months, after he has died. Christopher's family should be provided the contact information of a point person to whom they can reach out should such they experience such feelings and bereavement and counseling services be offered when deemed appropriate [40]. In other cases, doubt may lead to refusal to accept brain death when the diagnosis occurs. Objections may arise from specific religious beliefs or a belief that the patient can regain neurologic function. Such situations can place tremendous stress on families and care teams and often escalate to institutional legal experts and ethics committees, or even the courts. Should a family express disagreement with a brain death diagnosis, involve unit and institutional leadership early to determine a consensus approach. In some cases, it is best to be compassionately firm and emphasize that as difficult as it is to believe the child has died, there is a timeline in which the team plans to remove the ventilator. Some families will accept this plan when they realize they are not being asked to decide. In other cases, the objection may be more intractable or culturally rooted, or a family may even take legal action to block ventilator removal. In such cases, a decision will have to be made about whether to accommodate the objection or argue the case in court. In general, it is helpful to be aware of potential religious or cultural objections to the concept of brain death before proceeding with the testing, as well as particularities about the state's brain death laws. Currently there are three states with unique stipulations mandating families be provided with "reasonable accommodation" after brain death diagnosis, which affects the timing of ventilator discontinuation; these are New York, California and Illinois. New Jersey contains legislation stating that a patient shall not be declared brain dead should it violate a family's religious beliefs – a law that played a key role in the outcome of Jahi McMath's case [20]. Often the hospital ethics committee will be involved in conversations to resolve disagreement about the patient's status [40]. These cases can be traumatic for all parties involved and can create controversy in the public eye [20].

CONCLUSION

The concept of brain death has legally existed for over half a century, yet there remains significant confusion about its meaning among the public as well as some health professionals. In light of this, when a child is diagnosed with brain death, providers must be conscientious in their approach to disclosing this to families. This process can include many tenants of communicating difficult news more generally with modifications specific to brain death declaration. Communication about brain death is a special skill that can be acquired and practiced, and when effective, does a tremendous service to families who are experiencing the most traumatic event of their lives.

Table 1: Examples of NURSE statements for responding to emotion [44]

Naming	"I can see that you may be frustrated."
Understanding	"I can't imagine how difficult this must be."
Respecting	"You are an amazing advocate for your child."
Supporting	"We will be with you each step of the way."
Exploring	"Could you tell me more about what you mean?"

Table 2: Language to use and avoid when disclosing a brain death diagnosis

Consider Stating	Avoid Stating
"I am so sorry to say that your child is brain dead. That means he is dead."	"Your child is in a coma and is unlikely to recover."
"I know that your child is still warm and with a beating heart; this must seem very confusing. Right now, machines are maintaining his organs, but he is dead."	"Your child is brain dead and it is only the machines keeping him alive. He is on life support but he's as good as gone."
"You have decided that you would like your child to be an organ donor. We will explain to you what this process will look like. It is important to know that he is already dead, and he will be dead when his organs are procured."	"You have decided that you would like your child to be an organ donor. Right now we are maintaining him on life support. When his organs are ready to be procured, life support will be removed and he will die."

REFERENCES

1. De Georgia MA. History of brain death as death: 1968 to the present. Journal of Critical Care. 2014;29(4):673-678. doi:10.1016/j.jcrc.2014.04.015

2. Wijdicks EFM. Determining brain death in adults. 45(5):1003-1011.

3. Mathur M, Ashwal S. Pediatric Brain Death Determination. Semin Neurol. 2015;35(02):116-124. doi:10.1055/s-0035-1547540

4. Franz HG. Explaining Brain Death: A Critical Feature of the Donation Process. Journal of Transplant Coordination. 1997;7(1):8.

5. Siminoff LA, Burant C, Youngner SJ. Death and organ procurement: public beliefs and attitudes. Social Science & Medicine. 2004;59(11):2325-2334. doi:10.1016/j.socscimed.2004.03.029

6. Puri N, Puri V, Dellinger RP. History of Technology in the Intensive Care Unit. Critical Care Clinics. 2009;25(1):185-200. doi:10.1016/j.ccc.2008.12.002

7. Beck CS, Pritchard WH, Feil HS. Ventricular fibrillation of long duration abolished by electric shock. J Am Med Assoc. 1947;135(15):985. doi:10.1001/jama.1947.62890150005007a

8. Wijdicks EFM. The neurologist and Harvard criteria for brain death. Neurology. 2003;61(7):970-976. doi:10.1212/01.WNL.0000086804.18169.8D

9. Nakagawa TA, Ashwal S, Mathur M, et al. Guidelines for the determination of brain death in infants and children: An update of the 1987 Task Force recommendations*: Critical Care Medicine. 2011;39(9):2139-2155. doi:10.1097/CCM.0b013e31821f0d4f

10. Shewmon DA. The Brain and Somatic Integration: Insights Into the Standard Biological Rationale for Equating Brain Death With Death. The Journal of Medicine and Philosophy. 2001;26(5):457-478. doi:10.1076/jmep.26.5.457.3000

11. Goila AK, Pawar M. The diagnosis of brain death. Indian J Crit Care Med. 2009;13(1):7-11. doi:10.4103/0972-5229.53108

12. Guidelines for the determination of death. Report of the medical consultants on the diagnosis of death to the Pres-

ident's Commission for the Study of Ethical Problems in Medicine and Biomedical and Behavioral Research. JAMA. 1981;246(19):2184-2186.

13. Greer DM, Wang HH, Robinson JD, Varelas PN, Henderson GV, Wijdicks EFM. Variability of Brain Death Policies in the United States. JAMA Neurol. 2016;73(2):213. doi:10.1001/jamaneurol.2015.3943

14. Mathur M, Petersen L, Stadtler M, et al. Variability in pediatric brain deathdetermination and documentation in southern California. Pediatrics. 2008;121(5):988-993. doi:10.1542/peds.2007-1871

15. Russell JA, Epstein LG, Greer DM, Kirschen M, Rubin MA, Lewis A. Brain death, the determination of brain death, and member guidance for brain death accommodation requests: AAN position statement. Neurology. 2019;92(5):228-232. doi:10.1212/WNL.0000000000006750

16. Lewis A, Cahn-Fuller K, Caplan A. Shouldn't Dead Be Dead?: The Search for a Uniform Definition of Death. J Law Med Ethics. 2017;45(1):112-128. doi:10.1177/1073110517703105

17. Kilcullen JK. "As good as dead" and is that good enough? Public attitudes toward brain death. Journal of Critical Care. 2014;29(5):872-874. doi:10.1016/j.jcrc.2014.06.018

18. Jones AH, Dizon ZB, October TW. Investigation of Public Perception of Brain Death Using the Internet. Chest. 2018;154(2):286-292. doi:10.1016/j.chest.2018.01.021

19. Daoust A, Racine E. Depictions of 'brain death' in the media: medical and ethical implications. J Med Ethics. 2014;40(4):253-259. doi:10.1136/medethics-2012-101260

20. Luce JM. The Uncommon Case of Jahi McMath. Chest. 2015;147(4):1144-1151. doi:10.1378/chest.14-2227

21. Siminoff LA, Mercer MB, Arnold R. Families' understanding of brain death. Prog Transplant. 2003;13(3):218-224. doi:10.7182/prtr.13.3.314r1h430722176t

22. Sque M, Payne SA. Dissonant loss: The experiences of donor relatives. Social Science & Medicine. 1996;43(9):1359-1370. doi:10.1016/0277-9536(96)00002-0

23. Youngner SJ. How to Communicate Clearly about Brain Death and First-Person Consent to Donate. AMA J Ethics. 2016;18(2):108-114. doi:10.1001/journalofethics.2016.18.2.ecas2-1602

24. Long T, Sque M, Addington-Hall J. Conflict rationalisation: How family members cope with a diagnosis of brain stem death. Social Science & Medicine. 2008;67(2):253-261. doi:10.1016/j.socscimed.2008.03.039

25. Hickey M. What are the needs of families of critically ill patients? A review of the literature since 1976. Heart Lung. 1990;19(4):401-415.

26. Curtis JR. Communicating about end-of-life care with patients and families in the intensive care unit. Critical Care Clinics. 2004;20(3):363-380. doi:10.1016/j.ccc.2004.03.001

27. Lilly CM, De Meo DL, Sonna LA, et al. An intensive communication intervention for the critically ill. Am J Med. 2000;109(6):469-475. doi:10.1016/s0002-9343(00)00524-6

28. Balluffi A, Kassam-Adams N, Kazak A, Tucker M, Dominguez T, Helfaer M. Traumatic stress in parents of children admitted to the pediatric intensive care unit: Pediatric Crit-

ical Care Medicine. 2004;5(6):547-553. doi:10.1097/01. PCC.0000137354.19807.44

29. Danis M, Federman D, Fins JJ, et al. Incorporating palliative care into critical care education: principles, challenges, and opportunities. Crit Care Med. 1999;27(9):2005-2013. doi:10.1097/00003246-199909000-00047

30. Makoul G. The SEGUE Framework for teaching and assessing communication skills. Patient Educ Couns. 2001;45(1):23-34. doi:10.1016/s0738-3991(01)00136-7

31. Baile WF, Buckman R, Lenzi R, Glober G, Beale EA, Kudelka AP. SPIKES-A six-step protocol for delivering bad news: application to the patient with cancer. Oncologist. 2000;5(4):302-311. doi:10.1634/theoncologist.5-4-302

32. Norris WM, Wenrich MD, Nielsen EL, Treece PD, Jackson JC, Curtis JR. Communication about end-of-life care between language-discordant patients and clinicians: insights from medical interpreters. J Palliat Med. 2005;8(5):1016-1024. doi:10.1089/jpm.2005.8.1016

33. Maynard DW. How to tell patients bad news: the strategy of "forecasting." Cleve Clin J Med. 1997;64(4):181-182. doi:10.3949/ccjm.64.4.181

34. Sardell AN, Trierweiler SJ. Disclosing the cancer diagnosis. Procedures that influence patient hopefulness. Cancer. 1993;72(11):3355-3365. doi:10.1002/1097-0142(19931201)72:11<3355::aid-cncr2820721135>3.0.co;2-d

35. Kompanje EJO, de Groot YJ, Bakker J, Ijzermans JNM. A national multicenter trial on family presence during brain death determination: the FABRA study. Neurocrit Care. 2012;17(2):301-308. doi:10.1007/s12028-011-9636-2

36. Kirschen MP, Francoeur C, Murphy M, et al. Epidemiology of Brain Death in Pediatric Intensive Care Units in the United States. JAMA Pediatr. 2019;173(5):469. doi:10.1001/jamapediatrics.2019.0249

37. Responding to Emotion: Respecting. VitalTalk. Accessed July 6, 2020. https://www.vitaltalk.org/guides/responding-to-emotion-respecting/

38. October TW, Dizon ZB, Arnold RM, Rosenberg AR. Characteristics of Physician Empathetic Statements During Pediatric Intensive Care Conferences With Family Members: A Qualitative Study. JAMA Netw Open. 2018;1(3):e180351. doi:10.1001/jamanetworkopen.2018.0351

39. Institute of Medicine (US) Committee on Palliative and End-of-Life Care for Children and Their Families. When Children Die: Improving Palliative and End-of-Life Care for Children and Their Families. (Field MJ, Behrman RE, eds.). National Academies Press (US); 2003. Accessed July 5, 2020. http://www.ncbi.nlm.nih.gov/books/NBK220818/

40. Kompanje E. Families and Brain Death. Semin Neurol. 2015;35(02):169-173. doi:10.1055/s-0035-1547536

PEDIATRIC PALLIATIVE CARE FOR CHILDREN WITH NEUROLOGICAL DISORDERS

Caley Mikesell, BPH

School of Medicine, Universidad San Francisco de Quito, Quito, Ecuador

Michelle Grunauer, MD, PhD

Professor and Dean, Critical Care, Ethics, Palliative Care

School of Medicine at Universidad San Francisco de Quito

Academic Director and Attending Physician, Critical Care and Palliative Care

Hospital de los Valles, Quito, Ecuador

Professor (by courtesy), Johns Hopkins Carey Business School

Adjunct Clinical Professor, Zucker School of Medicine, Hofstra/Northwell

Quito, Ecuador

"How can we help you live the best possible day today?" —Atul Gawande, MD, MPH

Pediatric palliative care (PPC) is essential to incorporating humanism into the medical care of children with neurological conditions. At the core of palliative care (PC) is a humanistic reframing of the role of medicine, care, and healthcare personnel (HCPs). It recasts HCPs as specialized members of a multidisciplinary team, whose role is to help patients and families select the right care options in order to support their quality of life, hopes, and priorities for life given the reality of their circumstances.

Across his body of work, surgeon-public health researcher Atul Gawande [1] explains that PC models pause to ask patients and families fundamental questions that are often passed over in clinical settings: How can we help you have the best possible day today? What does the best possible day look like for you given your health?

Supporting the Protection of Children's Human Rights through Evidence-Based Care

Pediatric palliative care is a human right [2-4] as well as a foundational component of the best available standard of care for patients with life-limiting or life-threatening conditions [5]. PPC uses a holistic, multidisciplinary team-based treatment approach to evaluate, manage, and prevent diverse symptoms of suffering of patients and families [2-7]. PPC also focuses on creating opportunities to care for the needs of healthcare professionals who provide care to seriously ill children and their families.

PPC seeks to address "Total Pain," a term coined by Dame Cicely Saunders [8] to encapsulate the physical, psychosocial, ethical, spiritual/existential, cultural, familial, interpersonal, and other dimensions of suffering that patients with serious illnesses encounter. Modern palliative care also concerns itself with the role and care of the HCP team, death and bereavement considerations, care planning, care expectations, and logistical issues that impact the quality of life of patients, their families, and the professional teams that care for them [9-12].

Pediatric palliativist and global health researcher Justin Amery, provides the following examples [10] (adapted) to illustrate holistic dimensions of care:

- Physical — Pain and symptom management

- Psychological — Denial, collusion, depression, anxiety, etc.

- Social — Loneliness/isolation, stigma, community-related issues, difficulties with friends, classmates, and romantic partners.

- Spiritual — Existential crises, questions about one's purpose in life, difficulties related to one's legacy, the meaning of life, acceptance, and religious questions.

- Cultural — Cultural rites, interruption of "expected" timeline of life, religious issues, etc.

- Economic — Paying for care, planning for funeral expenses, managing sibling care amidst serious illness, dealing with work changes, and accommodating other financial needs.

- Familial — Creating memories with family, managing family conflict, dealing with conflicting needs/desires/beliefs/hopes, navigating denial, and coping with strong emotions of family members.

- Ethical — Navigating difficult issues related to end-of-life care, child's vs. family's desires, issues of consent, etc. DNRs, care decisions, end-of-life care, planning for the end of life, and other decisions.

While other branches of medicine may also consider diverse dimensions of patient wellbeing beyond procedural success or symptom management, an important factor which distinguishes PPC is its emphasis on quality of life over the extension of life [2,10]. PPC can and should be used in conjunction with curative care. However, it also encourages the patient-family unit as well as the professional care team to reflect on the goals of care as they work together to make decisions in planning and deciding what treatments to accept or forgo.

PPC is key to improving the quality of care and of life for patients suffering from over 400 conditions, including numerous neurological conditions [13]. Contrary to popular-conceptions, PPC should be integrated into treatment from the moment the diagnosis a life-limiting or life-threatening condition is made. It should be provided regardless of the disease stage, its projected trajectory, and whether or not disease-directed, curative treatment is given [4]. Evidence shows that seriously ill patients may reap greater benefits from the early application of PPC than beginning such care only once a terminal diagnosis has been confirmed [14].

Studies suggest that patients whose treatment includes the timely application of PC have better symptom management and pain control [6,10,15,16] more positive patient outcomes [15-17] and even increased patient survival times [6,17,18]. PPC is also associated with improved patient-HCP communication [15,16] as well as higher familial satisfaction with end-of-life care [19].

The clinical significance of PPC as a foundational component of the best available standard of care is so well-supported that international organizations have affirmed it as a human right. For example, the World Health Organization [4] describes palliative care for adults and children as follows:

World Health Organization's Definition of Palliative Care

"Palliative care is an approach that improves the quality of life of patients and their families facing the problems associated with life-threatening illness, through the prevention and relief of suffering by means of early identification and impeccable assessment and treatment of pain and other problems, physical, psychosocial and spiritual. Palliative care:

- provides relief from pain and other distressing symptoms;

- affirms life and regards dying as a normal process;

- intends neither to hasten or postpone death;

- integrates the psychological and spiritual aspects of patient care;

- offers a support system to help patients live as actively as possible until death;

- offers a support system to help the family cope during the patient's illness and in their own bereavement;

- uses a team approach to address the needs of patients and their families, including bereavement counselling, if indicated;

- will enhance quality of life, and may also positively influence the course of illness;

- is applicable early in the course of illness, in conjunction with other therapies that are intended to prolong life, such as chemotherapy or radiation therapy, and includes those investigations needed to better understand and manage distressing clinical complications."

WHO Definition of Palliative Care for Children

"Palliative care for children represents a special, albeit closely related field to adult palliative care. WHO's definition of palliative care appropriate for children and their families is as follows; the principles apply to other pediatric chronic disorders (WHO; 1998a):

- Palliative care for children is the active total care of the child's body, mind and spirit, and also involves giving support to the family.

- It begins when illness is diagnosed, and continues regardless of whether or not a child receives treatment directed at the disease.

- Health providers must evaluate and alleviate a child's physical, psychological, and social distress.

- Effective palliative care requires a broad multidisciplinary approach that includes the family and makes use of available community resources; it can be successfully implemented even if resources are limited.

- It can be provided in tertiary care facilities, in community health centers and even in children's homes."

Although its effectiveness in improving quality of life, maximizing quality of care, and supporting the wellbeing of professional care teams is well-documented [2,10,20]. PPC is inaccessible throughout most of the world. It is estimated that only about 10% of the children who require this type of care receive it each year [2].The confluence of a number of barriers create this reality, not the least of which is the absence of adequate educational infrastructure to train professionals in PPC and thereby expand access to it [3,10,16].

According to the Global Atlas of Palliative Care most of the world is underdeveloped in pediatric and adult palliative care provision, including the country of residence of the authors of this chapter (Ecuador). The lack of existing infrastructure, cultural support, and professionals to contextually-appropriate PPC training presents a challenge in increasing access to this specialty. However, as original research by the authors [2,21] as well as existing literature [10] has demonstrated, practitioners already demonstrate clinical competency in many of the fundamental building blocks to PPC.

Low-resource contexts are a long-way off from having the capacity necessary to build robust specialization programs and multiply specialized palliative care services in all local hospitals. However, we have a path forward to expanding PPC access in under-resourced settings. Integrating PPC into healthcare education, implementing PPC checklists and tasks, and training HCPs in PPC skills and philosophies has been shown to be an effective method to improve diverse indicators in pediatric intensive care units (PICU) and perhaps other clinical settings in low-resource contexts. In one study, a PICU team in Quito, Ecuador trained in an integrated model of care (IMOC) combining pediatric critical care and PPC skills saw a 5.2% decrease (from 10% to 4.8%) in annual unit mortality. Evidence of greater provision of holistic care, increased patient-family satisfaction, and greater familial involvement was also documented [21].

Expanding access to PPC through an IMOC is a cost-effective way to spread this essential specialty to areas in which it is not currently available. This model presents a way to protect neurologically-disabled children's human right to access the best available standard of care.

DECONSTRUCTING THE MEANING OF CARE, HCPS' ROLES, AND THE PATIENT

The foundational understandings of PPC represent a paradigmatic shift from many commonly held understandings of the goals of medical care, the role of healthcare professionals (HCPs), and the patient.

Care

Preventing death and extending patient survival time are the implicit goals of medical care in many clinical settings;

however, PPC more heavily emphasizes quality of life and patient goals. In PPC, the care team focuses on helping the patient-family unit to live the best quality of life for the longest time possible rather than seeking unlikely or impossible cures. PPC recognizes the damage of medical futility both to patients' quality of life and the healthcare system as a whole. It instead seeks to co-create solutions appropriate to each patient to allow them to live in accordance with their values, desires, and goals. It is worth noting that PPC can and should be provided concurrently with curative treatment [4,10] and that the early application of palliative medicine does not hasten death, but rather has been shown to extend survival time in some cases [10,17].

From the HCP perspective, this approach to care requires that death and incurable illness be reframed such that they are not understood as clinical failures. In palliative medicine, mortality and disease are understood as inevitable facts of life that must be accepted in order to develop care plans that allow patients to live comfortably and in ways that let them take part in activities that give their lives meaning.

The process of regoaling [22] is crucial in establishing realistic expectations for care and quality of life in the face of life-threatening and life-limiting conditions. Rather than relinquishing hope altogether when it becomes evident that beating death or illness is impossible, regoaling reframes patients' hope to focus on living and dying well despite their prognosis or diagnosis [6]. For example, seeking to control the symptoms and maximize the comfort of a child recently diagnosed with Batten's disease is a more appropriate and achievable goal than curing the illness.

HCPs' Roles

Palliative medicine also requires us to reimagine the role that HCPs play in medical care. PPC is based on a shared decision-making model that emphasizes communication, relationship-building, and care planning. There are widely differing perceptions of the appropriate role of physicians and medical information sharing across cultures [23,24]. However, PPC generally requires HCPs to adopt a collaborative model in which they accompany and guide patients and the care team rather than act as informative experts. Ultimately, this facilitates cooperation between the care team and the family to develop a care plan that balances evidenced-based medicine with patient goals and beliefs.

In one study comparing the communication styles of PICU and PPC physicians [25], intensivists were more likely to use language perceived by families as overly technical, communicating hopelessness, insensitive, and focused on their own work-related challenges. Contrastingly, palliativists were described as using supportive, hopeful, informative language that focused on quality of life and eliciting open-ended discussions with family.

Communication plays a significant role in medical care and patient-family satisfaction. Evidence suggests that the majority of patients want and expect their providers to initiate conversations related to care and end-of-life planning with them [26-28]. Furthermore, communication is one of the most important factors in how patients evaluate physicians and the care they receive [29]. However, most clinicians never receive instruction in how to share bad news, discuss end-of-life care, or conduct productive patient conversations [30]. PPC integrates evidence-based strategies in order to allow clinicians to assume this crucial but often neglected role in caring for seriously ill children and their families.

The Patient

PPC may also require we reconceptualize the focus of medical care: the patient. PPC uses a family-centered approach in which the most basic unit of care is considered to be the patient and their family. This approach values both patient autonomy as well as the importance of their most important relationships.

Evaluating patient competency, determining their role in medical decision-making, and resolving disagreements in care planning is inherently difficult with pediatric and adolescent patients. Some medical models strictly follow legally-established age-based guidelines in determining the role patients can adopt in their own care. However, PPC seeks to evaluate each case individually, considering factors like age, maturity, culture, disease, and disability to support patient wellness, consent, and autonomy in decision-making [10].

PPC's holistic, multidisciplinary approach demands a family-based focus. Especially for pediatric patients whose wellbeing largely depends on the care of their parents, elders, and community, family cannot be excluded if we are to deliver the best-available standard of care [10]. Clinicians can support the wellbeing of families through illness-specific education, inclusive care-planning conversations, psychological and spiritual care, and logistical support (e.g. translation services, allowing open-hours visiting policies in ICUs, providing break rooms for families, creating economic help opportunities, providing contact with diverse faith leaders, etc.). Another important aspect of family-centered care is considering the needs of often-neglected family members: caretakers, siblings, grandparents, and others.

Adequately supporting the patient-family unit requires a social-justice lens to appreciate challenges with which we may be unfamiliar and which are pervasive throughout medicine. For example, caretaking duties disproportionately fall to female family members. While many women adopt these roles in a way that are transformative and fulfilling for them, others face disproportionate combined burdens of family caretaking, work outside of the home, emotional labor, and inadequate support. Feminist perspectives in medical research can help us understand and work to prevent caretaker burnout and resolve these gender-related challenges [31]. Similarly, evidence shows the disproportionate undertreatment and undermedication of black patients and other minorities in diverse clinical settings [32]. Anti-racist perspectives in medical research can help us integrate checks and balances into protocols to strive for racial equity. Finally, disability scholars and others can help us understand the ways in which the stigmatization of disability affect our patients and may shape the type of care we feel comfortable providing (e.g. disabled adolescents and young adults are often excluded from sexual and relationship education at great cost to their wellbeing [33].

CLINICAL TOOLBOX

Integrating the ideals of humanism into a palliative care approach may seem like a lofty, esoteric ideal, but the following tools and strategies can help.

Resource Inventory

PPC's holistic, multidisciplinary, family-centered, quality-of-life-focused approach demands team coordination and collaboration. Especially in an IMOC, creating a PPC team does not require hiring a large group of specialists. Rather, an IMOC begins with taking an inventory of your available resources (human and otherwise) as well as those of each individual family and community. Knowing your colleagues' capacities, skills, and access to medical supplies is key to beginning necessary team-building, educational interventions, and division of PPC tasks [10].

Consider your team members' and institutions skills and resources—they need not be specialized to play an important role. Is a particular nurse skilled at talking to families? Does a certain physician have a gift at using games to involve children in care planning? Is a chaplain effective in resolving family conflicts? Note these valuable skills. As you complete your inventory, consider Amery's [10] categories (adapted by authors) and expand upon them as necessary as you assemble your team:

- Medical doctors: pediatricians, palliativists, intensivists, oncologists, other specialists, family care, etc.

- Nurses

- Community health workers

- Respiratory, occupational, speech, physical, and other therapists

- Mental health professionals

- Grief specialists

- Social workers and case workers

- Translators, interpreters

- Religious and spiritual leaders (in your institution and community)

- Elders

- Family members

- Contacts in local education system, teachers, guidance counselors, etc.

- Child life specialists

- Legal support

- Charitable funds

- Support groups

ACT Categories

Together for Short Lives, a leading UK charity for children with life-threatening and life-limiting conditions, created the ACT categories in order to help clinicians determine which patients can benefit from PPC [11]. A given condition may be catalogued according to different categories based on the trajectory of their disease, comorbidities, local medical resources, and other factors.

Categories of life-limiting and life-threatening conditions	
Category 1	Life-threatening conditions for which curative treatment may be feasible but can fail. Access to palliative care services may be necessary when treatment fails or during an acute crisis, irrespective of the duration of threat to life. On reaching long-term remission or following successful curative treatment there is no longer a need for palliative care services. Examples: cancer, irreversible organ failures of heart, liver, kidney.
Category 2	Conditions where premature death is inevitable. There may be long periods of intensive treatment aimed at prolonging life and allowing participation in normal activities. Examples: cystic fibrosis, Duchenne muscular dystrophy.

Category 3	Progressive conditions without curative treatment options. Treatment is exclusively palliative and may commonly extend over many years. Examples: Batten disease, mucopolysaccharidoses.
Category 4	Irreversible but non-progressive conditions causing severe disability, leading to susceptibility to health complications and likelihood of premature death. Examples: severe cerebral palsy, multiple disabilities such as following brain or spinal cord injury, complex health care needs, high risk of an unpredictable life-threatening event or episode.
A Core Care Pathway for Children with Life-limiting and Life-threatening Conditions by Together for Short Lives.	

Communication Algorithms and Tools

The importance of clinical communication to patient health and satisfaction is well-documented [2]. Keep in mind common hurdles in communicating with families and integrate these evidence-based algorithms into your team's training (adapted from the St. Judes' Quick Communication Reference Guide) [34]. Remember, although communication is often viewed as an innate "soft skill," clinicians are not born knowing how to lead difficult conversations and most medical schools do not teach these strategies, either. Integrating a PPC approach into the care of neurologically and otherwise disabled children necessarily requires training in clinical communication.

Common errors include:

- Giving too much information and too many details. Begin with an overview, be brief, and then allow a period of silence.

- Neglecting to ask the family about the information they need, assuming what the patient/family wants or needs to know.

- Excluding the child from care planning and decision-making conversations

- Excluding key family members, care team members, or others from decision-making

- Forcing the family to make a decision before they've had the opportunity to process the information.

General good communication guidelines incorporate the following:

- Establish goals focused on patient care using key questions:

  - What is a good day for your child? What is your child like as a person?

  - What have you heard from doctors about what's happening with your child? How has this experience been for you, your family, and your child?

  - Given what's happening with your child's condition, what is the most important goal for you? For your child? What is your top goal? What is your greatest hope?

  - What are your worries about your child's condition? What keeps you awake at night?

  - What gives you strength? Is that working well for you now?

- Ask permission to provide recommendations

  - Example phrase: Given what you've told me about what's happening with your child and your hopes for this situation, would it be helpful for me to share with you what I think about this situation?

  - Recommend goal-based plans. Review and monitor current treatments, exams, medications, etc. Periodically determine if these still fulfill patient/family goals. Make recommendations based on patient/family goals and incorporate the same words that they use ("Given what you've told me regarding your child's goals [name them], I would recommend...")

SPIKES

There are a number of helpful acronyms and methods used to help HCPs guide difficult care-planning conversations, including NURSE [34], WPC (Warn, Pause, Chunk) [10], PINCELES (for Spanish-speaking contexts) [34], and others. SPIKES was developed to deliver bad news [35], and the authors have found it to be particularly useful in training clinicians and medical students in low-resource contexts.

SPIKES—Algorithm to give bad news

Set-up

Review the clinical history, get to know current medical problems (e.g., clinical history, prognosis, treatment options). Prepare the setting. Find a private, quiet area, put your cellphone/pager on silent, have tissues ready, make sure you have enough chairs available, invite key people to be present, have translators/interpreters available if necessary. Have a meeting with the care team before initiating the family discussion. Coordinate team members that will be present in the meeting. Make certain that all team members agree on care recommendations and goals (e.g., What decisions do you hope to make today?) and decide who is going to lead the discussion. Discuss/coordinate a follow-up plan with the care team and family. Present all team members, their names, and their relationship with the patient at the beginning of the meeting.

Perception

Clarify the patient/family's perception and understanding of the medical situation. ("What have you heard about your child's condition?" or "What have other doctors told you about your child's illness?"). Ask-tell-ask. Ask the family to describe their current understanding of the problem. Do not interrupt. Seek emotional insight and information as the patient / family responds. Be prepared to repeat the information and present additional information if necessary.

Invitation

Explore how much information the patient and family want to know.

"Would it be okay for us to discuss the test results with you now?"

"How would you prefer medical information to be discussed in your family?"

"Some people prefer a global picture of what is happening, and others prefer to hear ever detail.

What do you prefer?"

Knowledge

Give medical information concisely, and then be quiet. Use a "warning shot" so that the patient and family members can prepare emotionally ("I have something serious that we need to discuss..." or "These tests did not show what we expected..."). Summarize the big picture in a few sentences. Just say it and then STOP ("Your cancer has spread to your liver and seems to be getting worse despite treatment"). Ask-Tell-Ask. Provide small bits of information about the situation or condition; provide more details once the family has had a chance to ask. Avoid medical jargon, use language that matches the family's level of understanding and education. Remember that even highly educated people with backgrounds in health sciences may be overwhelmed by technical details in the face of bad news.

Empathy

Respond to emotion. Expect the patient and family to have an emotional response. Use empathetic phrases to respond to emotions related to the news ("Hearing this must be shocking..."). Respond and validate emotions ("I can't imagine how difficult this must be..." or "I know this is not what you expected to hear today"). Name the emotions, especially if the patient or family is not responding verbally ("I can see that you are upset..."). Use phrases "I wish" ("I wish we had better news for you..."). Remain quiet and very attentive. Use pauses and wait quietly for the patient and family to respond.

Summarize

Discuss the next steps and a follow-up plan. Ask-Tell-Ask. Check the family's understanding ("We've talked about a lot today, could you tell me what you understand about what's going on now?"). Review options and ask permission to make treatment recommendations based on identified goals ("Would it be okay if I make a recommendation? Given what I have been told about your goals for _____, I would recommend..."). Summarize decisions and steps to follow ("Let's plan another meeting, I'll be here tomorrow but if you need someone from our team before, you can contact us").

Planning

Care planning is key to ensuring the continuity of holistic, family-centered care even in emergency situations. Amery's Golden Rules for PPC planning [10], hold true in emergency situations, Advanced Care Planning, as well as in general care planning:

- Don't panic
- Assess immaculately
- Hope for the best, prepare for the worst
- Treat what you can treat
- Communicate

Planning is largely contingent upon each individual patient's particular needs, culture, and familial situation. Plans should be available to all care providers and family members in the patient's medical file, in electronic medical file systems, school, home, and wherever else may be appropriate. They should also reflect patient-family goals and wishes and generally at least include the following (if applicable):

- Instructions to treat current and expected symptoms
- Resuscitation indications
- Discussions of patient goals, hopes, and wishes
- End-of-life plans
- Wills and legacy plans

Copies of these documents can be found in the Pediatric Palliative Care mobile application MedPal—CNN, available for free in GooglePlay and the Apple App Store (http://www.medpalcnn.org/en/). In addition to these documents, the care team should provide the family with the necessary medications, medical supplies, and education on how to use them if emergency or distressing symptoms strike while they are at home.

Symptom screening

A core tenet of PPC is impeccable assessment and symptom management. When possible, evidence-based, standardized assessment tools should be integrated into evaluation and applied regularly to monitor symptoms and adjust treatment as necessary. Standardized tools should be used because they incorporate evidence-based practice into evaluation, reduce the errors of subjective assessment, and create records of symptom evolution over time [10,36,37]. The FLACC, numeric/word symptom scales, Nonverbal Pain Scale (NVPS) for Nonverbal Patients, Baker-Wong Pain Scale, Rating of Perceived Dyspnea Scale, QUESTT tool, and numerous others to evaluate specific symptoms can be used.

Finally, it is crucial to consider patients' and family members' assessments of symptoms. Patients may underestimate and underreport chronic pain and other symptoms over time because they get used to them or don't wish to burden their loved ones by providing a distressing report. Family members and caretakers can often also provide important insight into patient progress. Compared to patients and family members, clinicians have been shown to be the least accurate in gauging patients' pain [10]. The limitations of these subjective evaluations further support the need to integrate evidence-based, standardized assessment tools into patient monitoring.

CONCLUSIONS

It is paramount that we reclaim Humanism in medicine and integrate it when considering the needs of our patients and families with neurological disabilities. A holistic approach to care implies that we ought to provide pharmacologic and non-pharmacological treatments and the impeccable management of symptoms. For the neuropediatric population, these include the management of Total Pain, seizures, spasticity, dyspnea, anxiety, constipation, end-of-life care, and grief. This should include advanced directives and conversations related to making difficult decisions related to hydration, nutrition, withholding and withdrawing treatment, as well as other ethical dilemmas. Discussing all treatment options goes well beyond the scope of this chapter. However, the authors developed a mobile application, MedPal-CNN, which is freely available on IOS and Android in English and Spanish (http://www.medpalcnn.org/en/). It addresses PPC and the specificities of neurological symptoms in PPC settings.

The American Academy of Pediatrics wisely states that the best possible life should be the goal for children with palliative care needs, even if their lives are short [38]. Neuropediatric health professionals are in the best position to apply palliative care skills through the trajectory of illness, even if they are seeking a cure. PPC can be integrated in all models of care, and by doing this we can provide a positive social and health impact for children and their families, most of whom might be dependent on technology to survive. When we think about the best approach for these children and their families, we need to make a commitment that consider that advances in technology as a mean of survival, must go hand in hand with advances in humanism for all children, even in the most remote and under-resourced places in the world.

References

1. Late Life: A Conversation With Atul Gawande 2016.

2. Grunauer M, Mikesell C. A Review of the Integrated Model of Care: An Opportunity to Respond to Extensive Palliative Care Needs in Pediatric Intensive Care Units in Under-Resourced Settings. Front Pediatr. 2018;6:3.

3. World Palliative Care Alliance, World Health Organization. Global Atlas of Palliative Care at the End of Life. London: Worldwide Palliative Care Alliance; 2014.

4. World Health Organization. WHO Definition of Palliative Care. 2019; https://www.who.int/cancer/palliative/definition/en/.

5. Chambers L. A Guide to Children's Palliative Care: Supporting babies, children and young people with life-limiting and life-threatening conditions and their families. 2018 ed. Bristol, England: Together for Short Lives; 2018.

6. Gans D, Kominski GF, Roby DH, et al. Better outcomes, lower costs: palliative care program reduces stress, costs of care for children with life-threatening conditions. Policy Brief UCLA Cent Health Policy Res. 2012(PB2012-3):1-8.

7. Curtis K, Foster K, Mitchell R, Van C. Models of Care Delivery for Families of Critically Ill Children: An Integrative Review of International Literature. J Pediatr Nurs. 2016;31(3):330-341.

8. Ong CK, Forbes D. Embracing Cicely Saunders's concept of total pain. BMJ. 2005;331(7516):576.

9. Loscalzo MJ. Palliative care: an historical perspective. Hematology Am Soc Hematol Educ Program. 2008:465.

10. Amery J. A Really Practical Handbook of Children's Palliative care for doctors and nurses Anywhere in the World. Morrisville: Lulu Publishing Services; 2016.

11. Together for Short Lives. A Framework for the Development of an Integrated Care Pathway for Children and Young People with Life Threatening or Life-Limiting Conditions and Their Families. 2013.

12. Rushton CH. A framework for integrated pediatric palliative care: being with dying. J Pediatr Nurs. 2005;20(5):311-325.

13. Hain, Devins. Directory of Life-Limiting conditions. 2014.

14. Gregoire MC, Frager G. Ensuring pain relief for children at the end of life. Pain Res Manag. 2006;11(3):163-171.

15. Somerville MA. Human rights and human ethics: health and health care. Death Talk: The Case Against Euthanasia and Physician-assisted Suicide. Montreal: McGill-Queen's University Press; 2001:327-344.

16. Human Rights Watch. "Please, do not make us suffer any more..." Access to Pain Treatment as a Human Right. Washington, DC: Human Rights Watch; March 2009 2009.

17. Boss R, Nelson J, Weissman D, et al. Integrating palliative care into the PICU: a report from the Improving Palliative Care in the ICU Advisory Board. Pediatr Crit Care Med. 2014;15(8):762-767.

18. Stewart MA. Effective physician-patient communication and health outcomes: a review. CMAJ. 1995;152(9):1423-1433.

19. Casarett D, Johnson M, Smith D, Richardson D. The optimal delivery of palliative care: a national comparison of the outcomes of consultation teams vs inpatient units. Arch Intern Med. 2011;171(7):649-655.

20. Brennan F. Palliative care as an international human right. J Pain Symptom Manage. 2007;33(5):494-499.

21. Biskup T, Phan P, Grunauer M. Lessons from the Design and Implementation of a Pediatric Critical Care and Emergency Medicine Training Program in a Low Resource Coun-

try-The South American Experience. J Pediatr Intensive Care. 2017;6(1):60-65.

22. Hill DL, Miller V, Walter JK, et al. Regoaling: a conceptual model of how parents of children with serious illness change medical care goals. BMC Palliat Care. 2014;13(1):9.

23. Levetown M, American Academy of Pediatrics Committee on B. Communicating with children and families: from everyday interactions to skill in conveying distressing information. Pediatrics. 2008;12(5):e1441-1460.

24. Searight HR, Gafford J. Cultural diversity at the end of life: issues and guidelines for family physicians. Am Fam Physician. 2005;71(3):515-522.

25. Ciriello AG, Dizon ZB, October TW. Speaking a Different Language: A Qualitative Analysis Comparing Language of Palliative Care and Pediatric Intensive Care Unit Physicians. Am J Hosp Palliat Care. 2018;35(3):384-389.

26. Balaban RB. A physician's guide to talking about end-of-life care. J Gen Intern Med. 2000;15(3):195-200.

27. Risk J, Mohammadi L, Rhee J, Walters L, Ward PR. Barriers, enablers and initiatives for uptake of advance care planning in general practice: a systematic review and critical interpretive synthesis. BMJ Open. 2019;9(9):e030275.

28. Reilly BM, Magnussen CR, Ross J, Ash J, Papa L, Wagner M. Can we talk? Inpatient discussions about advance directives in a community hospital. Attending physicians' attitudes, their inpatients' wishes, and reported experience. Arch Intern Med. 1994;154(20):2299-2308.

29. Berman AC, Chutka DS. Assessing effective physician-patient communication skills: "Are you listening to me, doc?". Korean J Med Educ. 2016;28(2):243-249.

30. Ha JF, Longnecker N. Doctor-patient communication: a review. Ochsner J. 2010;10(1):38-43.

31. Grunauer M, Mikesell C. Cuidados Paliativos Pediatricos. Medicina Familiar, reflexiones desde la práctica. Quito, Ecuador: World Health Organization, Pan-American Health Organization, Ministerio de la Salud Pública del Ecuador; 2017.

32. Johnson KS. Racial and ethnic disparities in palliative care. J Palliat Med. 2013;16(11):1329-1334.

33. Addlakha R, Price J, Heidari S. Disability and sexuality: claiming sexual and reproductive rights. Reprod Health Matters. 2017;25(50):4-9.

34. St. Judes' Children's Research Hospital, Universidad San Francisco de Quito, Hospital de los Valles- Unidad de Cuidados Pediátricos, Academia Ecuatorian de Medicina. Guía breve de comunicación. In: Universidad San Francisco de Quito, ed. Quito, Ecuador:1-4.

35. Rosenzweig MQ. Breaking bad news: a guide for effective and empathetic communication. Nurse Pract. 2012;37(2):1-4.

36. Giordano V, Edobor J, Deindl P, et al. Pain and Sedation Scales for Neonatal and Pediatric Patients in a Preverbal Stage of Development: A Systematic Review. JAMA Pediatr. 2019.

37. Franck LS, Bruce E. Putting pain assessment into practice: why is it so painful? Pain Res Manag. 2009;14(1):13-20.

38. Korones DN. Pediatric palliative care. Pediatr Rev. 2007;28(8):e46-56.

HUMANISTIC CARE IN CHILD NEUROLOGY: MOVING FROM LEBANON TO THE UNITED STATES.

Michel N. Fayad, MD
Assistant Professor of Neurology
Harvard Medical School
Staff Neurologist, Boston Children's Hospital

Some may say that pursuing humanistic care is a luxury, not afforded by developing countries, where resources are often lacking, and where many people still resort to folk medicine.

I would like to relate my personal experience of transitioning from practicing in a developing country (Lebanon) to the US. Obviously, the experience is probably different in other countries.

Growing up in Lebanon, especially after the age of 15, when the war in Lebanon started in 1975, went from a very easy and happy life to a very stressful situation with prolonged stays in the bomb shelters and avoiding going out (The COVID 19 is a bitter reminder of that time). I found a sense of purpose in the Lebanese Red Cross where I worked as a first-aid rescuer, moving wounded people across ceasefire lines, and staffing a field hospital built by the International Committee of the Red Cross. This gave me the first taste of humanistic care. I learned to look at the person and their suffering, and not at the religion or political stance.

What is considered humanistic care in Lebanon: There are some very basic issues that a provider faces, such as providing equal care to patients covered by medical insurance or self-payers and to patients (barely) covered by government medical insurance. At the same time, because of cultural attitudes, the personal interaction is much closer between providers and patients and their families, and people tend to become very familiar with each other. Most of my patients asked me questions about my family and children, the town I was from, and often tried to find common acquaintances. Providers are expected to give their patients their personal phone numbers and it is not uncommon to be called at night for questions that could have waited until the next day. Patients would expect their physician to answer their questions, rather than a nurse or even a covering on call physician. Also, patients expect their physician to advise them and most of the time, to make important decisions for them, decisions that we assume in the United States will be made by the patient and their family. If you give patients a choice between medications, or between different treatment options, they usually respond, "You are the doctor, you know better."

What is different in the US: The difference between patients with private medical insurance and government medical insurance is much less here. Despite all the shortcomings of Medicaid, I feel most patients have reasonable coverage. Very often, I am not aware of the type of medical insurance my patients have, unless I have to fill out paperwork, such as for a prior authorization. The interaction with patients and families is less personal, except for a few patients whom I have followed for years, as people in general expect and respect privacy. It is a mixed blessing because the interaction can be too "business"-like. As with many issues, the middle ground is best: It is preferable to establish a certain personal relationship with patients and families without too much familiarity. The fact that one is not on call 24/7, and that patients expect to have their questions answered by a nurse or a covering provider, allows us to have free time. Although I feel we should advise our patients about treatment plans, I prefer that the final decision be theirs.

In my practice at the American University of Beirut-Medical Center, I was able to treat patients coming from all over Lebanon and many countries in the Middle East. One of my duties was to give the Pediatrics and Neurology parts of the Medical Ethics course for the medical students.

Compared to my experience with Medical Ethics in the Ethics Advisory Committee at Boston Children's Hospital, the ethical issues in Lebanon had more to do with access to care and allocation of resources, whereas in the US, they have more to do with end of life decisions and cutting edge therapies.

The main barriers in practicing humanistic medicine after moving to the US were initially cultural. It took me some time to understand that patients and families were not distant, but respected my privacy, and I quickly came to appreciate it.

It was very rare for me to face bigotry or hostility because of my ethnicity or accent. Most people are very friendly, even though they expect and respect privacy. I have made very close relationships with some families whom I have followed for many years.

What I had to change when I arrived to the US: Upon arriving initially as a resident, I had to learn, in addition to medical knowledge and clinical skills, some very important cultural attitudes, including a less paternalistic approach to medical care. I had to recognize different priorities and expectations in different local and immigrant groups. I had very informative rotations in two inner city hospitals, in different private hospitals, on Navajo and Hopi reservations, and at a Veterans hospital, where I met people from different backgrounds and learned to respect their views.

Advice for physicians arriving to an industrialized country: We should learn about the culture and beliefs of the communities we live in, the different ethnic and racial groups, and the different immigrant groups. We should be less paternalistic with our patients and families. We should give our best advice and explain the facts as completely as possible, and then allow the patient and their family to make their own decisions.

HOW CURRENT GENERATIONS THINK ABOUT HUMANISM AS ESSENTIAL PART OF THE MEDICAL ART

Forrest P. Beaulieu, MD
PL-1, Pediatrics/Child Neurology
Children's Hospital of Philadelphia
Boston University School of Medicine

Commencement Address of the class of 2020

Looking back, we started medical school in the era of high-tech solutions – precision medicine, robotically assisted intervention, many incredible things that have and will continue to shape the landscape of medical practice over the course of our careers. We have algorithmic, evidence-based approaches in place for many of the problems we see in our day to day. In the past few months, this has paled in the face of a novel pandemic that has brought the country (and the globe) to its knees.

I don't think this is how any of us expected our fourth year to go. Many of us were hoping to be traveling, or brushing up on our skills before the start of intern year. I don't think anyone guessed that we would be stuck in our apartments (or our parents' homes), anxiously waiting to become a part of our nation's healthcare force while anticipating our webcam graduation – early graduation, I might add. But here we are.

Intern year was never going to be easy but starting our medical training in the throes of one of the worst crises in modern medical history is truly unprecedented. The best we can hope for is that, come July 1st, we will be dealing with the aftermath of a pandemic that has touched just about every life on the globe. In the worst case, we will be joining our profession at a time when our colleagues – and country – need us more than ever. Our skills will have to grow faster than those of any intern before, and our grit and endurance – traits I think we can all agree are particularly strong in the Boston Medical Center community – shall be engaged consistently and intensely – more than even at the most savage Prometric testing center.

Over these past four years, we have learned lifesaving skills, interviewing techniques, advanced anatomy, problem-solving strategies, and what seems like an enormous breadth of physiology and pharmacotherapy. Some of us may even remember vaccine schedules. We are knowledgeable, not just about the iceberg tip of medicine that we have uncovered thus far, but about the unending remainder of the undiscovered - a truth which has never been more painfully evident than today, as physicians around the world struggle with a novel disease on an epic scale.

The most important thing medical school has taught me is that even during crisis medicine is about people. Our job will be to meet people, hear their thoughts and their stories, and do our best to help them.

Of course, medicine isn't just about the person on the examining table – it's a team sport. To get to this point, we all have had the privilege of endless care, love, and support from family, friends, significant others, and mentors of every kind. We will need that more than ever, and we will need to create it anew - providing it to our new colleagues in intern year, building those relationships with nurses, therapists, and everyone else in our new homes come July.

Our role as physicians, in many cases, will be to deliver news to our patients. We will draw upon our repository of medical knowledge and seek diagnostic and therapeutic answers in order to treat each person to the best of our ability. This is critical. I have learned, though, that a physician is much more than an assigner of diagnoses and distributor of treatments – as physicians, we practice patient care. We employ our fund of emotional knowledge and social understanding to discern WHAT it is exactly that our patients need. In the future, it may not be novel therapies for a terrifying virus.

It's using our artistic skills, whether they're rudimentary or refined, to show the anatomy of what will be treated surgically. Maybe we schedule a patient in the latest possible slot, so that parents who work different shifts can both attend their child's appointment, or we ask whether someone has a refrigerator at home to properly store insulin. It may in fact be, no more and no less, a shoulder to cry on, a hand to hold, reassurance that "hey, we're in this together."

Being a person's physician - practicing true patient care – means caring for some of these less tangible but far more important facets of life.

We as physicians will have the enormous privilege of appreciating the full spectrum of what it is to be human, from the electric moments of happiness that may come only once or twice in a lifetime, to the crushing lows that can accompany truly bad news. Some patients we see will be having the worst day of their lives, while in the next room it may just be another Friday. We must learn to fine tune our demeanor, inject humor when appropriate, and use the rapport and relationships we will build to know what the person in front of us – whether in clinic or by webcam - best needs. As Sir William Osler once said, "The good physician treats the disease; the great physician treats the patient who has the disease." This stability and finesse, even in the face of chaos, is the most critical aspect of physician ship.

We are all human beings, with unique hopes, dreams, beliefs, and fears. No virus and no training program could ever take that away from us. Our existing roles as thinkers, teachers, learners, role models, family, friends, are all ours to keep and cultivate. Today we add a role that incorporates all facets of our training and personhood to date – physician.

At this critical inflection point in healthcare's history – the era of big data, of computer-assisted solutions, of genetically-matched therapies, and a virus that is wreaking worldwide havoc, we physicians are needed more than ever - as leaders, problem solvers, outside-the-box thinkers, advocates, and teachers. As healers. This frightening pandemic will have a permanent effect on this country and on healthcare as a whole. We will never be the same - and we have the once in a generation chance to build the future of American medicine. The panel of people for whom you will be caring in the next few months will need you more than they have ever needed a doctor before.

Class of 2020, I ask you to bring with you to residency your personality, your sense of humor, your curiosity, and your life experiences. But especially, bring your hope, because that may be what your patients and colleagues need most come July. Remember that you will not always be able to fix every problem, but you can always help. Some say it was Hippocrates who described the role of the physician as "to cure sometimes, to relieve often, and to comfort always." I ask you, my classmates, to join me in that mission. We will beat this thing. Boston University School of Medicine class of 2020, it has been a pleasure and an honor to be your classmate, and I look forward to being your colleague. Thank you. We're on to residency.

CHILD NEUROLOGISTS BETWEEN BURNOUT AND WELL-BEING

Alcy R. Torres, MD, FAAP
Associate Professor of Pediatrics and Neurology
Assistant Dean of Diversity and Inclusion
Director of the Pediatric Traumatic Injury, International and Bilingual Programs
Boston University School of Medicine
Boston Medical Center
Boston, MA, USA

Physicians burnout in the world has reached epidemic proportions is rising rapidly or do not burnout in another patient stable. It has negative impact this far-reaching includes car to the burnout physician us were less patients, coworkers, family members, close friends, has good organizations. Yet is not a lot of data or literature that was started either burnout in child neurologists or well-being.

In a review published by Rothenberger in 2017, he concluded that medical students physicians in training on practicing physicians are up significant risk of burnout and now exceeds 50%. Burnout is there unintended net result of most people, highly disruptive changes in society at large, the medical profession, on the health care system. Bold individual and organizational strategies have been only partially successful mitigating burnout on developing recipients were being among physicians. Tool highly effective strategies on aligning medicine alone organizational violence on enabling physicians to the goals 20% of the worker is to that part of that medical practice that is especially meaningful to them [1].

Physician burnout, a work-related syndrome involving emotional exhaustion, depersonalization and a sense of reduced personal accomplishment, is prevalent internationally. This problem represents a public health crisis with negative impacts on individual physicians, patients and healthcare organizations and systems. Drivers of this epidemic are largely rooted within healthcare organizations and systems and include excessive workloads, inefficient work processes, clerical burdens, work-home conflicts, lack of input or control for physicians with respect to issues affecting their work lives, organizational support structures and leadership culture [2]. Changes in the healthcare environment have created marked and growing external pressures. In addition, physicians are predisposed to burnout due to internal traits such as compulsiveness, guilt, and self-denial, and a medical culture that emphasizes perfectionism, denial of personal vulnerability, and delayed gratification [3]. Individual physician-level factors also play a role, with higher rates of burnout commonly reported in female and younger physicians. Effective solutions align with these drivers [2].

An online survey was distributed to 798 U.S. women neurologists through the closed Facebook group Women Neurologists Group. Burnout was assessed with the Mini-Z survey. Professional burnout and career dissatisfaction have high prevalence in women neurologists and threaten the future of the neurology workforce [4].

Burnout symptoms and career choice regret are prevalent among neurology postgraduates in China. Career choice regret is an important predictor of burnout. Further research on reducing burnout and career choice regret among neurology postgraduates is needed [5].

West et al., identified 2617 articles, of which 15 randomized trials including 716 physicians and 37 cohort studies including 2914 physicians met inclusion criteria. Overall burnout decreased from 54% to 44% (difference 10% [95% CI 5-14]; p<0·0001; I2=15%; 14 studies), emotional exhaustion score decreased from 23·82 points to 21·17 points (2·65 points [1·67-3·64]; p<0·0001; I2=82%; 40 studies), and depersonalization score decreased from 9·05 to 8·41 (0·64 points [0·15-1·14]; p=0·01; I2=58%; 36 studies). High emotional exhaustion decreased from 38% to 24% (14% [11-18]; p<0·0001; I2=0%; 21 studies) and high depersonalization decreased from 38% to 34% (4% [0-8]; p=0·04; I2=0%; 16 studies). This review indicated that literature indicates that both individual-focused and structural or organizational strategies can result in clinically meaningful reductions in burnout among physicians.

Horiguchi et al. evaluated the Mental Health of Physicians Specializing in the Field of Child Neurology. We assessed physicians working in the field of child neurology with the aim of improving the physicians' mental health. Our questionnaire included a burnout inventory and a general health questionnaire. We analyzed 29 responses from physicians in a variety of countries obtained through the Internet. According to their responses, 8 (27.5%) of the respondents had attained a burnout status, and 27 respondents (93.1%) had neurotic conditions. We found a greater percentage of physicians in poor mental health than we had found previously in assessments made in Japan. However, the respondents in the present survey had more positive styles for coping with stress. The length of time working as a physician affected respondents in Japan and internationally, whereas nationality or working environment (workplace, night shifts, and so on) did not. Consultants or mentors on work and assertive stress coping would be effective [7].

Specific solutions depending on the been suggested for example for excessive workflow: fair productivity targets, duty hour limits, appropriate distribution of job roles, part time choices, informed specialty choices, informed practice choices have been suggested.

For work inefficiency and lack of work support: Optimized electronic medical records, nonphysician staff support to offload clerical burdens, appropriate interpretation of regulatory requirements, appropriate interpretation of regulatory requirements, efficiency and skills training, prioritize tasks and delegate work appropriately [6].

For lack of work–home integration: Respect for home responsibilities in setting schedules for work and meeting, include all required work tasks within expected work hours, support flexible work schedules, including part-time employment, reflection on life priorities and values, attention to self-care [6].

For loss of control and autonomy: Physician engagement in establishing work requirements and structure, physician leadership and shared decision-making, stress management and resiliency training, positive coping strategies, mindfulness [6].

For loss of meaning from work: Promote shared core values, protect physician time with patients, promote physician communities, offer professional development opportunities, leadership training and awareness around physician burnout, positive psychology, reflection/self-awareness of most fulfilling work roles, mindfulness, engagement in physician small-group activities around shared work experiences [6].

But how these general concepts apply to child neurologists and more importantly what can we do to reverse a path that are leaving so many of our colleagues unhappy at the end of their careers? How can we change and give hope in a time in which we have no power? Who is looking out for us as a group? The first step is acceptance and understanding of the problem and some steps have been taking at least in certain societies to discuss about it but that is happening with no obstacles. Child neurologists know that some patients and some families overwhelmed with certain diagnosis like intellectual disability autism, refractory epilepsies, brain tumors or neurodegenerative disorders just to mention a few require more time, yet the business models that dominated medicine these days give us a certain amount of fixed time for every consultation or follow up in which impossible demands are imposed on caregivers as judged but the ways our patients could rank our performance regardless of the resources we are given. So to keep honest this discourse we need to get involved in our national organizations and through them demand changes are made immediately to the way our profession is carried out at the moment to prevent a future dehumanized environment in which medicine will become like any other services and the doctor patient relationship is exchanged for the merely customer relationship.

Although our understanding of physician burnout has advanced considerably in recent years, many gaps in our knowledge remain. Longitudinal studies of burnout's effects and the impact of interventions on both burnout and its effects are needed, as are studies of effective solutions implemented in combination. For medicine to fulfil its mission for patients and for public health, all stakeholders in healthcare delivery must work together to develop and implement effective remedies for physician burnout.

References

1. Rothenberger DA. Physician Burnout and Well-Being: A Systematic Review and Framework for Action. Dis Colon Rectum. 2017;60(6):567–576. doi:10.1097/DCR.0000000000000844

2. West CP, Dyrbye LN, Shanafelt TD. Physician burnout: contributors, consequences and solutions. J Intern Med. 2018;283(6):516–529. doi:10.1111/joim.12752

3. Gazelle G, Liebschutz JM, Riess H. Physician burnout: coaching a way out. J Gen Intern Med. 2015;30(4):508–513. doi:10.1007/s11606-014-3144-y

4. Moore LR, Ziegler C, Hessler A, Singhal D, LaFaver K. Burnout and Career Satisfaction in Women Neurologists in the United States. J Womens Health (Larchmt). 2019;28(4):515–525. doi:10.1089/jwh.2017.6888

5. Tian L, Pu J, Liu Y, et al. Relationship between burnout and career choice regret among Chinese neurology postgraduates. BMC Med Educ. 2019;19(1):162. Published 2019 May 22. doi:10.1186/s12909-019-1601-3

6. West CP, Dyrbye LN, Erwin PJ, Shanafelt TD. Interventions to prevent and reduce physician burnout: a systematic review and meta-analysis. Lancet. 2016;388(10057):2272–2281. doi:10.1016/S0140-6736(16)31279-X

7. Horiguchi T, Kaga M, Inagaki M, Uno A, Lasky R, Hecox K. An assessment of the mental health of physicians specializing in the field of child neurology. J Pediatr Nurs. 2003;18(1):70–74. doi:10.1053/jpdn.2003.16

HUMANISM IN THE PRACTICE OF CHILD NEUROLOGY: GLOBAL PERSPECTIVE, BARRIERS AND OPPORTUNITIES IN LOW RESOURCE SETTINGS

Sr Ornella Ciccone (SFMA) MD
Consultant Paediatric Neurologist
University Teaching Hospitals-Children's Hospital, Nationalist Road, Lusaka, Zambia
Istituto Serafico, Assisi, Italy

INTRODUCTION

The approach to human life in our medical practice is a "sacred space": a mix of known and unknown, measurable and unmeasurable, expected and unexpected. As much as scientific progress could allow medical society to know in greater details the genetic and molecular bases of physio-pathological pathways of human life, it would never be enough to unveil the deepest essence of a human being. Along history, philosophers, anthropologists and theologians have investigated the nature of a human life by accentuating, in different ways, the role of the body, the mind and the soul, but the definition of "human life" may never be complete and exhaustive. In opposition to a dualistic vision of body and soul, Christian anthropology affirms the substantial unity of body and soul: "embodied spirit" and "spiritualized body" [1,2].

The Indian greeting "Namaste: I bow to the divine that is in you," expresses the recognition of the sacredness of life, which is present in many cultures and religions [3]. In this vision, the value of a human life does not depend on the person's ability to produce and contribute to the society and neither on the level of pleasure or satisfaction that he or she may enjoy, but from the deep respect toward his or her Life originating from "Above." We need to acknowledge that if it may be easy for most people to "bow down" with great admiration in front of persons of great achievements, success, generosity or selfless service to humanity, the same sentiments and convictions may be greatly challenged by facing a person disfigured by sickness and multiple disabilities. At times, it may be difficult to recognize the "inner beauty" of people with severe behavioral and cognitive impairments without taking time to enter into contact with them, to understand their language and to listen with the "heart" to their sentiments and thoughts.

A certain ethic believes that a life signed by pain and suffering, unable to muster self-determination and independence, is not worthy to be lived or, by extreme, neither to be cared for. Quality of life is often the argument brought forward to justify this kind of vision: a sort of "compassion" for a life that is seen just as a painful and meaningless event. The questions might be: "What does quality of life really mean?" and "What makes the difference in a person's life, despite sickness and disability?"

In the practice of child neurology, we daily face these questions and sentiments. This short essay is an attempt to discuss some of the challenges and opportunities in practicing humanism in child neurology in low resource settings, with a holistic approach of care to children and families within their cultural, societal and religious contexts.

HUMANISM IN THE PRACTICE OF CHILD NEUROLOGY: BARRIERS AND OPPORTUNITIES IN LOW RESOURCE SETTINGS.

The "drama" of children with neurological conditions seems to be present with similar connotations across all cultures and socio-economical contexts. Stigma, misbeliefs, guilty feelings, isolation from family and society, crises in the parenting couple, and depression are common aspects of the life experience of parents with children with severe neuro-disabilities.

We all know the parents' challenge to accept a child's diagnosis for which we cannot offer a definitive cure or reverse the situation. The child's difficulties in feeding, sleeping, going to the toilet, communicating, moving, as well as the need for frequent hospitalizations and the overall uncertainty for the future, become such a burden for the child and the family that the situation cannot be faced without medical, spiritual, psychological and societal support. Empathic relationships between the physician, the child and the family play unique roles in the process of care: attentive listening, compassion, professionality and respect for the child and family's feelings and beliefs are the necessary base to build a "therapeutic alliance." Clinicians need to journey with parents, siblings and the same child from the communication of the diagnosis, to the implementation of therapeutic interventions and at times, to preparation for death. A "network of care," composed of health professionals, school teachers, friends, and religious and community leaders, is essential to offer the necessary human support to children and families.

Despite some common denominators, the possibility of holistic care for children with neurological disorders, both in terms of limitations and opportunities, is strongly influenced by financial resources, health and education systems, societal beliefs, faith, and family and community structures in different contexts around the world. Africa, in its complexity of cultural values, religions, high disparity of resources, and emerging medical society, represents a paradigm of both barriers and opportunities to providing care in developing countries. In South Saharan countries, the number of child neurologists is extremely low compared to the high incidence of pediatric neurological disorders [4].The most recent data from the WHO reports that there are less than 0.4 per 100,000 child neurologists globally, with 0.02 per 100,000 in LMIC [5]. Even though the impact on care of such an inadequate health system, with extremely limited diagnostic and therapeutic possibilities, is not the focus of the present work, we cannot avoid taking this element into account in discussing the humanistic approach to children with neurological disorders. Failure to receive specialized medical attention and to know what is determining the child's condition, open spaces of doubts, fears, and uncertainty in children and caregivers, and these emotions can lead to severe psychological distress. In many cultures and societies, any unknown "mysterious" sickness is explained as punishment, curse or possession by a "bad spirit." In many villages in rural areas of Africa, Latin America and Asia, people in need of medical care are mainly attended to by traditional healers or primary health care personnel with little or no understanding of neurological conditions. Very often, medical attention is greatly delayed and no explanation is given to the sick children and their families, other than societal and spiritual beliefs. The possibility of receiving an explanation of the child's sickness through an emphatic dialogue, adapted to the cultural level and sensibility of the family, is, in itself, a source of deliverance and the starting point for acceptance. The same failure to treat and relieve associated symptoms and comorbidities, such as pain, feeding and sleep difficulties, uncontrolled seizures, etc., due to limited available resources, aggravates the psychological and social consequences of the child's disability. As human beings, in whom physical, psychological and spiritual wellbeing are strongly interconnected, failure to provide the minimum needed medical care will automatically result in a condition of distress for which also spiritual and psychological interventions will have a minor impact. In poor health systems often overwhelmed by communicable disorders, the message that is frequently given to parents of children with neuro-disabilities is that the child has "brain damage" and there is "nothing more to do." This type of message will have a severe psychological impact on the child and the family leading, not only, to depression, but in some cases, to physical neglect. Families with severe financial constrains will often prioritize resources toward the healthy children and fail to provide adequate nutrition and care for the chronically sick child. The same education system, in most low resource settings, does not favor inclusion of children with neurological conditions.

Any government-run schools, with regular classrooms of 70-80 pupils and just one teacher, are unable to include children unable to move independently or in need of learning support. Some children with good cognitive abilities and just minor motor or language impairments are assigned to "special classes" together with children with severe mental disabilities: such a placement drastically lessens the possibility of their developing their potential. The few private schools that are able to offer more consistent support are extremely expensive and not affordable for the majority of families. In many rural regions, where there are not specials schools, children with disabilities will not be able to go to school at all. Access to other social groups in churches, sports and other recreational associations may be extremely limited due to physical barriers and the social and spiritual perception of a child with neurological impairments. The same communication, that is necessary, between the fragile health, education and social services, in order to create a favorable network of care for the children and their families, might be very difficult to establish in a poor resource setting. Traditional healers play an interesting role, and they are to be considered in the network of care: they are often the first contact for people experiencing "scaring" disorders like bizarre behaviors or seizures; they dedicate long spans of time in listening, getting involved in the affected families' dynamics, and being aware of the spiritual and emotional life of the people asking for their care.

Doctors and paramedical staff of overcrowded health facilities are unable to give time for listening and dialogue while traditional healers do. There are interesting experiences done by some neurology - epilepsy services in Africa in trying to interact with traditional leaders and include them in the network of care, but the "secrecy" that covers their practice and the preparation of herbal remedies, represent a great obstacle to a real collaboration [6,7].

Despite the many obstacles to the delivery of integrated - humanistic medical care, the cultural and societal set-up, still present in many low-income countries, may become an opportunity for the development of greatest support webs and the inclusion of children with neurological disorders, and their families, within the community. Rural communities and ancient societies, that are still deeply rooted in Nature, carry a culture of acceptance of, respect for, and interdependence on, Creation in her natural (visible) and supernatural (invisible) aspects. The controls and expectations over life, sickness and death, that characterize highly technological societies, are much less present in poor rural communities. Many of us might have experienced the differences, in the psychological and emotional reactions of caregivers coming from different cultures and socio-economical backgrounds, in front of a child's diagnosis that we cannot reverse. The pain and suffering envisioned in the future of the child may be exactly the same, but the acceptance of such events, within the course of Mother Nature and in the faith in God as Giver of Life, may be very different; simple, faith-rooted people recognize every human life, and any event of life, as gifts from Above that cannot be suppressed or manipulated by man's decisions. Another interesting opportunity of care in many poor resource settings is the "extended family." In many African countries a woman's children are the children of all the woman's sisters and a man's brothers are all fathers to the man's children. In contrast with nuclear families of the western world, the enlarged family may provide multiple caregivers for the sick child and reduce the risk for that child's institutionalization [8]. The strong sense of community and solidarity characteristic of many cultures in the southern hemisphere of the world may represent another great opportunity of inclusion for children with neurological disorders. The African saying, "I am as we are" expresses the meaning of human existence as part of a community and the obligation of every member to care for each other. These cultural and religious aspects represent a fertile background on which the medical society can carry out, or build upon, in order to sensitize, enhance awareness, and increase the empowerment of the communities to improve the care of children with neuro-disabilities. Finally, in the past years, there has been a growing interest in the practice of pediatric neurology in developing countries. The numerous training activities carried out by International Neurology Societies (WFN, ICNA etc..), with the goal of filling the gap in the number of child neurologists, represent an opportunity to integrate and promote humanism in the practice of child neurology as an integral part of the educational programs.

Experience in Zambia

My ten years' experience in Zambia, working with a local team of therapists and pediatricians in the effort to build up pediatric neurology clinics, neuro-rehabilitation and epilepsy services, both in urban and rural settings, has been a unique opportunity to experience barriers and the potentiality in the practice of humanism in child neurology in an African contest. Zambia is one of the countries in South Saharan Africa where most of the children with neurological disorders have little or no opportunities to access specialized medical centers and neuro-rehabilitations services. The country has a population of about 17 million people of which about 50% are under the age of 15 years [9,10]. For many years, visiting child neurologists from the USA were the only opportunity for the children, once referred to the Tertiary Care Hospital in Lusaka, to receive specialist care. When I first arrived in Zambia at the Pediatric Department of the University Teaching Hospital in 2010, my first impression was a high level of interest in pediatric neurology; at the same time, among the medical staff, however, the feeling of frustration was very evident, in light or their children with conditions for which they felt they could do very little. If this frustration was a widespread feeling in at the Tertiary Level Care Hospital, much higher was the powerless perception in local clinics and rural health centers.

In my years in Zambia, listening to parents of children with neuro-disabilities of all levels of educational and financial possibilities, I have collected so many stories in which they were told that the child's brain got spoiled and there was "nothing more that doctors could do." Other frequently heard, and very painful, stories were those of parents going up and down, to and from clinics, for several months, reporting abnormal movements and delayed development in the babies, without ever receiving any precise answer or diagnosis.

The establishment of the Developmental Intervention Clinic at the Paediatric Center of Excellence (CDC project) represented a unique opportunity for children with neurological disorders, of all socio-economic backgrounds, to receive multi-disciplinary assessments and interventions directed to the global needs of the children. It has been indeed an exciting experience to set up, together with a local team of therapists and young colleagues, a neurological service that could offer culturally adapted ways of communication and locally available interventions aimed to improve a child's and family's quality of life. The first step was an attentive listening to the child's and the parents' stories by different members of the team: children and caregivers were encouraged to speak their own languages and to freely express their feelings and beliefs. As a "western doctor," it was clear to me that working in isolation, without the support of the local team or directly giving my own medical explanation of the child's sickness, without listening or opposing parents' beliefs, would have just lead to a psychological barrier: my being identified as a foreign doctor unable to understand "what is going on in Africa." Despite the limited diagnostic tools, after an attentive history-taking and neurological evaluation, we could still explain to parents what may have caused the disease of the child and allow them to ask questions and express their doubts. One of the main goals during the child's assessment was to shift the attention of the caregivers from what the child "could not do" to what the child "was able to do," giving them motivations to interact more with the child and to stimulate his/her potential abilities. Culturally, most of the mothers and fathers in Zambia are not so used to talking to their babies and spending time playing with them; therefore, motivating caregivers to interact more with their children was a first necessary, and very possible, step to enhance children's potential and strengthen the bonding between them. Thorough a therapeutic alliance with the medical staff, many parents journeyed from fear and guilty feelings to love and passion, discovering the "great treasure" hidden in their child's sick body. Family-centered interventions, using local languages, songs and dances, were great means to empower parents to care for their children, by stimulating their abilities and integrating them in family's life. Preparation of local food and feeding techniques for dysphasic children that could respect the local feeding practices were among the goals of interventions. Sadly, it was not infrequent that poor mothers could not cope with the demand of care for the sick child, due to the pressure of feeding many other children also, and often such women were abandoned by the spouse because of the disabled child.

Despite the challenges of the educational system and available social services, the neuro-rehabilitation team tried to establish links with teachers and faith-based organizations to facilitate the integration of the children in schools and promote advocacy and sensitization within the community. One of the most interesting and effective interventions was the organization of "parents' support groups." Parents of children affected by epilepsy or autism organized themselves in "self-help" groups in which they could share problems and support each other psychologically, spiritually and in daily life (for example, helping each other to look after the children in case of emergencies or other needs). Children with epilepsy and their families are often isolated by the community because of the belief that the epilepsy is a "spiritual" and "contagious" disorder; the same applies to children affected by autism. Parents' support groups were also important to organize educational opportunities and awareness activities in the community.

Though these new services were just "drops in the ocean," they raised a new awareness and sensitivity toward children affected by neurological disorders among medical personnel, health authorities and some sectors of the society. More importantly, no "drop" is ever too small if it is able to make a single child's heart happy and loved.

Acknowledgements

The author would like to thank: Fr/Dr Rengo Pegoraro, Director of the "Lanza Foundation," Padua, Italy for the support received in writing this short essay; Dr Chipepo Kankasa and the Developmental Intervention Clinic's Staff, Paediatric Center of Excellence, UTHs, Zambia; children and families.

REFERENCES

1. Pontifical Biblical Commission. What is man? An itinerary of biblical anthropology. Vatican Publishing House, 2019

2. Ihor Boyko. The sense of life of a human being in a contemporary bioethical debate. Dissertatio at Doctoratum in Theologia Morali consequendum. Pontificia Universitas Lateranensis, Academia Alfonsiana, Institutum Superius Theologiae Moralis, Rome, 2006 K V Singh. Hindu Rites and Rituals: Origins and Meanings. Penguin Books, 2015

3. Jo Wilmshurst. Paediatric Neurology in Africa: Filling the Gap. Dev Med Child Neurol, 2017 Feb; 59(2):113.

4. Organization WFoNaWH. Atlas: country resources for neurologic disorders, 2017

5. Edward Kija. Traditional Healers and the Treatment of Epilepsy: An African Perspective; Epigraph Vol. 17 Issue 1, 2015

6. Andrea Sylvia Winkler et al. Attitudes Towards African Traditional Medicine and Christian Spiritual Healing Regarding Treatment of Epilepsy in a Rural Community of Northern Tanzania Afr J Tradit Complement Altern Med. 2009 Dec 30;7(2):162-70.

7. Better Care Network and United Nations Children's Fund (UNICEF); Making Decisions for the Better Care of Children; 5 Country Case Studies. October 2015

8. World Population Prospects 2019. United Nations Department of Economic and Social Affairs. 2019.

9. Zambia 2010 Census of Population and Housing; Central Statistical Office. December 2012.

Five Notable Ethics Issues Relevant to Child Neurologists During the COVID-19 Pandemic

A Message from the CNS Ethics Committee

William D. Graf, MD
Chair, CNS Ethics Committee
Connecticut Children's and the University of Connecticut
Farmington, CT

Leon G. Epstein, MD
Member and Past-Chair, CNS Ethics Committee
Northwestern University Feinberg School of Medicine/Ann &
Robert H. Lurie Children's Hospital of Chicago
Chicago, IL

Phillip L. Pearl, MD
President, CNS
Boston Children's Hospital and Harvard Medical School
Boston, MA

During times of societal upheaval, such as in war or pandemics, physicians take on leadership roles in their communities. Physician leadership is guided by the ethical values of the profession, the principles of medical practice, and a Code of Professional Conduct. This "Code" serves as a guide for professional ethics and physician behavior. Medical ethics traditions began in the era of Hippocrates, but a Code was first written in 1803 by the English physician-philosopher, Thomas Percival, and first adopted around the mid-19th century. This Code helped formalize the standards of conduct for physicians in relation to their patients, their fellow physicians, and the profession at large. The Code has evolved over time to align with the contemporary demands of medical practice. This Code distinguishes the words "must" (indicating a need for ethically obligatory actions), from the word "should" (indicating ethically permissible or strongly recommended actions). Professional actions are subject to exceptions under some special circumstances based on personal ethical judgment and discretion, but most actions are guided by a commitment to serve the best interests of patients in need. As during past pandemics, clinicians, nurses, and other healthcare workers belong to a group of essential personnel, called upon to lead a unified effort to prevent and treat clusters of infectious disease. In the current pandemic epidemiologists, infectious disease experts, and public officials indicate that we must prevent further outbreak of disease—in the short term through "social distancing" in an effort to decrease dissemination of the SARS-CoV-2 virus, diminish coronavirus disease (COVID-19), and avoid overwhelming hospitals.

Ethics Issue #1: Nonmaleficence and telemedicine. In contrast to past pandemics, modern communication technology, using HIPAA-compliant video-conferencing tools (or "telemedicine"), can help facilitate the social distancing of stable outpatients by caring for them remotely. In the prior SARS epidemic, up to 40% of infections were nosocomial and this pattern is repeating itself in the current SARS-CoV-2 pandemic. Based on the ethics principle of nonmaleficence, clinicians, nurses and other health professionals have a moral responsibility to inform patients about the risks of nosocomial infection and the need to prevent it. Strategic use of telemedicine during a pandemic is an ethical action, which should be valued and reimbursed by the health care system. Child neurologists should utilize telemedicine in clinical practices whenever possible during an epidemic or pandemic.

Ethics Issue #2: Protecting health care personnel. Physicians and other health care providers have an obligation to provide urgent medical care during disasters—an obligation even when there is a higher risk to the clinician's own safety, health or life. However, health care providers need to balance their obligations to patients, to themselves (and their families), and to future health care. Physicians and others in the health care workforce are limited resources in society. The risks of providing care to individual patients today should be evaluated against the ability to provide care for the next generation of patients. Whether clinicians can ethically refuse to provide care if personal protective equipment (PPE) is not available depends on several factors, including the anticipated level of risk. Some circumstances, unique to individual clinicians, may justify such a refusal (e.g. when clinicians have underlying health conditions that put them at much higher risk for a poor outcome if they were to become infected).

Ethics Issue #3: Veracity, fidelity, and autonomy. Veracity is the principle of telling the truth and is related to the principle of autonomy. Veracity is the basis of trust in the "doctor-patient" relationship (or in pediatrics, the "doctor child-parent/caregiver" triad relationship). Veracity enables meaningful treatment goals and expectations. Clinicians must be truthful about a diagnosis, the benefits and disadvantages of various treatment options, and their costs. Truthfulness allows patients to use their autonomy (or parents/caregivers to use their parental authority) to make decisions in their own (or their child's) best interest. The obligation of veracity, based on respect for patients and autonomy, is acknowledged in the Code. Clinicians should strive to prevent the distribution of misinformation or ineffective therapies during the COVID-19 pandemic.

Ethics issue #4: Allocating limited health care resources. Clinicians should be aware of society's limited health care resources and not squander those resources by providing nonessential or unnecessary care—especially during a viral pandemic. Criteria for allocating limited resources among patients in various contexts, including urgent triage situations (e.g. limited ventilators during a pandemic) may depend on the urgency of medical need; the likelihood and anticipated duration of benefit; and the likely outcome or change in quality of life. Health care professionals and institutions should:

1. give priority to patients for whom treatment will avoid premature death or extremely poor outcomes;

2. use objective, flexible, and transparent protocols to determine which patients will receive recourse when differences among patients are uncertain; and

3. require that allocation policies be explained when patient care is compromised due to limited resources. Guidance from the Code may help resolve the following ethical issues, which are emerging during the COVID-19 pandemic:

• Allocating personal protective equipment (PPE) among health care personnel

• Responsibilities of leaders of health care teams in the context of pandemic disease and the dilemma of needing to protect certain vulnerable physicians and other health care workers

• Considerations of stewardship in balancing the needs of individual patients and those of the community at large

Ethics Issue #5: Duties to community and society. During a viral pandemic, the idea of a health care "team" may encompass more than the traditional care teams of a health care organization. The professional community at large may need to function collectively as a "team" in providing care to the social and geographic communities in which they practice. Considering the financial barriers to health care access, physicians should promote access to health care for all individual patients, regardless of a patient's economic means. In view of this obligation, physicians (individually and collectively through their professional organizations, such as the CNS), should participate in the political process as advocates for patients (or support those who do) to diminish financial obstacles to necessary health care. All stakeholders in health care, including physicians, health facilities, health insurers, professional medical societies, and public policymakers must work together to ensure access to necessary health care for all people.

REFERENCES

1. American Academy of Neurology. The American Academy of Neurology code of professional conduct. Neurology. 1993;43:1257e1260.

2. Jonsen AR. A Short History of Medical Ethics. New York: Oxford University Press; 2000.

3. American Medical Association. AMA Code of medical ethics. Available at: https://www.ama-assn.org/topics/ama-code-medical-ethics. Accessed April 4, 2020.

4. Seto WH, Tsang D, Yung RW, et al. Effectiveness of precautions against droplets and contact in prevention of nosocomial transmission of severe acute respiratory syndrome (SARS). Lancet. 2003;361:1519e1520.

5. Berlinger N, Wynia M, Powell T, et al. Ethical Framework for health care Institutions Responding to Novel coronavirus SARS-CoV-2 (COVID-19). In: Guidelines for Institu-

tional Ethics Services Responding to COVID-19. Managing Uncertainty, Safeguarding Communities, Guiding Practice. The Hastings Center; 2020. Available at: https://www.the-hastingscenter.org/wp-content/uploads/ HastingsCenterCovidFramework2020.pdf.

6. White DB, Katz MH, Luce JM, Lo B. Who should receive life support during a public health emergency? Using ethical principles to improve allocation decisions. Ann Intern Med. 2009;150:132e138.

7. Wilkinson D. ICU triage in an impending crisis: uncertainty, pre-emption and preparation. J Med Ethics. 2020.

8. White DB, Lo B. A framework for rationing ventilators and critical care beds during the COVID-19 pandemic. JAMA. 2020.

9. Schiariti V. The human rights of children with disabilities during health emergencies: the challenge of COVID-19. Dev Med Child Neurol. 2020.

10. Vergano M, Bertolini G, Giannini A, et al. Clinical ethics recommendations for the allocation of intensive care treatments, in exceptional, resource-limited circumstances: SIAARTI. Available at: http://www.siaarti.it/SiteAssets/News/ COVID19%20-%20documenti%20SIAARTI/ SIAARTI%20-%20Covid-19%20-%20Clinical%20Ethics%20Reccomendations.pdf; 2020. Accessed April 4, 2020.

DELIVERING LIFE-ALTERING NEWS TO PARENTS-TO-BE

Margie A. Ream, MD PhD
Assistant Professor of Pediatrics
Division of Neurology
Nationwide Children's Hospital – The Ohio State University
Director of Nationwide Children's Hospital's Child Neurology Residency
Member of the Editorial Board of the Journal of Child Neurology

Pedro Weisleder, MD PhD
Professor of Pediatrics
Division of Neurology
Nationwide Children's Hospital – The Ohio State University
Director of Nationwide Children's Hospital's Center for Pediatric Bioethics
Seminars in Pediatric Neurology's Editor-in-Chief

NOTE

When writing about pre-natal diagnoses, it is hard to know when to call the fetus a baby and when to call the pregnant woman a mother, because in some instances, the pregnancy does not result in a live birth but in some of these same cases, the woman identifies as a mother even before bad news is received. We grappled with this conundrum while writing this chapter. In the 'real world,' one should address the woman by the name she prefers and try to avoid any terms that could contradict how the family actually feels, such as addressing the woman as "mom" or a male partner as "dad."

INTRODUCTION

Delivering bad news is an unavoidable responsibility that comes with the privilege of being a healthcare provider. In the realm of medicine, the term 'bad news' has classically been defined as that information which changes a patient's view of their future in a negative way [1]. Other authors have added that the information is life-altering, may engender a sense of hopelessness, runs the risk of upsetting an established lifestyle, limits a person's choices in life, and is expected to potentially have long-lasting cognitive, behavioral, and emotional consequences [2]. While one could associate the term 'bad news' with conditions that might shorten a person's life such as cancer or stroke, bad news could also include chronic conditions such as diabetes or epilepsy. As such, 'bad news' are not defined by the healthcare provider's beliefs, but by the patient's feelings [2].

A wide variety of clinical situations and physician-patient relationships require the communication of bad news and regardless of these factors, it can be a daunting task [3]. Delivering bad news as part of prenatal care, information that is mostly rooted on radiological studies, presents unique challenges. Herein we discuss an approach to delivering fetal bad news.

CASE EXAMPLE

A 26-year-old mother - G2, P1 - presented alone for a fetal medicine consultation with a neonatologist and a child neurologist to review the results of a fetal MRI. An interpreter assisted over the phone. The woman reported having had a healthy pregnancy until 30 weeks of gestation when an ultrasound identified abnormalities in the fetus' extremities. A fetal MRI, completed the following week, had not yet been discussed with the pregnant woman. In addition to the abnormalities in the fetus' extremities, abnormalities that raised suspicion for a neuromuscular disorder, the MRI revealed an intracranial cyst, polymicrogyria, and pulmonary hypoplasia. Understandably so, the woman was distraught by the news, and despite offerings to repeat the consultation when her husband was present or call him to discuss the results of the MRI, the pregnant woman declined further information and assistance. The woman presented in labor 2 weeks later, at 34 weeks gestation, and underwent an urgent Cesarean section. Shortly after birth, the parents opted to allow for the child's natural death, and the infant passed away within a few hours.

WHY FETAL NEUROLOGIC BAD NEWS IS DIFFERENT FROM OTHER MEDICAL BAD NEWS

Delivering bad news as part of prenatal care, information that is mostly rooted on radiological studies, presents unique challenges. First, an important member of the family, around whom the conversation gravitates, is not present [4]. Second, the pregnant woman suddenly becomes the intermediary between the fetus and the outside world. Third, delivering unexpected news about fetal anomalies often occurs between a family and specialists who have never met and may never meet again. Yet, despite this time-limited relationship, information that will impact the family for life – regardless of the pregnancy's outcome- needs to be conveyed. It is in such a context that clinicians need to deliver the news in a concise, respectful, and compassionate manner, lest the family harbor painful memories not only of the bad news, but of the manner in which is was delivered [4,5].

The impact of fetal bad news on a family is different from other medical bad news. Bad news in pregnancy relates to a future not yet realized and a patient not yet met by the family or medical providers. In contrast, a poor prognosis for an adult condition is more likely to imply the end of a reality or change

to an actualized way of life. A diagnosis of a chronic neurologic condition has many ramifications for a patient and family, including the implications of a "brain problem" on one's
identity. For example, in ancient times epilepsy was considered a spiritual condition, and such stigma is still attached to
the diagnosis [6]. Given that brain conditions can alter one's
essential being, personality and memory in ways that other
conditions do not, they can involve additional dread. Diseases related to the fetal brain can strike an even higher level of
anxiety and fear on the part of the expecting parents because
of additional guilt and hopes related to parenthood. A baby
represents the future and legacy of a family. Parents may or
may not have shared the fact of the pregnancy with family
and friends. As such, the parents-to-be must deal with grief
alone. In other cases, the parents-to-be must manage the expectations and sadness of family members who know about
the pregnancy. Regardless of the actions taken once the feared
diagnosis is made – e.g., continue or terminate the pregnancy
– parents-to-be feel intense grief.

MEDICAL FACTORS TO CONSIDER PRIOR TO DELIVERING FETAL BAD NEWS

Prenatal diagnoses are often suggested based on risk assessment rather than confirmative diagnostic tests. Understanding the specificity and sensitivity of common prenatal
tests is essential. Both biochemical and genetic testing using
cell-free fetal DNA (cffDNA) in maternal circulation provide
a risk assessment that is based on a variety of factors. For example, cffDNA can detect >98% of cases of fetal trisomy 18
and trisomy 21 with a 0.5% false-positive rate. However, the
positive predictive value of cffDNA for trisomy 21 is <50%
for a 20-year-old woman, while it is >95% for a 45-year-old
woman [7]. Definitive diagnosis of genetic disorders in a fetus
still requires fetal cells generally obtained via invasive testing (amniocentesis or chorionic villus sampling). These pro-

cedures carry a non-negligible risk of miscarriage. If invasive testing is offered, the woman should be encouraged to reflect on, and weigh in, the risk of the procedure vs. the probability of obtaining actionable information vs. information that would significantly alter her experience of the remainder of the pregnancy.

Genetic diagnoses during pregnancy should be considered carefully, not only due to the uncertainty of screening tests, but also due to the potential implications for future childbearing, for other children in the family, and for other relatives. Women require pre and post-test genetic counseling. Pregnant women may have anxiety at the time of the decision of whether or not to have testing and may have difficulty understanding the nuanced information surrounding risk. But as a general rule, women do not regret the choice to obtain screening tests [8].

For neurologic disorders, radiological studies are the primary means of evaluating fetuses. Ultrasound has been shown to be 88% sensitive for detecting CNS malformations [9]. Abnormal brain findings on ultrasound are the most common indication for fetal MRI [10]. MRI is superior to ultrasound due to the degree of resolution and structural detail it can provide. Technology that acquires images quickly and corrects for fetal movement results in images with a high level of resolution. However, fetal size and age, and maternal body habitus, can limit the images' quality. Specific abnormalities of the brain are best evaluated by MRI at different stages of fetal development. When reviewing diagnostic results, the limits of the medical information must be discussed [4].

There are times when a primarily neurologic diagnosis involves multiorgan system disease. Those instances may alter the birth plan and impact mother-infant bonding and breast feeding. The discussion of a diagnosis in a pregnancy that will be carried out should also include delivery room care, transfer plans for higher level of neonatal care, and the manner in which the baby's appearance could be affected. Providers should not assume that women want to breast feed, or even hold the child initially but providers should ask a woman's preference in a nonjudgmental manner.

PARENTAL FACTORS TO CONSIDER WHEN PREPARING TO DELIVER BAD NEWS

Parents differ in their expectations for, and connection to the developing fetus and they naturally differ in their comfort and willingness to discuss their emotions. From a mother's perspective, "maternal guilt" is an internal reality supported by external factors. As is evident, the fetus is dependent on the woman for its existence. That existence may be threatened by what are perceived as maternal choices. Media campaigns remind pregnant women to "make healthy choices," "don't smoke," and "don't drink." Taken to an extreme, these messages can be construed to mean that women have the sole responsibility for any unforeseen events that may affect the fetus. And while medical personnel know that in many instances such is not the case, the same cannot be said of the lay public. When hearing bad news, a pregnant woman may analyze her own behaviors, dissecting the recent past for any potential missteps for which she could blame herself [11]. Even medical providers may perpetuate this issue by repeatedly asking about smoking, drinking, medication and other toxic substances to which a fetus or baby may have been exposed, even if the diagnosis is not likely to be related to such factors [11].

While the pregnant woman's perspective has been a topic of discussion for centuries, the expectant father's perspective has received less attention from the literature, society and the medical field. A study in Sweden of the male partners of pregnant woman carrying fetuses with congenital heart disease found these men experienced intense emotion, the desire for joint decision making about the outcome of the pregnancy, and feeling emotionally neglected by medical personnel, all of this in the context of trying to set aside their own needs to support their partners [12]. Another study of men's experiences during fetal ultrasounds in which unexpected abnormalities were detected highlighted a "psychologic need" and ability to understand information provided to the couple. In an article titled "Facts first, then reaction," the authors found that when presented with bad news men tend to take on a role of "fact manager" and use these facts to gain a sense of control as well as to feel informed and better able to participate in subsequent decisions [13].

Parental decision-making related to pregnancy outcomes has many influences – social, psychological, religious, financial, among others. Parents often consider how having a child with life-threatening disabilities would impact the family, as well as considering what is the loving thing to do for the affected fetus [14].

HOW TO HAVE THE CONVERSATION

Prior to the consultation, the providers should ensure they have an accurate understanding of the diagnosis and options for treatment and intervention. Understanding local law can influence the available options. Providers should also understand their own emotions, and what situations they may find personally challenging. Unlike obstetricians and neonatologists, child neurologists can interpret fetal diagnoses in the context of the "life course perspective" [15,16].

When meeting with the family, provide introductions and establish the family's goals for the conversation. Many people are not familiar with the pediatric subspecialties or what a neonatal intensive care unit (NICU) is. When establishing goals, determine what the expectant mother already knows and understands, where she obtained this information, and if she has had personal experience with similar diagnoses. Offer to go through the available imaging – some parents will choose not to see it. Seeing the image of the fetus, in the context of fetal ultrasound has been shown to increase maternal-fetal attachment [17], which, depending on the choices the woman is facing, may or may not be welcomed.

Following a protocol for delivering bad news can help relieve physician anxiety and facilitate communication from the physician's perspective [5], however, we must be cautious as empathy and true communication may not follow a protocol [18,19]. When the patient is not alone, it is recommended that the physician identify the perspectives and concerns of all present [20].

The process of discussing bad news includes gathering information from the patient (what do they understand?), providing information based on what the patient wants, supporting the patient's emotional experience of the bad news and developing a plan to move forward based on the new information [21]. A six-step process (SPIKES) is widely taught and employed by physicians. The six steps include Setting up the interview, assessing the patient's Perception, obtaining an Invitation from the patient to give information, providing Knowledge and information, addressing the patient's Emotions, and summarizing and devising a strategy for next Steps [21].

When obstetricians and prenatal staff were interviewed regarding their experiences with giving bad news, they highlighted the need for professionals to demonstrate "proximity, empathy and assuredness" [22]. When parents were interviewed about their experience receiving bad news during fetal ultrasound, they identified with "vacillating between emotional confusion and sense of reality" [23]. When receiving a fetal diagnosis, shock and guilt are often the first feelings to arise and should be acknowledged by the consultants [4].

WHAT HAPPENS NEXT?

Families have individual approaches to interpreting and acting on bad news. In general, parental decision-making is influenced by hope, their personal morality, and perceived implications on their own and other's quality of life [14]. Overall, parents want to make the best decision possible with the information provided and to "have no regrets" once a course of action is decided [24]. With this goal in mind, Cote-Arsenault and Denney-Koelsch identified developmental tasks associated with a pregnancy that has involved bad news, specifically a lethal diagnosis for the baby. These tasks include understanding the condition, revising the goals of pregnancy, optimizing the time of pregnancy, advocating for the baby with integrity, and preparing for the birth and untimely death [24]. These developmental tasks likely apply to all recipients of fetal bad news albeit with some modifications based on expected outcomes.

Women who continue a pregnancy after an upsetting diagnosis move through emotional stages of shock, existential crisis, and life remodeling [25]. Woman who elect to terminate a pregnancy after the diagnosis of a significant fetal anomaly experience shock, intense physical and emotional pain, feelings of loss and longing for another child, fear about recurrence, and ambivalence [26].

ETHICAL ANALYSIS

If medical ethics should be a component of any patient-clinician interaction, the principles need to be at the forefront of conversations where life-altering news will be delivered. From the principles of veracity and transparency, to beneficence and non-maleficence, only a fully informed family can make decisions in its best interests.

As evident in the case presentation, the child had numerous abnormalities in several organ-systems. A question that comes to mind is: should the consultant share all information in one encounter, or should it be parceled out over several sessions? There is no simple answer because each situation is unique, and each family is unique. A recommended approach is to tell the family "I have several pieces of information to share with you. I can share them all today. Or if you prefer, we can schedule several visits." [4,5]. Following this approach affords the family an opportunity to decide the pace of the conversation, and upholds the family's right to know and the clinician's duty to be truthful.

As multiple authors have stated, a family who receives life-altering news will remember not only the information but the manner in which it was delivered [4,5]. Conveying life-altering news in a caring fashion and providing emotional support is the definition of the ethical principles of beneficence and avoiding harm.

In those instances where the family and the clinician don't share a common language, the information should be delivered through a professional interpreter. Relying on a family member to translate the clinician's words risks not knowing if all the information was communicated, how medical terminology was translated, and if the news was shared with the intended compassion. In addition, having a family member deliver the bad news places that person in the position of being the bearer of bad news. Such situation risks fracturing family relationships, and risks engendering feelings of hurt, anger, and guilt [27].

HOW STRESSFUL IS IT TO DELIVER BAD NEWS?

While receiving bad news can be devastating to the patient, having to do so, especially if frequently, also impacts the provider. Cohen et al., reported that healthcare providers who routinely deliver bad news experience psychological distress, exhibit signs of physiological stress, and endure high rates of compassion fatigue and job burnout [28,29]. These reactions are amplified for providers who are unfamiliar with the patient [30]. They are also heightened when, for one reason or another, the delivery of bad news must be delayed [31].

Weilenmann et al., reported that clinician distress can lead to guilt, anger, cynicism, doubt, hardening, poor performance, loss of objectivity, emotional detachment, and have a negative impact on patient outcomes and satisfaction rates [32]. For all of the aforementioned reasons, researchers have called for formal education on the delivery of distressing news [32]. The education needs to go beyond learning a script. It must also be focused on increasing clinicians' recognition of, reflection on, and management of emotion [33]. The use of one of such frameworks – SPIKES – has been shown to boost clinicians' confidence in their ability to deliver bad news, and has a positive effect on clinicians' well-being [5].

The conversation between specialists and expectant parents can relieve anxiety for both, "when they realize that an image or test result does not summarize the condition, existence or future of a human being" [4].

RECOMMENDATIONS GOING FORWARD

Parents of children who received life-limiting diagnoses during pregnancy believe that their "children are not a diagnosis" [34]. In the business of everyday practice and medical decisions supported by technology, the physician must remember that while delivering bad news may be a common part of medical practice, it is not a common part of the patient's experience. Accumulating the experience and knowledge for honest counseling, following a communication protocol while maintaining empathy and self-awareness, are essential components of the most humanistic of experiences that can paradoxically meet with a fetal diagnosis – the development of new life and the recognition of its limitation.

REFERENCES

1. Buckman R. Breaking bad news: why is it still so difficult? Br Med J (Clin Res Ed). 1984;288(6430):1597-1599.

2. Berkey FJ, Wiedemer JP, Vithalani ND. Delivering Bad or Life-Altering News. Am Fam Physician. 2018;98(2):99-104.

3. Monden KR, Gentry L, Cox TR. Delivering bad news to patients. Proc (Bayl Univ Med Cent). 2016;29(1):101-102.

4. Guerra FA, Mirlesse V, Baiao AE. Breaking bad news during prenatal care: a challenge to be tackled. Cien Saude Colet. 2011;16(5):2361-2367.

5. Johnson J, Panagioti M. Interventions to Improve the Breaking of Bad or Difficult News by Physicians, Medical Students, and Interns/Residents: A Systematic Review and Meta-Analysis. Acad Med. 2018;93(9):1400-1412.

6. Magiorkinis E, Sidiropoulou K, Diamantis A. Hallmarks in the history of epilepsy: epilepsy in antiquity. Epilepsy Behav. 2010;17(1):103-108.

7. Jelin AC, Sagaser KG, Wilkins-Haug L. Prenatal Genetic Testing Options. Pediatr Clin North Am. 2019;66(2):281-293.

8. Biesecker BB. The Psychological Well-being of Pregnant Women Undergoing Prenatal Testing and Screening: A Narrative Literature Review. Hastings Cent Rep. 2019;49 Suppl 1:S53-S60.

9. Grandjean H, Larroque D, Levi S. The performance of routine ultrasonographic screening of pregnancies in the Eurofetus Study. Am J Obstet Gynecol. 1999;181(2):446-454.

10. Peruzzi P, Corbitt RJ, Raffel C. Magnetic resonance imaging versus ultrasonography for the in utero evaluation of central nervous system anomalies. J Neurosurg Pediatr. 2010;6(4):340-345.

11. Landsman G. Reconstructing Motherhood and Disability in the Age of "Perfect" Babies. Routledge; 2008.

12. Carlsson T, Mattsson E. Emotional and cognitive experiences during the time of diagnosis and decision-making following a prenatal diagnosis: a qualitative study of males presented with congenital heart defect in the fetus carried by their pregnant partner. BMC Pregnancy Childbirth. 2018;18(1):26.

13. Ahman A, Lindgren P, Sarkadi A. Facts first, then reaction--expectant fathers' experiences of an ultrasound screening identifying soft markers. Midwifery. 2012;28(5):e667-675.

14. Blakeley C, Smith DM, Johnstone ED, Wittkowski A. Parental decision-making following a prenatal diagnosis that is lethal, life-limiting, or has long term implications for the future child and family: a meta-synthesis of qualitative literature. BMC Med Ethics. 2019;20(1):56.

15. Scher MS. Fetal neurology: Principles and practice with a life-course perspective. Handb Clin Neurol. 2019;162:1-29.

16. Scher MS. Fetal neurologic consultations. Pediatr Neurol. 2003;29(3):193-202.

17. Lerum CW, LoBiondo-Wood G. The relationship of maternal age, quickening, and physical symptoms of pregnancy to the development of maternal-fetal attachment. Birth. 1989;16(1):13-17.

18. Gardner C. Medicine's uncanny valley: the problem of standardising empathy. Lancet. 2015;386(9998):1032-1033.

19. Dean A, Willis S. The use of protocol in breaking bad news: evidence and ethos. Int J Palliat Nurs. 2016;22(6):265-271.

20. Lang F, Marvel K, Sanders D, et al. Interviewing when family members are present. Am Fam Physician. 2002;65(7):1351-1354.

21. Baile WF, Buckman R, Lenzi R, Glober G, Beale EA, Kudelka AP. SPIKES-A six-step protocol for delivering bad news: application to the patient with cancer. Oncologist. 2000;5(4):302-311.

22. Atienza-Carrasco J, Linares-Abad M, Padilla-Ruiz M, Morales-Gil IM. Breaking bad news to antenatal patients with strategies to lessen the pain: a qualitative study. Reprod Health. 2018;15(1):11.

23. Larsson AK, Svalenius EC, Lundqvist A, Dykes AK. Parents' experiences of an abnormal ultrasound examination - vacillating between emotional confusion and sense of reality. Reprod Health. 2010;7:10.

24. Cote-Arsenault D, Denney-Koelsch E. "Have no regrets:" Parents' experiences and developmental tasks in pregnancy with a lethal fetal diagnosis. Soc Sci Med. 2016;154:100-109.

25. Carlsson T, Starke V, Mattsson E. The emotional process from diagnosis to birth following a prenatal diagnosis of fetal anomaly: A qualitative study of messages in online discussion boards. Midwifery. 2017;48:53-59.

26. Carlsson T, Bergman G, Karlsson AM, Wadensten B, Mattsson E. Experiences of termination of pregnancy for a fetal anomaly: A qualitative study of virtual community messages. Midwifery. 2016;41:54-60.

27. Greiner AL, Conklin J. Breaking bad news to a pregnant woman with a fetal abnormality on ultrasound. Obstet Gynecol Surv. 2015;70(1):39-44.

28. Cohen L, Baile WF, Henninger E, et al. Physiological and psychological effects of delivering medical news using

a simulated physician-patient scenario. J Behav Med. 2003;26(5):459-471.

29. Sobczak K, Leoniuk K, Janaszczyk A. Delivering bad news: patient's perspective and opinions. Patient Prefer Adherence. 2018;12:2397-2404.

30. Hulsman RL, Pranger S, Koot S, Fabriek M, Karemaker JM, Smets EM. How stressful is doctor-patient communication? Physiological and psychological stress of medical students in simulated history taking and bad-news consultations. Int J Psychophysiol. 2010;77(1):26-34.

31. Shaw J, Brown R, Dunn S. The impact of delivery style on doctors' experience of stress during simulated bad news consultations. Patient Educ Couns. 2015;98(10):1255-1259.

32. Weilenmann S, Schnyder U, Parkinson B, Corda C, von Kanel R, Pfaltz MC. Emotion Transfer, Emotion Regulation, and Empathy-Related Processes in Physician-Patient Interactions and Their Association With Physician Well-Being: A Theoretical Model. Front Psychiatry. 2018;9:389.

33. Martin EB, Jr., Mazzola NM, Brandano J, Luff D, Zurakowski D, Meyer EC. Clinicians' recognition and management of emotions during difficult healthcare conversations. Patient Educ Couns. 2015;98(10):1248-1254.

34. Guon J, Wilfond BS, Farlow B, Brazg T, Janvier A. Our children are not a diagnosis: the experience of parents who continue their pregnancy after a prenatal diagnosis of trisomy 13 or 18. Am J Med Genet A. 2014;164A(2):308-318.

BREAKING BAD NEWS IN THE PEDIATRIC POPULATION

Zakir I. Shaikh, MBBS
Resident Physician
Department of Neurology
UMass Medical School
Worcester, MA

The word "Bad News" in itself generates a lot of negative emotions and perception amongst patients and their family, let alone the anxiety and discomfort faced by the physician while delivering this news. This essentially becomes more complicated while dealing with pediatric patients and their family. Numerous studies have demonstrated the magnitude of discomfort and stress physicians experienced while having this conversation. It is impossible to define exactly what "Bad News" actually means; it is highly subjective and sometimes news that is considered trivial by physicians can, in fact, be life-altering for some. Hence, extreme caution should be taken while delivering any kind of news. Special consideration, however, should be given to some "Bad News" that can significantly alter their life.

In this section we will discuss various problems encountered by pediatricians and various approaches to mitigate this problem.

PHYSICIAN PERSPECTIVE:

Even after years of medical training, physicians often find themselves stressed and fearful while delivering life-altering news. This stress exists beyond the actual conversation and there are fears of a "self-fulfilling prophecy," where there is a perception amongst physicians that early disclosure of a terminal illness may invoke a feeling of hopelessness amongst patients, lead to termination of all sort of treatment, opting for hospice/comfort care and may eventually lead to shorter survival. This is further complicated by fears of future litigation, cessation of care or change in provider.

PATIENT PERSPECTIVE:

In the last few decades with the advent of patient-centered care, more emphasis is given to providing all health-related information and having shared decision making, compared to the previous Paternalistic Patient Care model. Yet, there exist significant gaps in patient care and involvement in decision making. This has led to growing disappointment within patients and their families, further straining the patient-physician relationship. Sobszak et al., in his study showed that an underwhelming 47% of patients/families felt that information was given in a proper way. The following attributes were viewed negatively and lead to further strain in the patient-physician relationship: physician's behavior during the interaction, lack of physician's time and attention, lack of empathy and emotional support and withholding information/ providing wrong information.

BARRIERS TO BREAKING BAD NEWS

There are numerous barriers while delivering bad news, which can be broken down into physician-related factors, patient/family-related factors and facility-related factors.

PHYSICIAN-RELATED FACTORS:

Numerous studies have found that trainee residents/physicians most often identify a lack of formal training as one of the most important barriers in effective communication with patients and their families. Medical training often gets extremely gruesome and busy that minimal attention is given to training physicians in developing adequate communication skills. It is often assumed that physicians may develop communication skills with experience; however, this is not always true. This is also complicated by language barriers when both the physician and patient/family don't speak the same first language or share the same culture. In fact, discussions with the family are often so stressful that physicians often avoid having these talks. It is well-known that physicians are often overworked with significant time limitations, juggling between patient care and with increased documentation related workload, and that interactions with families often takes a backseat and becomes one of the least prioritized tasks for most physicians. All this time constraint leads to short, inappropriate communications and often perceived incompleteness by families. Excessive workload, time constraints caused unduly mental and physical fatigue leading to physician burnout and deprioritizing timely updates. Finally, the physician personality-related barrier significantly contributes to the ineffective delivery of life-altering information.

PATIENT/FAMILY RELATED BARRIER:

Hospitals and health care facilities tend to a wide variety of populations of different colors, religions, cultures, nationalities, and beliefs. To deal with this cultural diversity, physicians are often trained with cultural competence, which often leads to stereotyping beliefs and characteristics attributed to specific cultures, leading to assumptions while communicating and delivering life-altering news. To mitigate this, there is increasing emphasis on cultural humility rather than competence.

WAYS TO DELIVER LIFE-ALTERING NEWS/BAD NEWS:

There are a number of proposed modules developed by various organizations to facilitate the delivery of "bad news."

However, a dedicated tool for the pediatric population hasn't been developed yet. The most widely used tool is the SPIKES module, which has been endorsed by the AAP. We will discuss the SPIKE module in length and briefly look at alternate modules, like ABCDE and PEARLS.

SPIKES

SPIKES is a six-step approach for "breaking bad news," which was first introduced by Baile et al., primarily for cancer patients. It is now a widely used technique by most practitioners. We will discuss the application of this technique in the pediatric population. The mnemonic SPIKES: Setting up, Perception, Invitation, Knowledge, Emotions, Strategy, and Summary provides an easy and sophisticated way of handling this extremely complicated process.

S - setting

Giving life-altering information to the family is extremely private and sensitive. It is important to ensure that it is done under appropriate physical set-up. It is important to pre-plan about the place, time, presence of the right people and minimizing interruption. Adequate mental preparation by rehearsing the choice of words and topics to be discussed eases up the initiation of the interview. Physicians must chart review beforehand and make a mental note of the topics that need to be discussed. The physical setting is equally important. It is never appropriate to give any news in the hallways or other inappropriate places where discussions can be uncomfortable and can also lead to a potential threat to patient privacy. Physicians should make themselves available for adequate time and make sure that the family meeting is not cut short prematurely. It is understandable that an emergency may arise and an on-call physician may have to attend these calls; hence, meetings should be held at times when they are fully available. The physician should ensure that his/her phone/pager is silent to minimize interruptions. The next important step is to make sure that the right number of the patient's family members and treatment team is present while delivering this news. Involving the pediatric patient in such discussions should be decided on a case-by-case basis. In a complex scenario where there is a dispute between biological/foster parents vs. legal guardians, care must be taken while disclosing information to appropriate health care agents. In a multidisciplinary team, it should be ensured that respective consultants are present during the discussion. For example, while having a risk vs. benefit discussion about a terminal cancer, an oncologist should be present to ensure that the right information is delivered. It should be ensured that the same information is delivered to the family by different health care physicians involved in the care. Once the physical set-up and number of personnel involved in the meeting are determined, physicians should make sure to have a proper introduction of all the people involved and should try to build a rapport with the family before initiating a discussion.

P - perception

The next step is to get a sense of the patient/family's education and perception regarding the patient's ailment and its seriousness. Always begin with an open-ended question; for example, ask, "What exactly do you think is going on with you?" or "What and how much do you know about your illness?" Physicians must allow the patient/family to complete fully and correct any misinformation or misunderstandings. It is important to assess the level of understanding that the patient/family demonstrate, and the information should be modified to their level of comprehension. Physicians should assess early signs of denial, misunderstandings and unrealistic expectations.

I - invitation

Having assessed the patient's/family's perception, the next step is to determine how much information and in what way, they would like to obtain the information. It is important to respect patient/family's autonomy; however this can become challenging in pediatric patients. It is important to know why a patient or family refused to get more information and they should be counseled on the importance of receiving life-altering details.

K - knowledge

It is now important to provide information so that a well-informed decision is made by a patient/family in terms of their care. Always summarize the events briefly leading up to this point. Information should be relayed in simple language by using non-technical terms and avoiding medical jargon. Emphasis should be put on appreciating the emotional aspect of the situation and avoiding excessive bluntness. Avoid using words such as "bad news," which creates a general sense of negativity. Warning shots should be given in the anticipation of upcoming "bad news," preventing shock at a later time. Give information in pieces and take pauses in between, allowing the patient/family to process fully the information. Make sure that all important news is given without missing any piece. Avoid building up suspense, as that only worsens this already uncomfortable discussion.

E- emotions

It is expected to have an emotional outburst after receiving all the information, and the patient and their family should be given adequate time to recover from this news and to respond. Use humble statements demonstrating to the patient that his/her feelings are important. Addressing the patient with nonverbal communication consists of observing the sadness or tearfulness. When emotions are not clear, ask exploratory questions- help to understand. If physicians do not understand the reason for the emotion, ask again. Give the patient/family a brief period to express their feelings. Physicians can use connecting communication/statements so that patients may come to know you can relate to their emotions and cause of emotions. Use NURSE technique as outlined later to show empathy.

S - strategy and summary

Set to close the interview and prepare a plan for referrals, further diagnostic tests, and treatment options. Confirm with the patient/family whether they want any clarification and if any additional question arises, offer a means of communication. Physicians should avoid negative phrases, which may leave patients abandoned. Offer the agenda of the next meeting to the patient. Use PEARLS tool as outlined later in shared decision making.

PEARLS

PEARLS tool reflects an objective of making clinical decisions, teamwork, communication skills, interprofessional alliance. The four distinct phases included in debriefing the process are reactions, descriptions, analysis and summary phases. PEARLS is one of the methods used to answer the patient suffering from an unexpected, shocking, heartbreaking disease outcome with many complex questions.

P-Partnership

"Let's deal with this together" like statements can be used, which emphasizes that physicians and patients/families are tackling together to resolve his/her health problem.

E-Empathy

Physicians putting their feelings into words may show understanding and compassion towards a patient's illness. If the patient is angry or sad, the physician should try to understand the reason behind, be their support and assure them that the problem can be solved.

A-Apology

The family may be angry, upset, frustrated. Let them know that the care provider is also worried.

R-Respect

"I respect your courage and decision, you have been standing hard in this." Such a statement can be used by a physician to show respect for a patient/family's fear and concern.

L-Legitimization

Physicians can justify the response or feelings of patients. Let them know that their behavior is expected and normal.

S-Support

Educate them about the disease and related treatment. Let the patient/family know that their care provider is always in support as much as s/he can.

NURSE technique to express empathy:

Naming may describe the emotions of the patient's family. Emotions may possibly vary with treatment and the patient's condition. Physicians could show that it's absolutely normal having emotional reactions.

Understanding how the treatment will affect the child's life, and family as well, and it was quite difficult for them.

Respecting that it must be a massive amount for them to deal with and physicians should appreciate the way they handled their child and his/her treatment.

Supporting them in all stages of treatment and let them know that the physician and team are always helping hands for the child and their treatment

Exploring the patient's family more about physicians' involvement in treatment side effects and effects of it on children.

ABCDE PROTOCOL:

Advanced preparation	Physicians must review the history of the patient, prepare mentally and emotionally. On the basis of the patient's family desire, support could be arranged. The knowledge of the patient's family about their child's illness is determined.
Build a therapeutic environment/ relationship	Physicians and teams can ensure privacy and adequate time. Provide seating arrangements for everyone. Maintain eye contact. If appropriate, a person delivering news can sit close enough to touch the patient.
Communicate well	Use general language which can be understood by a news receiver. Medical jargon should be avoided. Maintaining silence physicians can move at the child's pace.
Deal with patient and family reactions	As soon as the bad or life-altering news is delivered, emotions may arise. Address such emotions. Can express empathy, listen to the broken emotions actively and respect the feelings.

Encourage and validate emotions	The patient's family may have misinformation. Correct it. Physicians may explore what life-altering or bad news means to the patient's family. Physicians should be cognizant of their emotions and belonging staff.

CONCLUSION:

A combination of the modules mentioned above can be used by clinicians to facilitate smooth delivery of "bad news." However, one must realize that this two-way communication has numerous barriers and factors that can complicate the discussion. In the end, one must keep in mind about the human factor and oneself in the patient's shoes while delivering any life-altering news. Also, early dedicated training would further help bridge gaps and achieve a true patient-centric model of care.

PART 4

GLOBAL HUMANISTIC STORIES IN CHILD NEUROLOGY

FEEL SAFE AND TRUST DOCTORS

Roxana Orbe, MD
Child and Adolescents Psychiatry Resident
Hospital General de Niños Pedro de Elizalde
Buenos Aires, Argentina

During my first year in Child/Adolescents Psychiatry residency, I had the opportunity to work with a fifteen-year-old patient, who had recently been diagnosed with her first psychotic episode. She presented with paranoid delusions, and visual and kinesthetic hallucinations associated with physical assaults by third parties that were non-existent. Like many mental health cases, this was complicated by a devastating family and social reality. Her only adult reference was her mother, who had exerted physical and psychological violence towards her for several years.

At the first meeting in outpatient, she was suspicious and reluctant to bond with me. The dynamics of the encounters were based on her denying to dialogue and refusing to carry out any activity that we proposed. This attitude was maintained throughout what seemed to me as an endless month.

With time and work and after she saw that her problems did not cause me fear or rejection, she dropped her defenses and allowed me to enter the world of her delusions. As the sessions progressed, the patient was able to tell that the violence continued to occur but she didn´t have the confidence to confess it until that day. Although the case was being followed up by local agencies and the corresponding measures were taken, it seemed to me that my work as a doctor was insufficient, since the pharmacological treatment and therapy were not solving the conflictive family background.

In the months that followed, the patient had a relapse and had to be hospitalized again. I clearly remember that her fantasy about hospitalization was based on us being in the hospital together, with us talking until everything improved.

This episode made me wonder about the bond we had made: was it too close, too empathetic; and if so, was that wrong? It felt that in some way the professional line of the doctor-patient relationship had blurred.

After deep thoughts I came to the conclusion that the patient had somehow searched for refuge from her overwhelming world in our relationship. This became a great responsibility, but at the same time I was happy to help her through this moment in her life that caused her so much pain. I contemplated that, if I found myself in the same situation, I would like a doctor to accompany me without reservation, with dedication, empathy, and compassion.

The patient was transferred to a children's home where the follow-up of her case was carried out by the psychiatrist in charge. In our last meeting, she told me that she knew that she could share her thoughts and emotions with other professionals because she learned to feel safe and trust doctors. To me, it taught me that in the face of someone who suffers you can never give too much.

NEVER FORGET THE PARENTS

Shen Yan-Wen, MD PhD
Pediatric Neurologist
Department of Pedeatric
the First Medical Center of PLA General Hospital
Beijing, China

Under the same blue sky, lives different people, they seem coming from the same world but also from a totally different world, they seemed to know each other well and also know nothing about each other. It is very unimaginable for us to map up the world in those severe mental retarded children. How do these kids with deficits in intelligence feel the world? What is the world like in their mind? Can they actually also think but in different ways? If low intelligence and coma meant that they had no idea about happiness and sorrow, if there were conflicts between those who could sense the world and think like a healthy human and those who could not, who could be in the first place we could give up? Is it all right and justice when we make sure all lives live but on the other way make the lives of others worse? And are the choices we made all right even for those who couldn't think for themselves? It has been eight years when I decided to be a pediatrician majored in pediatric neurology and began to deal with neurologic problems in kids, to get to know many of these families with many stories, many questions about what humanism is and how we make it during medical practice still confuse me.

When I was a kid, I was always curious about the world, how I came out and grew up, how different people think, why we could feel happy sometimes, and angry the other time. After growing up, biology became my favorite subject in high school and neurology naturally became a subject that attracted me to university. But eight years ago, when I decided to choose pediatric neurology as my field, I still surprised many of my friends. The majority of them thought it to be really hard work because the parents of the pediatric neurologic diseases were the hardest to deal with just like the diseases. In this most famous pediatric center in the northeast part of China, there were many different wards in the pediatric department, neonatal wards, respiratory and endocrine wards, gastroenterology ward, hematology ward, pediatric urology ward, general pediatric surgery ward, pediatric orthopedics ward, pediatric neurology ward and so on. And the pediatric teaching was among the best around China. Despite the different voices from my friends, I still insisted on the decision. To me, it was full of challenges. It was a place you could meet a lot of strange undiagnosed diseases and a lot of syndromes and I imagined it to be a rather interesting ward with a lot of smart doctors also. And seeking for this self-fulfillment to settle a very complex problem can appear unconsciously and are common among neurologists. The first few months' studies of internship did look up really happy and exciting, it was the first time I got to know different facial palsy, many kinds of pediatric epilepsy and different neurologic syndromes. Soon I got to know why my senior friends suggested me not try this field.

In my first year of internship, I had met the father shouting at me because his 2-year-

old son who had a febrile seizure a day before got fever again. Despite my patient explaining the disease, he was just hard to calm down until the body temperature of the son become normal. I had met the mother holding her son who got epilepsy and rushed into the office at night to beg me for an EEG examination and I refused because of no reservation. And the mother insulted me as a bad doctor. The parents of refractory epilepsy kids hold the kids in their arms and sat in the doctors' office threat us that if the seizures of the kids could not be stopped they could have killed the doctors and nurses. Things like these took place now and then. Conflicts seemed more common in this ward compared with other pediatric wards. Most of the parents of the kids in the pediatric neuro-logic ward were more or less irritable or some degree of de-pressed, and to some degree, much hard to handle. What was unlucky for me was that the relationship between doctors and patients was also very bad during my first few years studying and working in pediatric neurology, which made the situation worse.

I did feel regret about my choice many times earlier. You worked very hard and tried your best to diagnose and treat these kids but parents seemed never really satisfied or about the cost or about the prognosis or both or more. And many times you just tried your best but still couldn't find out the etiology or you found it out finally but had to tell parents that there was nothing you can do to cure the disease. And sometimes you just don't know how to tell parents. Both of the pressure from parents and your own occupational expectations may disap-point yourself as a young doctor newly in this field. However, things become different as the longer I work in this ward and understand the disease and the dilemma of the parents, and the longer I work the better I understand why some of them become so irrational. What's more, not all parents were like that. And one would learn to be tolerant of these poor people and would know that more understanding to the living peo-ple but not focus on finding out what and how to actually get self-fulfillment. These were very different children and their parents were living a very difficult way compared with fami-lies with other diseases. And I gradually noticed that in many situations mothers are victims that were too much ignored by society and these families are really in great need for care and help. Understanding is more treasure as what a pediatric neu-rologist can do that finding out the criminals of the diseases, which make one look like a very great neurologist.

The diseases one can meet in pediatric neurology are epilepsy, encephalitis, mental retardation, autism, and many genetic disorders, and so on. For the patients with convulsion, it is impossible for you to predict when and where a next seizure attack would take place. For newly diagnosed parents, the fears are deep in the heart and can drive one craze sometimes. The situation becomes worse because of discrimination. Even though things have changed a lot with medical development, the traditional impression of ominous or evil-like feeling for epilepsy, what is also known as "Yang Dianfeng" still exists. People are fearing about these diseases. For mental retardation or congenital neurologic malformation with low intelligence, people look down on these groups. All people like smart kids and beautiful kids, nobody was born to like the kids with abnormal appearance who can't even respond to you and can't look at you or listen to you. And for autism kids' mothers, they are more likely to be blamed for inappropriate guidance or not enough care for the kids. At that time, in a traditional Chinese family, the mother was usually the first one to be blamed. Sexual discrimination never totally disappears even now. As a female, giving birth to healthy kids and raise them to successful adulthood is always regarded as inborn tasks for a mother.

Eight years before, I met a couple in the neurology ward with a boy around 4-5 years old. The boy had refractory seizures with severe mental retardation and could not take care of himself. We had tried some AEDs (antiepileptic drugs) but they were of little help to control the seizures. We tried to assess the disease but it was very hard to find out clues. One day the mother found me and had a talk with me. She told me that because of the disease, the couple gave up jobs and took a turn to take care of the daily life of the kid. The whole big family thought it disgraceful for such a prestigious family with no history of neuro system diseases to give birth to such a freak, the mother was the one to be blamed. The father refused to get a divorce from the mother. The grandpa and grandma were very rich and provided financial support for them but they had to live with the grandparents as an additional condition and kept it a secret that there was such a boy in the family. However, one day the mother occasionally found out that the grandma sometimes hid the AEDs and replace the drugs for the kid, and she had an argument with the grandma but was of no use. After then, the grandma even forced to give the kid treatment of folk prescription. The mother thought the irregular treatment was the key problem but she had no right of speech and decision because they could lose the financial support and treatment of the kid needed money. The father had already decided to work again and the mother still stays at home to make her effort to protect the kid as she could. But the money the father earned was far from enough. She begged me to have a talk with the grandma about the disease and the importance of some examination and how a kid could benefit from appropriate AEDs but kept it a secret that she had found me and pretended that I didn't know all about these. It actually shocked me and the first time I noticed that there were things even more important than providing the right diagnosis. The mother wept as she told me how difficult she was and how she hoped that I could help because I am the doctor of her only boy. I couldn't imagine how difficult for a woman to live in a family that gave birth to severe neurologic disabled children. And she was not the only mother that suffered a lot. I had met many divorced mothers taking care of their sick children and some of them were unable to get financial support from the children's fathers. Two years ago, a boy with Dravet syndrome (a severe epileptic encephalopathy) was admitted because of an encephalopathy attack triggered by acute severe infection and septic shock state. The kid had no insurance and the treatment cost a lot.

Government support was far from enough. The father divorced the mother and remarried a young wife and had a healthy daughter. During the 3-4 weeks in hospital, the father just showed up one time and did not pay for the fees. He was ashamed of his son and not even wanted to talk with the doctors. In many families, mothers seem to suffer more. When genetic studies become cheaper and more popular, sometimes the genetic examination, which supports a bad gene inherited from the father, may help ease the burden of mothers.

Besides the possible sexual discrimination, most of the neurologic diseases kids and their families also suffer from discrimination from the communities and society. It is known that epilepsy and some other neurologic problems tend to happen in poor families or in developing countries, which make the survival of the families even harder when the society does not provide enough support and working opportunities, which may also facilitate the parents to take care of the kids. And there are really very few non-profit organizations that may help take care of those severe mental deficits occasionally for the parents. I traveled to Japan to visit Shizuoka Institute of Epilepsy and Neurological Disorders, which was famous for comprehensive care for epilepsy. However, the special school next to the epilepsy center would not accept those with severe mental retardation that had to take care of all the time too.

Other aspects of the discrimination sometimes show itself as sympathy but end up in fewer chances to these groups when come to taking action. The majority of us are actually rather realistic and good at risk control since it is a human instinct to avoid disadvantages. Most of the children with neurologic problems are actually less likely to be accepted by some good school.

People may feel regret and pity for these kids with epilepsy or autism especially those with intelligent deficiency but many of them do not really accept that their kids play together with those patients. The reason maybe they are afraid the kids might get frightened if the partner had a seizure attack before other kids or their kids may be hurt by unexpected incidences. And most parents' hope by finding a better partner it may help with their kids' growing. From this aspect and also unacceptance of the fact that their own kids are worse than others, some of the parents also refuse to send kids to a special school.

The most difficult part that parents of many kids with neurologic diseases face which I noticed during my eight years of experience working in this field in China is actually lack of support in spirit. As a pediatrician, the hospital I work for also receives many acute leukemia kids, which is also a severe disease. Compared with the parents of severe neurology deficits, leukemia parents tend to receive more donations especially when they show the smiles of the kids. The arousing of the feeling of sympathy and willingness to provide help is comparatively easier for kids with normal appearance and when the disease can be cured. It is another aspect of human instinct.

People need feedback as an encouragement to continue their kindness. And it is actually the same situation for many neurologic deficit parents. I had many talks with many different parents of acute leukemia or other diseases, the most impressive thing was that many of them told me despite how hard life was for them when they come back home and when the kids looked into their eyes when they hear love from their kids though they were so small and weak, they felt full of strength and made up their mind to carry on. But this kind of feedback was in many cases lacked and unable for those severe intelligence deficits. Many of these patients with severe neurologic diseases can't feel the exhausting tiredness of their parents and can't provide feedback. In China, these patients are usually sent to the grandparents and raised by those elderly.

If the grandparents are not in good health or have already passed away, the burden came back to parents. Lacking social support and the contradiction of earning money and taking care of the kids together with discriminations from perhaps communities or inner from families, life becomes extremely difficult for them. You sometimes just can't expect how life the kids may have even though for severe intelligence disorder they may not feel sad and not even know what sad is. A parent told me once that there was once a foreign businessman who wanted to buy his grandson who had refractory epilepsy the corpus callosum dissection surgery. And he refused.

I couldn't help think of organ trading and reminded him that it was forbidden by law that buying a person even though he may not have normal thinking as a completed individual. Some of the parents told me that they hope the kids may die peacefully earlier because life was too hard for these kids also. For chronic progressive diseases like progressive leukopathy and some incurable metabolic diseases, the progress of seeing their own children dying is rather heartbreaking and not so many chances that the parents can tell out how they feel or any chances to take a break from the fear for infection or many other incidences. When I was still an internee, I still remembered that one day my teacher murmur and like talking to herself that she happens to meet a mother of a severe encephalopathy boy she diagnosed and treated before, she asked the situation of the boy and the mother told her that the kid had passed away already. My teacher thought that if taking good care of, the boy might have a chance to survive even longer life. Malnutrition, unproper nursing, anyway, there were many ways the life could leave in peace and not be accused of being murder, right? I couldn't understand why my teacher didn't ask for details of the death of the boy if she was confused with the cause of death. And how could she be so calm? It had been nearly eight years and I have seen too many desperate parents. I am a pediatric neurologist, protecting these kids is the thing I regarded as a job. Even though I have noticed the dilemma of the parents and try to help as my best, besides trying my best to accurately diagnose and proper medical support, give the parents more encouragement and understanding during my work. However, as a doctor what you can do is rather limited. And most of the hardest part of life the parents had to come across by themselves. Sometimes I get confused and can't help doubt that does maintain life outweigh all the other? Does requiring those who can feel can think to give up all for those who had no ability to think to feel really morally correct because life is equal and does it equally for parents to suffer all just because they give birth to these kids? If not, does let life gone really justified itself?

I got a confirmation from a Japanese mother this year on my journey to visit a hospital. The boy got influenza when two years old. Influenza induced a severe infection-related encephalopathy and from then on the boy lost a chance of developing to a person who could be able to survive independently. I met him lying on a chair and couldn't speak and had the chorus and suspected mild seizures. I noticed that there were smiles on the mother's face and while I was talking to the mother the boy sometimes making weird sounds. The mother laughed and explained to me that her son felt nice to know me and helped wept away the saliva on his face. And she told me she felt satisfied with life now with her son still alive although fear could come out sometimes. And the people she met are very nice to her and her son. So you see, happiness exists in one's heart and strengthens from feedbacks from other human beings. By helping the parents to regain the ability to feel happiness is a very important way you help the neurologic disorders. The humanism of the medical field should not be fully focused on patients only but also on the family behind him or her. Less discrimination, more help, most importantly mental support to let them feel about understanding and love and kindness are extremely important.

Love and acceptance of the parents of these kids protect the kids best, but the parents need our support to maintain their love. They are the ones who suffer most because they think normally feel normally even though the kids are the ones who get sick. And they are the ones making up the most important part of those bitter lives but not doctors, nurses, neighbors, or other strangers, or even the government. Caring for parents in many situations equal to caring for these helpless small lives.

IF A PERSON SUFFERS, WE ALL SUFFER TOGETHER

Juan David Naranjo, MD
Pontificia Universidad Católica del Ecuador
Quito, Ecuador

In my last year of medical school, while I was at PICU, in one of the biggest hospitals in Ecuador, I met a 4-year-old girl with refractory status epilepticus. I remembered seeing her convulse episodically for several days. The medical limitations we had coming from a developing country made her management extremely challenging and frustrating.

Seeing her during the episodes with her eyes completely lost was very difficult for me since in my own experience I had lived closely how hard it is to see someone having a seizure. I saw reflected in her eyes my younger sister with Angelman Syndrome and the memories of my childhood, while she was convulsing, were terrifying. On the other hand, I was thrilled by the care that her mother was giving to her. I remember her voice speaking with so much love and asking her to be strong and fight to get better. This touched the deepest part of my being, reflecting my mother's voice and my own as caregivers. Trying as much as possible that my emotions do not affect my work as a doctor, but at the same time, allowing myself to experience my feelings and my humanity to the fullest. This allowed me to discover empathy from a compassionate point of view. I remember that it was that awareness of compassion that gave me the energy necessary to try to give the best medical care possible. I was studying more and more about her pathology, working extra hours and managing the acquisition of medications that my institution didn't have.

I was changed of medical service following my studies schedule so I could not continue being in touch with the patient, but months later in a grand round while presenting about the use of ketogenic diet for seizure management, the patient's case was presented, and I was able to witness the improvement she had to have since the last time I saw her. She was able to walk almost with no difficulties, she looked like a healthy girl and although she was still in the recovery process, she looked strong and happy. Again I experienced compassion but this time from another perspective. As the renowned author Milan Kundera explains, the term "compassion" varies according to the etymological origin; for example, in languages derived from Latin, compassion comes from suffering. But in languages such as German or Polish, it is derived from feeling and this in Kundera's own words: "to have compassion (co-feeling) means not only to be able to live with the other's misfortune but also to feel with him any emotion- joy, anxiety, happiness, pain." This compassion led me to feel the joy of her recovery and the peace on her mother's face. I could understand that empathy can extend the limits of pain and suffering, and put ourselves in our patient´s shoes also means to feel their desire to live, get better, and to be happy. I realize that many times we can be doctors but also patients or caregivers, and that allow ourselves to appreciate empathy from an intimate perspective with our own existence and the connection with others that bond that allows us to experience compassion in all specters of human feelings and emotions. If a person suffers, we all suffer together, but also if one is happy, we can all share his or her own happiness.

THE VILLAGE OF HAPPINESS, ITS SOUL

Joseph R. Deacon III, Ph.D., LP, BCBA-D
Retired, Supervising Psychologist/Director of Research
Pauls Valley State School, Pauls Valley, OK
J. Iverson Riddle Developmental Center, Morganton, NC, US.
Member of American Association on Intellectual and Developmental Disabilities

The story that I have attached was related to me numerous times as a child. It is found in a book entitled, The Village of Happiness. The book was published in 1934. If you are interested and wish to know and read more about this amazing book here is the available link. https://www.disabilitymuseum.org/dhm/lib/detail.html?id=1748&page=all.

The director referred to in the story is Edward R. Johnstone. He was director of the Vineland Training School in Vineland, New Jersey for nearly 50 years. Extensive research and service programs were developed with his guidance and he was twice president of what is currently known as the American Association on Intellectual and Developmental Disabilities. He was best known as Prof. Johnstone to families and staff at the Vineland Training School. I became quite familiar with the depth of his character and faith through many stories provided by both of my parents. During the 1930s, 40s, and early 50s, my father was initially supervisor of the boys' division and eventually Assistant Superintendent at the Vineland Training School. My mother was a research assistant under the supervision of Dr. Edgar Doll at the school during the same time period.

One reason I have always held great interest in this story stems from my feelings that many professionals seem to feel the need to focus heavily upon economic contributions when highlighting what individuals with intellectual disabilities may furnish to society. Interestingly, I have found this much more common among persons employed in the field of intellectual disabilities than among persons employed in the field of those who work with individuals with intellectual disabilities. Some attention to economic contribution is obviously necessary based on our societal interests and concerns. However, I think there have been perhaps excessive efforts to shy away from any discussion of spiritual insights that individuals with intellectual disabilities may provide. I think this story suggests benefits to be gleaned from humbly observing individuals identified as persons with intellectual disabilities and respecting the spiritual insights they have to offer. Perhaps more attention to spiritual benefits would be more productive in gaining respect and dignity for these individuals than emphasizing solely how good they are for the economy.

Another story I would like to present involves one of the many experiences my father had with Prof. Johnstone. It also reflects on the character of the director. Dr. Johnstone was certainly one who would not be included in any segments of the TV show in which owners or bosses of companies go undercover to experience the work setting. A need for such action would most likely have seemed ludicrous to Prof. Johnstone. He made the rounds of the school several times a day, every day of the week, helped with the church service on Sunday mornings, and taste-tested the food in the kitchen of each cottage while sitting down at the table with the children. He would also share time with staff over coffee during their breaks at the employee cafeteria or his office, which always had an open door. The story involving my father relates to the campus softball teams and the simple rule laid down by Prof. Johnstone," Happiness first, all else follows." He meant that before anything could be done to assist with improving an individual's mental or physical challenges, he must be made happy. My father, who was superintendent of a state residential facility and a longtime member of the American Association on Intellectual and Developmental Disabilities, reflected me that at national meetings over the years he heard others criticize what they described as a sugarcoated approach. My father suggested that those who were critical we're actually the naïve ones with respect to the true substance of this rule. He applied its powerful message throughout his career. I have felt that this concept of happiness first and all else follows was actually an early presentation of what applied behavior analysis may today call behavioral momentum. In any case, the following story describes my father's early experience regarding the application of this rule through some guidance from Prof. Johnstone.

Evening entertainment at the Vineland Training School during warm months often involved various resident softball teams challenging each other or an employee softball team. On this one evening, Prof. Johnstone made his usual visit to watch the game while making his evening rounds. My father played on the employee's softball team. The next day Prof. Johnstone stopped to speak with my father while crossing the campus. They discussed the business of the day and before separating Prof. asked about the outcome of the previous evening's softball game. My father reported that there was much excitement. All patrons had a wonderful time cheering as well as sharing refreshments during the game. My father said that Prof. Johnstone was, of course, glad to hear a fun time had been had by all. Before separating to follow their morning schedules Professor Johnstone had a follow-up question with respect to the outcome of the game. My father reflected that it was a rousing game. The evening was extended into extra innings during which the employee team was eventually able to win by one run. Prof. Johnstone kindly looked at my father down and said, "Well, don't let it happen again."

The third story I experienced at a small church in Tuscaloosa, Alabama during graduate school and is a story about the "widow's mite." The church had a building assigned as a shelter for those in need. The minister had recently given attention to the church needing some funds in addition to the member's usual tithing in order to make some repairs to that building. During the sermon a few weeks later the minister had a confession. The minister placed what appeared to be a heavy paper bag on the pulpit and said he would be writing a check to the church equal to the amount of the contribution made by one of the members from the congregation. He was going to keep the contribution the individual had made. The contribution was from a woman who lived near the church but had resided for years at the state school for individuals with intellectual disabilities in Tuscaloosa. She had been saving pennies in a paper bag until she heard the church needed money.

A HOPE CAN RAISE MANY SPIRITS

Dr Javeria Raza Alvi
Fellow Pediatric Neurology
Department of Pediatric Neurology
The Children's Hospital & Institute of Child Health, Lahore, Pakistan

Dr Tipu Sultan
Professor of Pediatric Neurology
Institute of Child Health
Children Hospital, Lahore, Pakistan
National Delegate AOCNA
Secretary General, Pakistan Pediatric Association

When a child is entering their teens, parents have big dreams for them, and certainly the adolescent themselves too. Maybe they want to be astronaut or engineer or just wants to help the dad at his farm; like the twelve years old Meer, student of grade 7 and the only brother of five sisters. Everything was going well until the day when a call came from the school informing his parents that his class performance had been steadily declining and if everything was alright at home. Worried parents asked Meer if there was something bothering him? But it wasn't clear until he started to fall on the ground just like that. The parents took him to a general physician who referred him to the pediatric neurology department for consultation considering it a drop attack. I, after detailed history and examination, explained to the parents that this was a different type of seizure and the disease was progressing for which he required admission and thorough investigation. Neuroimaging, electroencephalography was performed which showed a typical pattern and considering the previous history of measles infection, anti-measles antibodies were checked in cerebrospinal fluid. The mother had the results when I went to see Meer, lying in his bed, dependent on his parents for everything as if he was entering his childhood again not teens, unfamiliar with his surroundings, and a vacant look on his face. I still remember her mother asking me "Positive can still be wrong?" The anti-measles antibodies came out to be positive.

I was quiet for a few minutes, thinking of words and courage to break the news. Subacute sclerosing panencephalitis, a devastating disease, which in this child was progressing and the outcome weren't looking favorable. I could see denial in the parent's eyes as if they were hit by a truck. All possible treatment was started and the parents were explained about the nature of disease, its course, possible options, complications, and the long term outcome. Daily I would go to them and they would ask me "are you sure?" His father came to me and out of helplessness said, "We will take him home only when he gets better." I had no answer to give them at that moment but I gave them time to apprehend the situation themselves. Side by side, our team explained the steps of home care and it built their confidence as well. The day he was being discharged, the mother shook my hand with a smile, gave me lots of prayers, and said we will meet again.

The hope I saw in her eyes was something I have never seen in a case like this. A few days later, they came back. Meer was static regarding his health but I could see how optimistic the parents were. The dreams were still big and hopes were sky-high. I listened to their questions and

concerns patiently for as long as they wanted and answered all their queries. On one side, I thought to myself that all I could do is to listen and give them advice but on the brighter side, I believed that in certain neurological conditions of children, the outcome is guarded, but helping the parents to keep the hope is very important, even for treatment outcomes. Hope keeps them motivated. While leaving the hospital, his father said that he would invite me to his farm where Meer wants to work with him once he is better and ambulatory. And I silently in my heart said Amen.

Unfortunately, subacute sclerosing panencephalitis a progressive neurological disorder with a dreaded outcome. The families of these patients have a lot of physical, psychological, and emotional stresses to endure and a great deal of external support is required to cope up with these stresses. Being a doctor we could lessen the suffering by not only answering their medical concerns but also psychological, emotional, and other sources of distress, including normal reactions to living with a progressive and disabling illness.

"Being human is given, but keeping our humanity is a choice"

Names have been altered to maintain confidentiality.

HUMANISM IN NEUROPEDIATRICS, THE VISION OF A CUBAN SPECIALIST

Nicolas Garofalo Gomez, MD, PhD
Second Degree Specialist in Neurology
Associate Professor
Neuro Pediatrics Service
Instituto de Neurologia y Neurocirugia de Cuba

Humanism in medicine is essential for the best development of health professionals. In our specialty, dedicated to the care and treatment of children and adolescents with neurological diseases, a high dose of humanism is required among its professionals.

Since 2001 until today I have worked as a specialist in Neurology in the Neuropediatrics Service of the Institute of Neurology and Neurosurgery of Cuba. This Service belongs to the third level of medical assistance in my country, and it cares for children and adolescents nationwide. After the completion of my studies in Medicine, I started a Neurology residency at this Institute, and at the end of it, I began my work in this important service.

In my professional training, the medical teachers have had a primordial role, both during the medical career and in residence. To them, always my eternal gratitude and respect. During these 20 years, I have been able to attend multiple and varied cases, all without exception have nurtured my preparation and knowledge, we owe it to them and they mark the path of our work and their sacrifice to provide the best of our preparation.

As an essential part of the professional development process, I have been able to participate in various national and international events and also provide medical attention in different parts of Latin America, and also training in developed countries like Europe and the USA.

In one-way or another, all the experiences I have lived in these 20 years have marked me. Listing them all would make this report very extensive, so for the sake of the synthesis, I will present only two cases, which due to the context in which the office visits developed, I have never been able to forget.

In 2008, as a part of a comprehensive study of people with developmental disabilities, I worked as a neuro pediatrician together with a group of other Cuban specialists. There I provided specialized assistance through consultation of child neurology, which allowed me to offer more comprehensive care to a number of Venezuelan children and teens detected during the study.

The first case was a preschool kid, referred for evaluation by present an overall delay in neurodevelopment and an exaggerated growth of the head circumference. The clinical examination confirmed macrocephaly with craniofacial disproportion, frontal bulge and flattened occiput, venous engorgement, and sunset eye sign. It was not difficult to diagnose that the child had macrocephaly with intracranial hypertension and that a neuroimaging study was necessary to rule out hydrocephalus, with a clinical suspicion of possible stenosis of aqueduct of Silvius. I explained to the child's mother that it was necessary to carry out these tests on the child because, if my diagnostic suspicion is confirmed, he would have to get surgery (ventricle-peritoneal shunt), which would save his life. To my surprise, the mother refused to have the child investigated and treated, she said that if God she wanted her son to be like this, she couldn't do anything. I tried to explain what would happen if she didn't intervene, which could lead to the death of the child, and she kept her position. I have to confess that I'm not part of any religion, but in that instant, it occurred to me to say is that I was there because God had placed me in this place to save the child. Thus, the mother agreed to start the process for the study and treatment of her son, and I was much more relieved, even though for work reasons, I could not continue working on the case.

The other case was a schoolboy with epilepsy and intellectual disability. After finish the questioning and the physical exam, I was able to diagnose that he was having focal impaired awareness seizures and required antiepileptic drugs but he did not take them because he had never attended a neuro pediatrician. I decided to start treatment with carbamazepine. After writing the method and the way the drug is administered, I realized that the mother did not understand my prescription, and I asked her if she how to read, she replied no. It was shocking for me, that has never happened to me in Cuba. I had to draw a circle that simulated the tablet and marks how they had to divide it according to the dose that corresponded to the child. It was in this way that the mother understood how to apply the prescribed treatment.

With the presentation of these two cases, I want to convey the idea of the way in which the patients and relatives we serve can influence our way to address their care. For this, humanism is essential, and trying to put ourselves in the patients' place is also important. It doesn't matter where we were born, where we grew up, and in which schools we trained, if we have that humanist training, we will always be in a better position to provide the best of our knowledge for the greatest benefit of our children and adolescents.

GIFTS

David L. Coulter, MD.
Associate Professor of Neurology at Harvard Medical School
Senior Associate at Boston Children's Hospital
Boston Children's Hospital
Boston, Massachusetts

I have a patient whose parents are very Christian. Both parents are from Africa. Her father was a military professor in the Army and now works for Raytheon. They named their daughter Rhema, which means (in Hebrew) "The spoken language of God." So it was ironic that their daughter became unable to speak. The school thought she was intellectually disabled and autistic. But then her mother provided her with a keyboard. Pretty soon she was able to type out full sentences with no assistance from anyone. She was doing grade-level work in school using her communication system.

I observed this in clinic. I would ask her a question and she would independently type out a full answer with no coaching, facilitating or prompting from anyone. Her mother and I agreed that the language of God is not always spoken or audible but is present if we know how to listen for it. I am sure that all children are "Gifts" when we are prepared to celebrate them for who they are.

SARA'S STORY

Dr J.M.F. Niermeijer MD PhD
Pediatric Neurologist
Department of Neurology
ETZ St Elisabeth Twee Steden Hospital
Tilburg, The Netherlands

Dr. Mariette Debeij,
Pediatric neurologist at Kempenhaeghe
Academic Centre for Epileptology University of Maastricht
Heeze, The Netherlands

Marjon Milatz
Teacher and Ambulatory Educationalist at Educational Center of Expertise De Berkenschutse
Heeze, The Netherlands
A special Ambulatory Educationalist School Guidance service for children with epilepsy

Meet Sara.........

In 2016 Sara was diagnosed with absence epilepsy at the age of 4,5 years. Until then she had been completely healthy and had even never visited a hospital. She visited a regular school and was a cheerful little girl. For Sara and her parents, a journey full of challenges followed. Fortunately, they did not stand alone in this journey.

Their pediatric neurologist, who worked in a regional teaching hospital in Tilburg, the Netherlands, started treatment of epilepsy. Treatment consisted of an explanation about the type of epilepsy and the possibility of a trial with daily anti-epileptic drugs. In addition to this, the impact of the diagnosis was addressed from a humanistic perspective. Being a paroxysmal disorder, that can happen at any moment, it has an impact on many aspects of life. Parents and other caretakers and teachers have full responsibility for the well-being of a child. With this diagnosis this responsibility changes. For the child itself, the reaction of the parents and caretakers decides the amount of impact on daily life. Also, the reaction of the teacher and the peers in the classroom decide how stressful the child experiences the fact that she has epilepsy. All aspects of life can change due to the diagnosis of epilepsy.

In order to assist Sara and her parents in this process, guidance by a team of educational specialists with expertise in epilepsy, outside the hospital was started. This service is obtainable for all school children in the Netherlands: a special ambulatory educationalist school guidance service for children with epilepsy.

For Sara, this additional guidance service was very necessary, as the diagnosis of epilepsy brought a lot of insecurity for her and her parents.

The diagnosis of epilepsy caused a decline in self-confidence for Sara and thereby a decline in her school results. Sara stood at the beginning of her school development, all kinds of activities for reading and mathematics and preparatory writing skills.

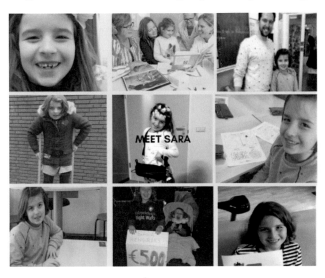

An absence seizure may look small, and not harmful. However, imagine that you have to be constantly busy putting together the pieces of a puzzle, to sort out what the teacher has instructed you to do, or which word your spelling test was about. Imagine that much of the information at school comes in tiny fragments, and not in the fluent way your peers pick up the information.

In some instances, you don't even notice that you have missed some parts of essential information and you do not ask questions. As soon as you realize this is the case, your self-confidence in the functioning of your brain and body and hereby your self-esteem are harmed. You suddenly realize you cannot trust your body or brain anymore, you cannot trust your experiences anymore.

Your balance in life is weakened. You and your parents start to get worried.

There are suddenly certain rules and restrictions that prevent you to freely enjoy outdoor activities such as swimming or climbing, or taking part in gymnastics at school.

These safety rules force you to accept and adapt, in your family, in your social surroundings, while playing with friends and at school.

Pediatric neurologists in the Netherlands can work together with a special team of ambulatory educationalists who are specially trained for the guidance of children with epilepsy at school and have knowledge about epilepsy and the effects it has on the learning process. This group of educationalists reaches out to children with epilepsy and their caretakers at school. Thereby their interventions can make a full circle from hospital to home.

As soon as a child is diagnosed with epilepsy, a referral to the educationalist service is started, so that the socio-emotional pitfalls of the diagnosis of epilepsy can also be addressed as soon as possible, in order to prevent unnecessary delay of making emergency protocols at school, answer questions from teachers, so that there is no unnecessary anxiety in the classroom or insecurity of the teacher who suddenly has a child with epilepsy in the classroom. In this way, stigmatization can be reduced as well. This reduces anxiety in the child and the parents.

In addition, the service consists of the possibility to observe the pupil in the classroom for the presence of absence seizures and how to deal with this. It is complementary to the necessary hospital visits and checkups, and even reduces anxiety about that part of the process.

Sara's story continues...

In the meantime, an ambulatory educationalist was involved in Sara's school. Mainly for observing Sara during class, to advise the teacher and to support in any relevant questions from the school.

The ambulatory educationalist had short conversations with Sara on questions she had: "What is happening in my head? Why is my brain not functioning the way it should, compared to other children? Why do I have to put more effort into everything I do and still not seeing the aimed results?" Sara and the ambulatory educationalist talked about brains, how they can work faster and better, how they can grow by practice and determination.

Sara is not only an epilepsy patient, but she is also a girl with many talents. She is the boss of her own thoughts and can decide on what she thinks and does.

The ambulatory educationalist started the conversation with the teacher and the parents of Sara to discuss and advise on how to make it easier for Sara to follow the class. They also made agreements to enable Sara to experience success in school tasks, to improve her self-esteem and motivation.

Advice on small adjustments for the teacher was for example:

- Reaching out to Sara individually after instructing the class in general, to make sure Sara has understood the instructions and knows what to do

- Dividing tasks into smaller or shorter pieces, to make it less complex

- Sara needed more support in practicing reading skills, she experienced more difficulty in the automation of letters.

Also thinking along with the parents on pro-actively preventing any difficulties during her scholar development.

The ambulatory educationalist continued supporting the parents with their questions. Together with the teacher and internal supervisor they framed the educational needs for Sara. What kinds of skills are needed from the teacher and how can these skills be improved? The teacher was actively thinking along and being very creative in drafting possible solutions and small supportive tools to improve Sara's ability to learn.

IMPACT ON FAMILY AND SOCIAL LIFE, BY SARA'S PARENTS.

As a result of Sara's epilepsy, it felt necessary to quit my job. We didn't have a family to rely on, so we had to manage it ourselves. Besides that, it also influenced Sara's social contacts with friends. It is not visual on the outside if somebody has epilepsy.

Sometimes she felt an outsider when she was not asked to play with other children, or when other children made fun of her because she had more trouble with reading and writing. Also, other parents didn't invite her because they were afraid of a possible seizure. There are even children with epilepsy and emergency medication who are refused at certain schools, unbelievable... When she had active epilepsy, she was not allowed to go outside cycling or to play in the street on her own.

Rosie, her little sister, was not yet born when Sara was diagnosed with epilepsy. She never saw and experienced an actual seizure of Sara but she was aware of the tension and sadness of Sara and her parents. There was a lot of talking about Sara's school and epilepsy.

Rosie had to adjust to the situation and she did wonderfully well. Getting diagnosed with epilepsy is a diagnose for the complete family and everybody has to deal with it. It's in many little things...

At a certain moment, the pediatric neurologist referred Sara to a specialized Academic Centre for Epileptology, since the medication was not sufficient in preventing seizures. There also was an indication for a long video EEG registration to get a good impression of the frequency of absence seizures, and the influence of these seizures on her functioning. The pediatric neurologist of the Academic Centre of Epileptology has reviewed the medical treatment, the development in school and at home. A nurse specialized in epilepsy, visited Sara's home twice to support in some practical tips. How could the parents deal with epilepsy at home? The issues Sara encountered at school, were also experienced at home. How could her parents deal with the exhaustion of Sara after a day at school and how can they deal with the process of putting her to bed in the evening? The Anti-epileptic drugs (AED) caused side effects: She needed more time during the evening to prepare for bed and she had some difficulty getting things done in the right order.

The neuropsychological examination was conducted to show the strengths and weaknesses in cognitive functioning and attention span of Sara. Together with all professionals that were involved, the parents, the teachers, and the educationalist, practical agreements were made, based upon the outcomes of the examinations. This plan aided the improvement of Sara's wellbeing, her educational and social development.

To improve Sara's confidence, she was referred to a medical psychologist at the regional teaching hospital. Together with the psychologist, Sara was able to share her thoughts and questions. Also, Sara's parents could express their feelings and concerns during these conversations. The main goal was to strengthen the wellbeing of Sara and her parents.

Complementary to the psychological support, video interaction guidance was started by the ambulatory educationalist. Short video recordings of Sara were made during class to find out what's going well, what makes Sara happy, and what makes her stronger. Each week Sara chose two videos, which made her proud. The ambulatory educationalist edited these videos into a short movie to show Sara all the things that are going well as a reminder. Sara is very creative and made a token (a kind of necklace), to remember all the good things she achieved so far.

After 30 months, at the age of 7, Sara and her parents received the wonderful news that they could start reducing the dosage of the anti-epileptic medication. However, this also created a certain tension: how would she react to this change? Luckily Sara was reacting very well; she is now seizure-free for more than a year. She is relieved from the impact of epilepsy on her daily life. As a celebration of this milestone, Sara shared treats in her class at school and went on a trip with her family.

Due to her epilepsy, Sara remained an extra year in the same grade. For closure, the ambulatory educationalist visited

Sara's class once more to observe and have a chat with Sara. She is a happy and relaxed girl who is feeling well. Sara is now able to finish her scholarly tasks in time, do some extra work, and knows how to stand firm in life. (Below mentioned quotes from Sara reflect on how she is doing at the present moment.)

All involved practitioners are proud of the treatment process, guidance, and support of Sara and her parents in the past years. While looking at Sara they see a resilient girl who is facing her future with confidence together with her parents and her 4-year-old sister.

By using each other's qualities, knowledge, and strengths the practitioners and Sara's parents were able to create a full circle of support around Sara. They covered all areas of humanity: physical health, personal identity, development, relations, social functioning, psychological health, cognitive functioning, and behavior.

The "epilepsy iceberg" is used as a model to explain which factors play a role in children with epilepsy in daily functioning at school: the iceberg illustrates that there is a lot more going on below the surface.

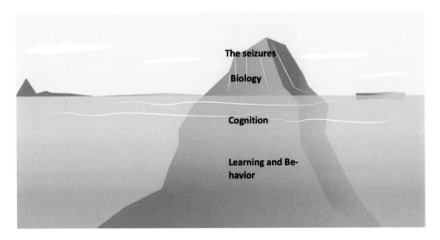

The humanities are about what it is to be human. As health care professionals we constantly have to be triggered to understand what the effects of a disease are on all areas of being human. By making yourself realize the impact of a disease on all areas of life, you realize how much work there is to do with your patient to make life work again.

As Professor Raymond Tallis stated as follows (Philosophy Now, 2009): "there is a distinction between the epileptic fit, and the person who has the fit, and the actions by which he tries to cope with it." It is in this complex constellation that we tried to make all factors work together, to reach synergy at last, in an important period of the development of a young child, the period of learning how to read and write. Also, a period in which children need to experience success in scholarly tasks to build self-esteem that is necessary for future functioning.

If we keep a close eye on the human factor in our day-to-day health care practice, as we have tried to show in this paper, it is possible to empower patients and their caretakers. This results in a very rewarding experience.

Quotes from Sara and her parents....

Parents: "We worried a lot, so it was very helpful to have the guidance of a pediatric neurologist who is providing more than just the medication"

Parents: "All practitioners focused solely on Sara's needs and wellbeing"

Parents: "Sara felt lousy, she just wanted to be just like her friends. She gained a lot in meeting the other children with epilepsy. Having EEG threads on her head during breakfast at the Academical Centre for Epileptology together with the other children makes her feel like she is not alone anymore"

Parents: "We appreciated the complete approach. We didn't have to invent it all by ourselves. The care for children with epilepsy in the Netherlands is well organized which helps in preventing problems. Everybody in this process just cared for Sara and her wellbeing"

Sara: "Mathematics is going much better, as well as language education, orthography, and writing. Reading, I love it, all those books! I also want to write a book again. Yesterday evening I was reading and writing. I was in a wonderful fantasy world. Reading is so nice, once you get better at it"

Sara: "I am so happy to go to school. I am hoping to go to school. Sometimes I wish schooldays would last a little longer. Comprehensive reading is very easy and fun to do. In crafts, I can make very creative objects."

Sara: "Sometimes I rate myself with an 8 or a 9 and sometimes a 6. For instance, when I'm a bit upset while waking up. I try to think of something nice. When I think positively, I start to smile, which is the advice I got from my teacher. I have to say it out loud and it works! I am very happy when I rate myself a 10. You can see it in my eyes. My eyes are very cheerful."

We, as practitioners involved, are very grateful for Sara and her parents for giving their permission for publication of their story.

REBECCA, THE PREMATURE "CONVERSATIONALIST"

Oscar Ignacio Doldán Pérez
Intensive Care Pediatrician
La Costa Medical Center
Asunción Paraguay

There are uncountable cases of premature children that I have assisted in the last four decades while working in pediatrics, but I have to recognize that this story has left a print in my memory because of the surprising reaction that little Rebecca had from her neonatal habitat. A unique experience, worthy of the figure in the annal of neonatal neurodevelopment.

HYPERTENSIVE STORM

The pregnancy of Marta, the young future mother, was 27 weeks old, meaning that she still had a long way to run to reach her happy ending.

It was a cold and stormy day in winter, with a stubborn drizzle, when the unexpected, dreadful eclampsia of pregnancy appeared. This unleashed her blood pressure through the clouds, accompanied by seizures and loss of consciousness. So there was no other option than to take her urgently to the operating room to advance the premature cesarean delivery.

LITTLEST REBECCA

The tiny baby was born on the 8th of June of 2004 at 10:45 AM, with a weight of 1.080 grams, that after the consequent physiological weight loss, added to the few calories that she initially received, became 920 scrawny grams.

While checking on her, I noted the authenticity of her scarce 27 weeks of gestational age, which were calculated obstetrically, meaning that her immaturity was to the point where she was not that far away from the limit compatible with life.

Despite her great prematurity, Rebecca showed great strength, and, for everyone's happiness, she didn't require a ventilator, something that was unusual for babies with extreme prematurity.

ENDURANCE RACE

That's when we started this stoic race, a long and exhausting journey that I had to go through with the afflicted parents, dodging every obstacle that was presented, with an itinerary plagued with physical, emotional, and economic wear. That "Neonatal Crisis Track" would last no less than 72 days, a true marathon where resistance was key, not speed.

There was a tight-knit relationship that doctors and parents shared, which increased a little with the two daily reports and even more when there was a setback, but no one was expecting that the little girl, from her minuscule and not so comfortable radiant heat crib, also participated in the daily conversation.

HEY, REBECCA. CAN YOU HEAR ME?

Days became weeks, and weeks became months. Like the petals that fall from the trees during autumn, the pages from the calendar also fell, putting a light on the "maturational flight" of the little girl.

One day, while I was giving one of the two daily reports with meticulously explained details to the parents, Marta interrupted me abruptly exclaiming:

"Doctor! Rebecca is listening to everything you are saying!"

I smiled, looking at her with a most compassionate look that I could do, and patted her back trying to explain to her that it was not possible.

But the mother insisted vigorously:

-"I'm telling you she recognizes your voice!" Marta repeated stubbornly. To prove her that those were mere hallucinations of an anxious mother, I agreed to discard her -- for me -- fictional illusions: I started to speak for a certain time frame, following this with a long silence, then I started to speak again and then a long pause, I would retake my chat and then sudden silence...

What we found with this simple test was extraordinary and I never saw something that resembled it: every time I spoke, the baby was still, with a frown and a stare, but when I stopped she returned to her normal attitude. With every cycle of this talk-silence experiment, the corporal language repeated time and time again. With palpable proof, I had to admit the prodigy of this event, which I did not find it in any neonatology treatise.

IMMATURE BODY, MATURE BRAIN

Hours and hours of daily talk with the parents had an amazing and almost unbelievable impact on the small and immature brain of the small patient, who, in her characteristic frog position that is typical of extremely premature babies, assimilated everything that was being discussed from inside the incubator and -- in her own way -- talked back me.

HAPPY ENDING

Rebecca spent two months and a half hospitalized in the Neonatal Intensive Care Unit of the now gone Hospital Frances and were discharged with 1.995 grams. At home, she reached two kilos and achieved a convenient growth and development, without any motor or intellectual sequel.

Years later her sister Alethia came, also premature, but with better weight and older gestational age. She was in the Neonatal Intensive Care Unit of the La Costa Medical Center for a short period and soon the Lopez Quintana family was happily reunited.

15-YEAR-OLD FUTURE PEDIATRICIAN

She turned 15 on 8 June of 2019! Her family organized a big party in which there was a lot to celebrate. The parent asked me to record a video message, which was played in the event, where I testified about her neonatal adventure and her posterior growth and development in all these years of pediatric follow-ups. A fair recognition for this beautiful and happy young lady that neurologically came out "whole" of a highly risky extreme prematurity.

In her film tribute the image of the little girl with whom I "had conversations" since her tender neonatal stage swirled in my memory.

Her parent told me that she wants to be a pediatrician... and it's not for less, having into account that since an early age she already participated in medical records.

THE HAPPINESS OF THE SAD CHILD

Dr.Oscar Ignacio Doldán Pérez
Intensive Care Pediatrician
La Costa Medical Center
Asunción Paraguay

This is a story so sad that it destroys the soul.

Diego, almost 4-years-old, was with his parents riding an ox-drawn cart. Suddenly, one of the oxen reared up and the little boy fell to the ground headfirst, leaving him a paraplegic.

He was hospitalized in Medical Emergencies and my wife Malú, in her capacity as neuro-pediatrician of the institution, visited him every day. The boy -- and his parents -- was undergoing though an inconsolable sadness and started having constant fevers of unknown origin that presented daily.

On his birthday, we went with my daughter Anita to choose two gifts for him, one from Malú and the other from Doctor Gómez, the head of the Intensive Care Unit. We brought him a colorful and huge plastic truck and a police van that was a real cliché. The smile in Diego's face was the first since a long time ago.

In all the days that followed, the two vehicles were "parked" to both sides of his head.

After that, the fevers ceased to happen. Mysteries of medicine.

AN UNEXPECTED REQUEST

Ronnie E. Baticulon, MD
Pediatric Neurosurgeon
Division of Neurosurgery, Department of Neurosciences
Philippine General Hospital
Associate Professor of Anatomy
University of the Philippines Manila

On the day I met her for the first time, I had heard her screams before I actually saw her. She kept saying "Noooo! Noooo!" with a shrill voice that reverberated throughout the waiting area, just outside my clinic in Philippine General Hospital, where I see pediatric neurosurgery patients on Saturdays. She contorted her body into grotesque curves and flailed her arms and legs in all directions with as much resistance as a four-year-old could muster, her family overwrought as they attempted to restrain her. There's no need for that, I gestured to them, and I stayed a full meter away from my patient. Her eyes were fierce but they were filled with tears, and only after seeing both my hands held up did she stop, abruptly lying motionless like a rechargeable toy whose batteries had run out. The sobbing, however, persisted. In any other circumstance, she would have been dismissed by passersby as a spoiled brat. I knew that above all, she was just scared to see the doctor. Me. It was clear I would not be able to perform a neurologic examination that morning.

Ofelia had a brain tumor the size of a golf ball in her cerebellum. Two months earlier she almost died when the tumor completely occluded the flow of her cerebrospinal fluid; the resulting acute rise in pressure inside her head caused her to stop breathing for a full minute. If it weren't for emergency surgery to drain the excess brain fluid, her life would have ended that day. Luckily, she regained consciousness, and so after two days, her attending neurosurgeon decided to convert the tube sticking out of her head into a more permanent diversion, a ventriculoperitoneal (VP) shunt. She was discharged fully awake, in time to celebrate her birthday, and not a month later, she was back to singing "Let It Go," channeling Elsa as if all she had was viral tonsillitis.

Except she still needed brain surgery to take her tumor out. The shunt only addressed hydrocephalus, a symptom. The tumor would continue to grow if we did not do anything about it, and though we had a narrow list of possibilities, it would be unwise to do outright chemotherapy or radiation therapy without knowing what kind of tumor it was. Surgery offered Ofelia the greatest possibility of a cure. I explained this to her mother, as her grandmother, uncle, aunt, and every other family member inside the clinic listened, periodically holding their breaths or nodding in unison.

When I asked why the patient wasn't in the room, they told me the girl had developed a phobia of doctors and nurses. Her admission in the previous two hospitals had caused so much emotional trauma, no person in white could come near her, be it for blood extraction or vital signs monitoring. This wasn't unusual, and not a first for me, either. Precisely the reason why I don't wear my white coat in the clinic or when doing rounds. After reviewing her CT scan and MRI films and deciding that it was indeed a tumor that could be resected, I stepped outside the room with her family, and that led to our first encounter, sans the human touch ever important to neurology clinicians. Her mother agreed to have the surgery done as soon as possible. That left me a little over a week to figure out how I would be able to examine my patient.

A considerable part of pediatric neurosurgery happens outside the operating room. After all, how do you tell children that you need to get inside their heads to take out a brain tumor? How do you convince a boy or a girl to lie still for a few minutes, even endure an ounce of sharp pain, so that you could take off a wound dressing and inspect your post-op site? How do you break the news that they would not be allowed to watch cartoons on their iPad, hold their favorite toys, or see their friends for a few days after their operation? How much truth should you tell them, how much truth could they handle, and how much truth would they care about?

The first high five, fist bump, flying kiss, or freely given hug is always a milestone. The skill is in earning children's trust without ever forgetting, or worse, compromising their vulnerability. It is a skill only acquired by reading their books, watching their films and TV shows, speaking their language, and playing their games—essentially reawakening your child self—something I have gotten better with through several years of treating children of all ages, but admittedly, have not yet fully learned. I have yet to have children of my own.

Even till the day I first operated on Ofelia, I could not come near her without eliciting a vile reaction. I had to settle with observing from afar as she interacted with her mother and family, paying close attention to how she grasped her plastic toys or stood up and walked to reach them. In the operating room, the pediatric anesthesiologist had to draw faces on a family of inflated hand gloves. It was Papa Glove, Mama Glove, and their four kids who put her at ease and convinced her to breathe through a transparent mask until she fell asleep from the anesthetic. The ingenuity brought relief to the neurosurgeon, too.

Over several hours, as Ofelia lay face down, unconscious and immobile, I excised her brain tumor. When she woke up in the recovery room, we made sure her mother was at her side. She did not seem to have any new neurologic deficit. If this were a feel-good story, I would have ended the narrative right there at that moment, with hugs, kisses, and maybe even sparkles, but this isn't.

When you've operated on hundreds of your own patients and taken care of thousands of others, you become familiar with the sinking feeling you get upon seeing a sign—no matter how subtle—that heralds a surgical complication. It may be a one-point drop in consciousness level that nobody else noticed, a clumsy hand movement you catch from the periphery of your vision, slight redness on one end of your incision, or any other exam finding prompted by discomfort that your patient casually mentions as you are about to reach for the doorknob to make your exit.

The reaction is instantaneous: your eyes lose fixation, you feel a pounding in your chest, and a bitter taste creeps from the back of your throat, as disbelief, denial, and dread hurtle towards you. Suddenly all you want is for everything around you to stop moving and keep silent, a time-freeze so you could sit down, process all information, and decide, without interruption, how to address the problem and what course of action is best for your patient. The answer to the latter is not always the easiest alternative for the surgeon, especially when you've already given yourself a pat on the back; previously thinking everything had gone well. Sometimes you just need a moment to sigh unnoticed, because in the next one you would have to explain to your patient's family why and what to expect, at which point your gaze must not wander, your voice must not tremble, and your knees must not buckle. You do what you have to do.

Twice this happened to me while taking care of Ofelia, each instance just a few days before I thought she would be going home. Persistent fever that, was the first sign. The sight of cloudy cerebrospinal fluid aspirated from her VP shunt only confirmed what I had feared. She developed a surgical site infection and I needed to remove her VP shunt, otherwise, the intravenous antibiotics we were giving her would be useless. And second, a mild limitation in eye movement and facial weakness I observed three days before she was supposed to complete her antibiotic regimen. I filled out her CT scan request form with a heavy hand; I knew what I would see on her images. The hydrocephalus recurred, and back to the operating room we went, this time to insert an endoscope and create an alternate route for her brain fluid.

"Nagkulang ata ako sa dasal sa batang ito (My prayers for this child must not have been enough)," I told her neurologist in frustration when we saw each other in the nurse's station.

Complications notwithstanding, an unexpected good came out of these agonizing weeks, with long nights spent trying to figure out what more I could do to make her better. After her second surgery, a relatively short procedure, when Ofelia became lucid enough to talk to her mother in the recovery room, she made her first request. It was not to ask for food or water but, "Gusto ko kargahin ako ni Doc. (I want Doc to carry me in his arms.)"

I was next to her, writing my post-op note when she said this. I was surprised. Still, I put my blue pen down and obliged, and when I did, she pleaded, "Balik na tayo sa room. (Please bring me back to my room.)"

"Hala Doc, anong binigay ni'yo sa kanya? (Oh no, Doc, what medication had you given her?)" her mother teased, also perplexed at this spontaneous 180-degree turn in our patient-doctor relationship. She had to snap a photo to capture the moment.

From that day onward, it seemed all four walls of Ofelia's fort had collapsed. Or at least, the gates were opened for me. Whenever I saw her in a bad mood during rounds at the end of the day, I would whisper to her with a cupped right hand, "Sinong nang-away sa iyo? (Who made you feel this way?)"

and she whispered back her descriptions of the nurses who extracted her blood or reinserted her intravenous line. She told me the names of her toys and introduced her Disney princesses. She handed me paper money so I could buy miniature cakes and cans of soda from the play grocery she set up in her room.

Whereas before she had always sulked when I entered, refusing to even acknowledge my presence, now she welcomed me with a constant smile. If I came at the right time, she would set up her plastic dinnerware and we would dine together in her restaurant. It amazed the nurses and other doctors to see me carrying her along the hospital corridors when she hated to be touched by everybody else. I became my patient's ally, confidante, protector, and I daresay her favorite loyal shopper/diner.

In the days leading to her discharge from the hospital, after three surgeries that spanned almost two months, my child patient asked me repeatedly, "Sasama ka ba sa amin pauwi? (Are you coming home with us?)" to which I replied, "Bakit? Gusto mong sumakay sa kotse ko 'no? (Why? Do you wish to ride in my car?)"

Indeed, we had come a long way from the screaming child and the doctor who had to hold up his hands in surrender. I was not completely certain what I did right.

As an outpatient, Ofelia completed a course of radiation therapy to prevent her tumor from coming back. Remarkably, she tolerated the daily procedure without any form of sedation. I praised her for her bravery and asked her to tell me what it was like. She got to celebrate Christmas and New Year's Day with her family, and her three-month brain MRI came back negative for any tumor.

I was wrong to assume that the princess finally got her happy ending. Cancer can be a traitor, and it could not care less how old you are.

As innocuous as symptoms could go, this time it was back pain. Especially when walking. A week at the most, vague is a lousy description, but that was the best one I could elicit as we sat in my clinic.

"Masakit ba ang ulo mo? (Do you have a headache?)"

She shook her head left and right.

I asked her to squeeze my fingers with both hands, try to kick while I push back her legs. There it was. Weakness. Minimal, but undeniable.

Once more, that sinking feeling I knew all too well.

I spoke to Ofelia's neurologist after her visit and relayed my suspicion. A week later, an MRI of her back showed that the entire length of her spinal cord was covered in a tumor, when her previous imaging studies and laboratory workups did not show any evidence of this at all. Her kind of tumor had two variants; the way it was behaving, hers was the more aggressive type. This time, I could not offer any form of surgery to help Ofelia without causing more disability. Why did every conceivable misfortune have to happen to this child?

Ofelia died ten months after I first met her, three months after we diagnosed disseminated disease, and a few weeks short of her and her mother's planned migration to another country. They were merely waiting for Ofelia's visa. As fate would have it, the family had to prepare for a departure markedly different from what they had anticipated.

I was not ready, either. The day after she died, as I was about to start my car to leave the university-hospital complex where I worked, I received messages of gratitude from her family in my Instagram account, and they included, among others, a photo of the time she asked me to carry her in the recovery room. She must have been scared of all the monitor beeps, the hustle and bustle of patients being wheeled in and out, and I was someone familiar. She knew her doctor would not hurt her, and that would go down in memory as one of my proudest moments as a neurosurgeon.

I pulled a toy figure of Batman riding his Batmobile from the central console and rested him on the steering wheel. It was one of those toys you could get with a Jollibee (most popular fast-food chain in the Philippines) kiddie meal, a token from Ofelia that she gave herself in a sealed brown bag. It dawned on me that I would never see her again in the clinic, where each visit commenced with the little girl marching into the room with a giggle, after which she would hand me a sugary treat, usually a piece of chocolate, followed by the persistent question, "Kailan ka na pupunta sa amin? (When are you visiting our house?)" I was told every time she had a follow-up with me, Ofelia would wake up early, excited as if she were visiting Disneyland. Once, her visit was heralded by a phone call, "Papunta na kami diyan, hintayin mo ako! (We're coming today, wait for me!)"

In the driver's seat, delaying my drive home, I grieved for Ofelia. I admitted to myself, I would miss her and her silliness. I wondered, too, why I was deeply affected by this loss. Would it have been preferable to have kept my distance all throughout, if that were even possible? I could only arrive at the conclusion that in my everyday attempt to earn her trust, in caring for her for almost a year, I allowed myself to be vulnerable, too. I suppose you could file this under work hazards when treating children.

Too often you read about patient testimonials stating how this doctor "changed my life forever." The reciprocal is also true. Every patient interaction influences all others that come after, some just more than the others. Batman would never leave my car.

That last time Ofelia and I spoke, she was seated on her hospital bed, having dinner next to her mother. With a nasal cannula to supply oxygen and aid her breathing, she would not look up, seemingly more interested in playing with the morsels of food on her plate than talking to her doctor.

"Puwede ba akong bumili sa tindahan mo? (May I buy from your store?)" I asked, seeing all her plastic toys in the corner.

"Sarado na... (It's already closed.)"

"Ha? Kailan magbubukas ulit? (Is that so? When will it open again?)"

"Bukas. (Tomorrow.)"

Tomorrow, as it turned out, meant never.

HUMANISM AND CHILD NEUROLOGY

"In order to comprehend anything human, be it personal, or collective, it is necessary to tell its history.... Life turns a small degree of transparency in the presence of historical reason"

Ortega y Gasset

Mendoza Cruz Joel Fernando, MD
Pediatrician Neurologist.
Head of the Neurology Service of the Morelia Children's Hospital.
Associate Professor of Neurology
Member of the Bioethics Committee of the Morelia Children's Hospital
Founder of the School for Parents of the Morelia Children's Hospital
Founding Member of the Mexican Society of Pediatric Neurology.
Founding Member of the Michoacan Neuroscience Society.
ICNA member since 1985.

Yes, there is a reason behind our desire to be a doctor, I think that the main one could be the desire to serve, among others, but it is this noble purpose that can be accompanied by new reasons not to lose direction. Finding an honest and noble doctor occurs more easily to find in an honest and nobleman. Many of these values are latent in every human being, but it is necessary to be close to good examples and wise teachers. Nothing seems to mature prematurely and following the opinions of Orson Welles, nor does the mind mature before its time.

When do we start being humans? and when do we stop being it?. Dr. Ignacio Chávez, humanist, doctor, and teacher said that a doctor must be above all a cultured person, because it is there, through the culture that you come to understand a man. In the medical school of the city where I live, Morelia, –one of the most beautiful cities in Mexico--, I found examples of consistent doctors, with ethics and the desire to train other doctors, focused on the patient and not in disease, as William Osler recommended. This training, unfortunately, not lavished in classrooms, is in contact with patients, when they have these opportunities to open ourselves to receiving the intimacy of the sick.

To get to Child Neurology surely there are many ways, I have had to go into it by serendipity, I was looking to be a neurologist and I have presented the option to focus on this branch of pediatrics, incidentally, emerging in Mexico. The academic preparation is long, but if the pleasure of caring for children is the engine, the chore is facilitated. I started the road with a maxim under my arm: -all that it is worth doing, it is worth doing well. The training centers in this specialty, located in large cities and endowed with many resources, dazzle you, attracting you without realizing it, little by little you move away from the patient and focus in diseases, their nuances and the countless studies of all kinds which you can have to check them, in addition to the profusion of articles of disclosure in the specialty, which seems to drown you. It's like a powerful siren's call. I returned to the place where I was trained, and entered a small public children's hospital, with few resources and many patients, that was my commitment. A short time later one of my most dear teachers gave me a very valuable lesson, which has allowed me to develop my work. Dr. Francisco Esquivel asked me, "How are you doing in your Dr. Mendoza hospital?", I made a precise count of all the deficiencies in terms of technology, spaces, and supplies for laboratory and radiological studies, etc., he listened quietly and, in the end, he said to me

"A sick person can lack everything, except his doctor." Those words woke me up and brought me back to the center of my vocation as a doctor, the sick. I was then able to be attentive to the needs, deficiencies, pains, and wishes of children and parents, I returned to the soul of medicine, the doctor-patient relationship and I remembered the words of Luis Portes, the medical consultation is nothing more than confidence in front of conscience, and in the center, like a lighthouse, the clinic. "You can study medicine deeply and become wise, but without the clinic, you cannot become a doctor." So knowing about medicine is not the same as being a doctor, all this said by Esquivel the master.

One day, while my office was getting ready for that day's work, I went out to the waiting room and I sat next to the parents and patients scheduled, it occurred to me then ask them: how was the diagnosis of your children given to you? I was frozen, surprised with the answers received, "The doctor was insensitive," "It caused me a lot of pain," "I was left without hope," "I couldn't understand anything" and thus the worst ways of making a diagnosis started piling up.

I imagined that parents received the diagnoses as if it was a sentence and their children entered the cells, without hope or future. This is how the school for parents, which is now turning 30 years, started. I've spent many hours of consultation caring for parents and treating neurological illnesses in their children. Another maxim: if we can instruct the parents, all the children will improve, that is, information is the best tool to equip parents of the necessary knowledge and achieve a better understanding of the problem, eliminate the guilt. On the other hand, our closeness and willingness to dispel all the doubts will win their confidence and strengthen their spirit in the task of the recovery of their children, because if the pessimism or discouragement invade, the risk of failure increases; -we can be victims of our own predictions-. At least we should give them hope and joy, since everything we do will be made of ourselves, of our faith, enthusiasm, and love for families.

By focusing our attention not so much on the disease but on the child, and insist that we are treating human beings, we can help them understand that dignity is necessary to live and that in principle must arise from the parents because, without that recognition, children are left helpless. We are the ones who provide a good dose of the acceptance and recognition of that value of the child, by treating them with affection and compassion. Irvin Yalom tells us, the relationship is what heals.

We can say that we are born human and we develop within an environment of relationships of human dimensions. Imagine parents facing the loss that represents the son with a disability, no doubt they may soon realize or suspect that something is wrong with the children and the denial will be immediate. To get out of the doubt, I am sure that first of all, they are not looking for a wise doctor, they are looking for the human being which they presuppose will guide them in their search for relief. This is the test we go through every day, although our Mexican health system has changed parents, making them demanding and defensive, our prudence, patience and affection, skills that the doctor must have, will manage to dissipate the resistance. Accompany the parents in the difficult acceptance of their child's problem. Carl Jung wrote: "Know all the theories, master, all the techniques, but as you touch a human soul be just another human soul." I remember that in the modest hospital where I work, serving low-income and needy people, I heard the director saying that the medicine of the poor was the worst medicine, that made me angry and frustrated, finally, during a conference in which he would present a topic later I had the opportunity to tell him: the medicine of the poor in spirit, is undoubtedly the worst kind of medicine.

In our environment, there are factors that lead us to the dehumanization of medical attention. Technocracy, which favors rigid forms and measures medical attention in terms of times and quantity, which seeks effectiveness and efficiency and only that. The Health Industry, which strives to turn patients into clients and doctors in workers and thus distributes poverty both in quality of care and in treatment. On the other hand, irrational worshiped sometimes, privileging the method in which multiple studies are carried out and omits the essential critical assessment regarding its utility in the environment in which medicine is practiced, these studies convert objects into subjects and transmute them into percentages. Not everything in medicine is based on this type of evidence. "Put in a static way what is dynamic, acquires in our imagination, qualities (dimensions), which they really lack." R Tagore in 1940. Finally, everything that keeps the doctor away from reading and continuous contact with all the people in his environment will result in distancing from the most human thing that we have, the relationships, I think on screens of all kinds, which invite us to leisure and loss of the objectivity of everything around us, pushes us not to question anything and to take as real what is virtual, which are not realities.

So we must be vigilant, focused, and doomed to read the history of medicine, medical ethics and to have time to review our behavior, because this is how human height is measured, in our behavior with the weakest.

Here is a brief story of one of the ways of understanding, living, and giving in pediatric neurology. Humanism is the center of medical work, that's how I lived it through contact with my teachers and then in daily contact with parents and children. Every day we must remember that we work with small human beings who require everyone to make them recognize how valuable their lives are. Without humanism, you are only an employee of medicine. It is in poverty where more signs of daily gratitude are given to doctors as a way to repay them, with the consequent joy of the heart of those who know how to receive it.

"Life is given to us, we earn it by giving it." R Tagore.

With gratitude to the International Child Neurology Association for their invitation.

HUMANISM IN CLINICAL PRACTICE – MUSINGS OF A CHILD NEUROLOGIST FROM INDIA

K P Vinayan, MD, DNB, DM
Professor and Head
Department of Pediatric Neurology
Amrita Institute of Medical Sciences
Amrita University
Cochin, Kerala, India
Convenor, Pediatric Neurology sub section, Indian Academy of Neurology
Member, Commission for Diagnostic Methods, International League Against Epilepsy (ILAE)
Member, Asian Epilepsy Academy (ASEPA)
Treasurer, Indian Epilepsy Society

How do human relations work out? Communication skills of the concerned individuals shared cultural values, as well as religious beliefs, might be the major contributing factors. Improving these innate personal attributes along with consciously trying to reach out for the identification of common grounds will help in fostering fruitful relationships. However, the success of some interactions might also be based on a gestalt feeling of wellbeing on both ends. Even then, we might be able to pick up some common factors retrospectively on a purely reductionist paradigm. According to some schools in ancient Indian philosophy, this type of justification by conscious explicit reasoning merely follows the subconscious intuitive actions and not vice versa.

In clinical practice also, the same principles hold true. After all, if you take out the medical jargon and technicalities, the interaction between the patient and physician is a very special form of human relationship based on mutual consent. Like in any other intimate relationship, unrealistic expectations, let down feelings, reversible and irreversible breach of trust, and many other complex emotions might spoil the show of this bonding. Over time, repeated close and intense patient-doctor interactions have the potential to mutually influence their individual beliefs and value systems. Every physician, worth his name will have several patient-related stories that had impacted his approach to life and profession. On the other hand, all of us have heard much patient folklore about physicians, their clinical skills, and empathetic interactions.

In the practice of pediatric specialties, the parents and immediate caregivers take the surrogate role on behalf of the affected child. They feel for the child and most often act in the best interests of the child. In countries like India, extended families also might play a major role in the decision-making and care of children. In such a scenario, the physician may have to accommodate many more people, their expectations, and value systems during the clinical interactions. Challenge is even more in the practice of child neurology, where chronic functional impairments are the norm, needing long-term support and care. An end of life paradigm, which is in vogue in the formal palliative medicine, may not completely work out in child neurology. Without any proper training in fostering humanistic skills, most of the child neurologists end up using their intuitive brain networks, while engaging with the affected families.

Do we have a magic lamp that will help the physician deliver humanistic care in child neurology? I feel it is definitely paternalistic to view the family and the caregivers as the vulnerable side in child neurology practice. Developing one-sided management plans for the child without paying attention to the emotional status, value systems, and expectations of the caregivers is not humanistic at all. Even though difficult, we can try to literally step into their shoes and empathize with them. In child neurology, we see many children with chronic functional and neurological impairments, which might make their parents inherently jittery and unstable. It becomes exceedingly difficult to agree upon shared and realistic clinical goals in such a setting. There is even a chance that the family might openly accuse the medical system and the physician for the perceived improper care and lack of improvement in clinical status. Definitely, this might have the potential to adversely affect the morale of the medical team with long term implications for the care of similarly affected children.

I work as an academic child neurologist in charge of a busy clinical division in a university hospital in India. Our patient care services are really overcrowded with very minimal supporting staff. As a result, quality time for ensuring proper humanistic interactions with patients and families is not built into the consultation process. In spite of all these, a strong attachment may develop with many families during long term follow up visits. Over these years, I have been part of many care teams for a large number of children with acute neurological insults like encephalitis or refractory status epilepticus who after a fairly prolonged and heroic medical struggle, are left with major neurological deficits. Many of these children improve over the long term and make a meaningful clinical recovery. However, some will end up with permanent neurological sequelae with severe functional impairments. The social welfare system is very inadequate or non-existent in our country and the families literally struggle to take care of the affected children. In the long term, many of them experience severe emotional burn out as well as a financial drain.

As the primary physician engaging these families, I had often wondered whether it was proper on our part to salvage these children during the acute phase when we perceived that there was a relatively high chance for severe neurological deficits in the long term.

Like the caregivers burn out, child neurologists are prone to experience feelings of helplessness and low self- esteem, while taking care of their patients. Sometimes, terrible self-doubt may arise with the perception of our services as being merely palliative with very limited options for curative treatment. Working for long hours, I have personally gone through these low phases, many times during my professional career. Sometimes, humanistic gestures from my patients and their families have helped me come out of those periods faster and concentrate on the work at hand with renewed vigor.

I still remember one particular family of an infant who had an early onset developmental -epileptic encephalopathy with prolonged seizures and seizure clusters. He used to have very frequent admissions through the emergency needing prolonged intensive care. Finally seizures got controlled over some months. However, his development got plateaued. As per the routine departmental protocol, the family was counseled about the guarded seizure and developmental outcomes. However, the overall perception among the members of the care team was that the family, especially the mother, was not willing to accept the suggested care plan, which was aimed at achieving realistic clinical goals. They did not come back for regular follow up visits for some time. After around one year, the boy was brought back to our services with a recurrence of seizures. By then, he had picked up some early motor milestones. However, the cognitive and social milestones were significantly affected. It was one of those low days as mentioned earlier and I was seriously reflecting on the limitations of the available therapeutic interventions in complex early-onset epilepsies.

While going through the personal records, I noted that after going home, the family had renamed the boy with my first name. On further inquiry, the mother responded that all the immediate family members jointly made a decision to name the boy after the physician who saved him! I was really surprised and shocked to hear that. From my professional perspective, his clinical status was not at all encouraging. It was sure that he would certainly have multiple disabilities in the future, which the family might have to endure. However, the mother was so happy at the signs of neurodevelopmental progress in him. According to her, even that developmental status was not expected during the previous stormy periods of seizure emergencies. She used to wonder whether he would succumb to one of those episodes. The family was attributing all the little gains in the child to our treatment and was very thankful for all the efforts of our team. I became really perplexed and was not sure whether to confront her then with my viewpoint. As a physician, I would have definitely liked to make her understand the status of her child in realistic clinical terms. However, on a personal level, I was really humbled and touched by her gesture.

At that point, I really felt the physician-patient relationship as a very complex social interaction between equal individuals with very different worldviews and not something to be manipulated by the physicians as commonly perceived in the medical circles. As in any human relationship, mutual respect with empathy as well as reciprocity might probably hold the key for success here.

Namaste

EXEMPLARY PARENTS

Dr.Oscar Ignacio Doldán Pérez
Intensive Care Pediatrician
La Costa Medical Center
Asunción Paraguay

In my four decades as a pediatrician, I have learned to value the parents (I'm referring to the father-mother pairing) of my little patients, many of them touching heroism in extreme situations. This story, which occurred in the middle of the 90s, moved me deeply when they accepted progressively an unexpected condition and a difficult contingency that presented later on, without forgetting other families with similar experiences.

LABOUR AT THE WOLVE'S HOUR

The placid dream I was in, late at night, was interrupted abruptly when my cousin-gynecologist "chose" me to be the one to be in charge of a normally scheduled childbirth, in the now disappeared Hospital Frances. With iterative yawns and still sleepy, I made it to the delivery room, in what looked like it was going to be a birth more from the hundreds I already had under my belt. But this case would be very special because of the later connotations that would make it an exceptional story.

GRIEF IN THE EARLY MORNING

Everything went by normally, the baby emerged without problems, crying vigorous, but... wait a minute! I stood stiffly watching him closely. The obstetrician noticed my immobility:

"What is it, Oscar?" He asked me in a muffled voice and questioning gaze so that the new mother would not notice. I did not reply with words, but I gestured facial expressions denoting that "something" was not right: the boy had obvious dysmorphic features, which undoubtedly corresponded to Down syndrome, which had not been detected prenatally.

DISTRESSING QUESTION

After the immediate care of the newborn, I called the father to award adjoining, to explain to him that his child had clear indications of a genetic alteration; so visible that confirmatory testing was just a routine to be done to confirm the unquestionable. The new father literally collapsed, he watched me fixedly with a scrutinizing look, he asked me a stammering question that I had never heard before: "Doctor ... you ... have you ever done something wrong?" My answer came out spontaneously: "I've been wrong a thousand times, and I know I'll make a million mistakes in more than one diagnosis! Medicine is not an exact science and all doctors fail continuously," and I added: "The best doctor is the one who makes the least mistake! By the way, we are going to do a genetic study to confirm your child's diagnosis," I said, trying to sound as comforting as possible.

TAKING CARE

The infant was discharged. Happily, he did not have a cardiac malformation, a very frequent situation in this genopathy. In the office controls, I could perceive the enormous amount of affection that both parents gave to the son, who went unto growing up in a family atmosphere of great human warmth. Also, as compensation from nature, these boys are characterized by being extremely affectionate and awaken an immeasurable tenderness. Years later, a little brother came to join the happy home.

LEADING PARENTS IN SOLIDARITY

Not only they welcomed this child with great love, providing all the treatments of early stimulation needed in these cases, but with the passage of the time, they led the "Association of Parents with Down Syndrome," in which, thanks to the union of families with similar circumstances, they were able to share experiences and unite in a solidary commonwealth, which linked common concerns. But life would have a new surprise in store for them, a hard test that they also had to bravely face.

A FEARFUL EVIL

It is known that carriers of trisomy 21 have less immunity and are exposed to acquired diseases. Almost leaving the preschool stage, a terrible diagnosis invaded their lives: acute leukemia. The parents did lose hope and subjected their beloved son to harsh chemotherapy treatments with the faith set in healing. The situation was controlled with the attack dose, and the parents now decided to take another step forward in their laudable intentions.

ALTRUISM WITHOUT LIMITS

Faced with this new situation, the parents reconsidered the meritorious project of sharing with their peers, their "route companions" on this path strewn with fences, and they surprisingly organized the Down Child Parenting Group with Leukemia! They plausibly helped other parents with great generosity, with the aim of mitigating their painful experiences. The wise nature rewarded so much nobility and granted them the definitive cure of their beloved child.

PERSONAL PARAGUAYAN MARCH

End of March 1999. One of the first chemotherapy sessions coincided with the social-political outbreak called "Paraguayan March." While our little patient-hero was waging his own revolution at the Private Children's Institute, just a few blocks from there, they detonated the first bursts that killed young immolated lives for our incipient democracy, which is not yet consolidated. Today, that child is already a young adult who got ahead thanks to his exemplary parents and his own personal effort. Hopefully, our country will continue with the same principles.

THE BRIEF STORY OF CHULITO

For Elsa, that MOTHER.

Mario Tomas Rodríguez, MD
Consultant Physician in Child Neurology
Former Head of Pediatrics Service, and Teaching and Research
Hospital General de Agudos de Lanus.Buenos Aires Argentina
Director of Degree of University Specialist in Pediatrics
Children's Medicine Academic discipline. Universidad Nacional de Buenos Aires
Full Member of the Argentine Society of Children's Neurology

The second Saturday of each month had been chosen for us to meet at the hospital.

The man who would later be my teacher had had the generosity of coming to hang out on those days, so that's when we talked about those patients, his opinion seemed necessary for the diagnosis and treatment.

Nicolas, the doctor on call on Friday nights, yelled from the door.

-"There is this crazy [1] child again in the waiting room, what a mess! Did you give him anything?"

Chulito, my little patient, was seen from afar, ran and bumped into the other kids, doors and windows, chairs and toys in the waiting room, it like a tornado and his screams could be heard from afar.

Elsa, his mother, was always attentive to stop him, caring, but never too soft. When Chulito approached the window that overlooked the yard, the expression on her face changed, her eyes blackened and her shallow cheekbones burned with fear, but she never screamed at him, she ran, caught him and showered him is kisses between his screams and kicks.

Come on, my naughty Chulito, what is the doctor going to say! she would say, in her characteristic low voice directly into the boy's ear and gave him a loud kiss on his coarse and tuberous skin.

Look, sir, the mother would always tell me: read books, they weigh less in your head than in your arms, my mom was right, I kept collecting books for a while and I don't even want to think about what's going to take me to put them in the moving truck.

-"Say, sir, have you read all your books? And of course, your head does not weigh more because of that, right? You... don't speak a lot, my mom always told me I talk too much, you know, I think I got used to it when I started working at a hair salon. How that guy talks way too much in there! It's worse than at the dentist because your see, dentists talk and talk but they also answer themselves, that's because the patients are there with their mouth wide open and fearing the dental drill, they can't even say a word... That's why dentists and hairdressers speak so much. Ah! I almost forgot, today among the books I found this rosary. The stones are very yellowish, worn, it seems that it used a lot, my grandmother taught me to pray when I was a kid, my granny prayed a lot, pebble by pebble... The prayer I liked the most, every time I remember it, it makes me feel funny in my chest, was the one that said 'Hail Mary, full of grace, the Lord is with thee; blessed art thou among women, and blessed is the fruit of thy womb, Jesus.' I didn't understand it at first, but then my grandma explained it to me. Clear as the lemon tree in my house, that one gives lemons. Women bear the fruit, which is the children, in their belly. My Granny said that the father gives his own, but the mother bears the fruit. I always pray with a rosary, as well as this one. It's really worn out! I can see that you used it heavily You... pray?"

That second Saturday of the month, my teacher confirmed my presumption about Chulito.

I had been struck by the lanceolate spots on his skin, his behavior, his way of speaking, his face, with those little marks outstanding on his skin and his fingers and some other features that I kept discovering as I dealt more with him.

Elsa looked at me in amazement. Her eyes seemed full of nights, the sallow skin of her face muted, pale and sweaty, the doof of the calvary, unintentionally and to my regret, began to open.

He can't be cured then, Doctor. It must come down to his father's family; he has a nephew who's the same as Chulito. No, what am I saying? He's not the same, that child does not walk and is prostrate, but look at Chulito, nobody can stop him. So it comes from the father's side, then? Chulito's face is his father's portrait. You see, Doctor, he has that curly hair, just like my husband. His mouth, his nose. But not his eyes, those look like mines! That ruffian, my Chulito!

Elsa was silent for a few seconds, thinking about what she was going to say next.

Maybe it's from his father's side, but I had him inside me, I made him like that, he's my fruit, Doctor. You can look at it from any angle you want, Chulito, however, is my fruit.

The crisis of epileptic seizures, in the hospital bed, with a jolt after another, did not stop. The screeching of the bed, by its shaking, could be heard from afar. Chulito despaired. He was old enough to be in a bed, but his disease had produced a change in his contexture, so it was preferable to put him to bed in one of those metal cribs with sidebars that could be raised and prevented anyone who was there from falling to the floor. If we put him to bed in a single bed, his seizures were such that they would have fired him to the ground. The sound that the metal made with each shake was disturbing.

Those are intrants, right, Doctor?

Elsa said with her sallow face bathed in sweat and tears.

Andrés Grieco, a second-year resident, impeccable, managed the syringe, and when he heard "intrants," he said quietly and almost robotically "Subintrants.. the crisis" The glance I gave him was enough. He lowered his head and continued with his task.

Rude brat, I thought, who are you trying to correct?

Be as it may, Chulito had been shaking for a long time without rest. The rales of his breathing filled the room. Just the nurse's footsteps, a few other sounds, and our voices, occasionally cut off the purr of his lungs and the squeak of the bed shaking from the seizures.

At last, a long, dull sound (like the tiredness of an old engine), marked the end of the crisis. Chulito, lean and twisted, drooling profusely, fell asleep, full of punctures and caressed softly and tenderly by Elsa, who she let out tiny moans and suppressed sighs.

So, Doctor, it comes from the father's side?

I think I told you several years ago about my husband's nephew, he had something like that but he was bedridden! And you see, Doctor! Chulito used to run and break so much stuff, I remember pleading with him just so he would stop, that cute and loud Chulito is now in that chair we made for him, bah! It was made by Omar, my husband.

No! Social work is gone.

You already asked me that, Doctor, Elsa said with a mocking smile but nice.

And at night I sleep with him.

He doesn't take up any space in the bed.

I'm so scared that something will happen to him, you know?

Sometimes his entire body shakes, other times is just his face, mouth, and hands.

Then it stops as if nothing.

Ah! Did you see his mouth?

It started little by little and now it is so crooked that it seems that the ear it is going to go inside.

There is no case, Doctor, Chulito is not going anymore.

He no long attends School 501. [2]

Yes, I know that you said it was good for him to go to that school, but he doesn't learn anything! Who is going to teach him?

He doesn't stop all day, it seems that he flies through the patio or through the classroom, he runs and takes what he can, and don't even make me start on what happens when the crisis comes back.

Also, you see, in that school there is everything and I am afraid that the Chulito will do something to those boys, poor things!

He's already around 6 and he wants me to tell him, he doesn't learn.

Do you remember that Saturday at the Hospital? That day that you brought another doctor with you. The one with the pipe, remember? Well, while I was talking and talking softly to you! Chulito bit him!

Do you remember now?

He didn't like him.

Bah, he just lets you check on him!

He does everything just so they can't work on him! He also nibbled at the one that was here on Friday, the one that calls him blondie, [3]

Why do they call him blondie? Chulito is not blond, his hair is brown, it doesn't even look like a redhead, although the red-heads are quite restless, just like my Chulito.

And this piece was the matrimonial. But when Chulito began to get worse, I put it together for him.

I sleep with him, he hardly takes up anything in bed!

I think I already told you. Although he is old, his body is that of a small child.

Is it the disease?

See that big window, Omar put it, so Chulito could see the backyard, which is about forty meters by eight, and that tree is good, no like the one in the front which is a paradise, where the birds don't make nests because that tree is bitter.

Although Omar says that it gives good shade and that if he takes out a branch it could be used to hunt butterflies.

Chulito is going to hunt butterflies!

Instead, this one at the bottom is nice. Nice shade, very bushy.

Every afternoon a mockingbird comes and sings a long time.

I wish you could see Chulito, he likes it a lot!

You wouldn't believe me! But he tells me.

The same way the tells me about you coming to check on him.

I put the sprinkler on the grass and after a while the mockingbird comes.

I put the microwave and this other oven here in his room.

I cook everything from here.

It is more comfortable this way.

And it's just the two of us...

Chulito is an early bird.

I make everything a smoothie.

Everything.

He eats me less and less by the day, but I insist.

I'm not very fond of the mouth thing going on, but hey!

I think he doesn't eat because he is inside all day.

What can I do!

That way no one is hungry. Right, Doctor?

The day you gave him that other pill, the yellow one, his crisis became less and less frequent.

He hardly has any of the longer ones, the little ones and the shakes still happen from time to time.

I put that other pill, the blue one, under the tongue.

Bah! I can! And immediately they pass.

On Tuesday at gastro they told me they want to put something in his belly to feed it.

Button, a button they call it. [4]

I look at Chulito and say button! You are going to be a button! You know why, don't you Doctor? About the button, I mean... [5]

and a faint but mischievous smile crossed his face and narrowed his black eyes.

No, look, I don't want that, the button thing, while I still have my force I will feed him his food. I'll continue making everything into a smoothie, everything.

If not then what am I going to do with the microwave and oven?

I have nothing to do but to just take care of Chulito.

Chulito left the special school.

Rather, the school left him.

Who could keep that little indomitable boy, who threw everything to the ground, who had a crisis of epilepsy all the time, who did not speak and growled like an animal?

Confined to his wheelchair.

To make matters worse he had already bitten several boys and teachers.

The director called Elsa and without hindrance he expelled him.

I think Elsa appreciated it.

She suffered horrors bringing him and even more taking him back home.

The attempt lasted two or three years, I don't remember correctly, but as Chulito grew, so did the problems to retain him into that school.

Only Elsa and her persistent will, could with him.

Only the journey to the asphalt a hundred meters from Chulito's house, it became a tremendous problem just to get him there.

On rainy days the wheelchair Omar made for him would sink into the mud and there was no one who has enough force to move it.

Then only in arms could they cover that journey, to the asphalt and from there to the bus, or the solidarity of a neighbor who took them to the school.

Elsa had already given up her efforts in countless offices municipal to get help, she put her body, what she had of strength, and her tenacity, which was endless.

In October of that year I saw him again, it had been a long time since I had visited.

For those mysterious things about diseases, Chulito didn't have as many crises and even less of the "big ones" as Elsa used to say.

She handled the medication with more experience than anyone.

Chulito's deterioration was evident.

He sunk between impeccable white pillows and slept many hours a day.

This whole room was for him alone, the bed with very white sheets gently wrapped him.

Almost starch-free [6] so it doesn't hurt him.

The thing in Chulito's back, in his bum, [7] has healed.

Look, I cried so much because of it.

And nobody has attended him, no other doctor I mean, because he hasn't had any crisis,

Bah! I always ask for you. You know, Chuli loves no one but you.

It was difficult to understand and bear that responsibility, but as soon as I entered the room, Chulito that seemed submerged in a world of supports, gently opened his little eye on the "good" side as Elsa said to the half-paralyzed body of her son.

The black iris could be confused with the blackness of his pupil giving the sensation of a huge eye peering around him.

A diaper covered his body, filled with hard, blackened hair that it stood with a hairy little column and encircled his navel.

Breathing really loud, while his wet cough sounded in the room.

Chulito perceived my arrival.

His dry, extremely dry skin, and the lethargy of his consciousness, denoted the worst.

He didn't shake his head when I ruffled his thick hair with my fingers as a way of greeting, but his breathing changed rhythm and a sound deep and smooth sound came from his lips.

He doesn't eat anything, Doctor.

It doesn't even drink anything.

That's why I called you.

He doesn't want anyone to check on him, just you.

Elsa said, with slow and shaky sobs.

That night, as I left, the last words of Elsa on the porch of her house were stuck in my head.

Chulito is not ok, Doctor. He's fucked, doctor.

Then, a slight smile crossed her angular face, she asserted ...

Other times he was also in very bad shape but he came out alive.

How can I know, but we will not admit him in the hospital anymore, doctor, God have mercy, he will lye here, in his little house.

Is that ok, doctor?

He already told me that he wants to say goodbye to you.

I called Mercedes, Elsa's midwife, who lived in the house in front of Chulito's and who was a nurse.

I'll get an IV access, Doctor.

She said from the door.

Do we pass a normal saline one and another of glucose and so?

Mercedes's customary voice said.

Chulito did not complain about the punctures on his right hand when Mercedes applied it to pass the liquid. Just a brief purr and he returned to his lethargy, while a trickle of blood flowed slowly from his forearm and stained the sheet white.

That Sunday in October was sunny.

The breeze hardly moved the leaves of the trees and the sun licked over everything that made up the neighborhood.

A thousand laps I imposed before leaving the house for Chulito, were few.

I knew it was all over, but I refused to be present.

My own excuses fueled my anxiety.

Around noon and without pretexts, I headed for the house.

When I reached the beginning of the dirt road, I noticed the two tremendous ditches that lined the street, dirty, blackened, where Elsa had told me about the times that Chulito had fallen. Ditches that, on hot nights, bordering the sidewalk, were a house for a thousand and one singing frogs.

Many neighbors crowded around the house, the men were the shadow of paradise and the women were in the middle of the street, in the sun, which, although warm, was almost annoying, with their hands wrapped in their aprons, talking quietly, while the kids ran and skipped the ditch skillfully.

I thought sadly.

Everything is over! and a sense of relief washed over me.

An immense tenderness invaded my soul.

I was driving the car very slowly so as not to lift as much dirt and I made my way through the neighbors.

I parked in front of the house, at the dirt entrance that worked as a bridge, which Omar had made over the ditch.

I had not yet got out of the car when moved and pushing aside the plastic curtain into thin slices, which covered the entrance, Elsa went out into the street and shouted,

Thank goodness, Doctor, you've arrived! Chulito is in really bad shape, but he is waiting for you to say goodbye!

Chulito had been on the verge of dying for several hours.

Upon entering his room I automatically took my stethoscope and reclining on the bed, I placed it on his chest.

My other hand brushed Chulito's "good" hand and I perceived a slight movement of his fingers trying to squeeze mine.

Her heart was beating slow, cottony, without cadence, like stumbling.

He breathed with deep rales and long pauses.

You see, Doctor. He was waiting for you to say goodbye, he told me that he wanted to do it, Elsa said.

The IV is not even passing anymore, but the arm is not swollen, it is no longer circulating!

As the minutes ticked by, his heart slowed down even more.

It became slower and slower.

Increasingly dull.

Then he let out a long gasp, choppy and sad ... very sad, accompanied by his last heartbeat.

The fingers of the "good" hand began to loosen, releasing mine.

Without crying and with an accustomed movement, Elsa took the Chulito's inert head and with a smooth and accurate movement, took out the rosary that hung from his neck.

She opened one of my hands, placed it in my palm, and closed my fingers on the rosary.

He wanted this to be yours.

It is a little wasted from praying so much.

It always accompanied him.

He didn't even take it off to bathe.

And now that he has said goodbye to you, you can have it.

He no longer needs it.

Keep it.

Those were Elsa's last words to me.

Chulito abandoned life little by little.

He crawled toward death without regrets.

A cruel hereditary disease made sure that happened.

He lived a little more than two decades with his hemiplegia in tow,

... with the obscenity of his tremendous convulsions,

... with a slow and sustained tumor in his brain that was finishing him

And with Elsa's unconditional love.

THE 'F-WORDS' IN CHILDHOOD DISABILITY: I SWEAR THIS IS HOW WE SHOULD THINK!

P. Rosenbaum
CanChild Centre for Childhood Disability Research, McMaster University, Hamilton, ON, Canada

J. W. Gorter
CanChild Centre for Childhood Disability Research, McMaster University, Hamilton, ON, Canada
NetChild Network for Childhood Disability Research, Utrecht, the Netherlands

ABSTRACT

The 21st century is witnessing a sea change in our thinking about 'disability.' Nowhere are these developments more apparent than in the field of childhood disability, where traditional biomedical concepts are being incorporated into – but expanded considerably by – new ways of formulating ideas about children, child development, social-ecological forces in the lives of children with chronic conditions and their families, and 'points of entry' for professionals to be helpful. In this paper, we have tried to package a set of ideas, grounded in the World Health Organization's International Classification of Functioning, Disability and Health (the ICF), into a series of what we have called 'F-words' in child neurodisability – function, family, fitness, fun, friends and future. We hope this will be an appealing way for people to incorporate these concepts into every aspect of clinical service, research and advocacy regarding disabled children and their families.

INTRODUCTION

Childhood disabilities are conditions that do, or are highly likely to, affect the trajectories of children's development into adulthood. Many have a neurological basis and are commonly referred to as 'neurodevelopmental' disabilities (or simply as 'neurodisabilities'). Additional impairments often include musculoskeletal conditions or genetic syndromes, and cognitive, behavioral and communication disorders, reflecting the complexity of most of these conditions.

The field of childhood disability (what we like to refer to as 'applied child development') is still in its infancy as an academic discipline. For this reason, traditional views of childhood disability have been influenced very strongly by approaches taught and practiced in biomedicine, built to a large extent on the way health problems are managed in acute care medicine. Think, for example, of how we manage the sudden onset of acute chest pain: we take a history, examine the patient, 'rule out' competing possibilities in order to make the right (specific) diagnosis, find the right treatment, intervene and watch the evolution of the illness after treatment. In this way of thinking, we work towards 'fixing' (one of the 'F-words' traditionally used in childhood disability, as elsewhere). 'Fixing' refers to the expectation that the appropriate diagnosis will lead to the right interventions and that the underlying biomedical impairments will be ameliorated to the patient's advantage. Of course, in acute situations the time course of events is usually rapid and outcomes can often be assessed in days or weeks.

We believe that there are a number of significant limitations to the idea of 'fixing' in childhood disability. First, although we often forget this, in our field there is much less precision regarding many of the common 'diagnoses' we make. 'Cerebral palsy' (CP) and 'autism spectrum disorder' (ASD) appear to be specific terms, but in reality they describe a rather heterogeneous group of conditions that can impact on the development of children's function for a variety of biological reasons, with a very wide range of effects.

Second, the 'treatments' we have available may at times address signs and symptoms underlying biomedical aspects of the condition (as is the case, e.g. with botulinum toxin to manage spasticity, or anticonvulsants for seizure disorders); however, given both the limited understanding and the complexity of the biomedical underpinnings of conditions like CP and ASD, and the paucity of specific 'treatments', we have very few opportunities to 'treat' bio medically to prevent or cure the conditions. Even for the treatment of something as obvious as muscle weakness in CP, we still have insufficient evidence to support or refute the efficacy of muscle-strengthening exercises in children with CP (Verschuren et al. 2011).

Third, even when it is possible to affect the biomedical 'impairments' of these conditions, there are often, at best, limited connections between changes in how the body works and the functional outcomes of those changes (Wright et al. 2007). Fourth, the course of development is usually rapid, while the effects of many of our treatments are relatively slow. Against the background of natural changes influenced by growth and development, it is challenging to detect causal connections between interventions and outcomes that can be attributed to those treatments.

The good news is that in the 21st century there are important new ideas about health and childhood disability that are helping us to expand our thinking. International health experts recently published a discussion paper about the limitations of the current World Health Organization (WHO) definition of health and proposed a new, more dynamic and empowering definition: 'health is the ability to adapt and to self-manage' (Huber et al. 2011). Informed by our own 'development', the evolution of the field, endless discussion with colleagues and over two decades' of childhood disability research at CanChild and more recently NetChild, we have formulated these ideas as a set of six 'F-words', presented in a way that people will hopefully find both fun and memorable. Our purpose is to encourage people in the childhood disability field to apply these concepts in their work with children with disabilities and their families.

Background to the F-words: The International Classification of Functioning, Health and Disabilities (ICF) 2001

In 2001, the World Health Organization (2001) published a set of ideas about how we might think about health. These ideas, refining the WHO's original (World Health Organization 1980) International Classification of Impairment, Disability and Handicap (ICIDH), are meant to apply to all of us, and not just to people with 'disabilities'. The ICF provides both a detailed classification of aspects of people's health and function, and a pictorial framework that brings these ideas together. In this sense, we see it as a 'rule-in' approach, in contrast to the way acute issues are assessed. The ICF was published a decade ago, and represents the work of professionals and health consumers from around the world, but is still not as widely known and applied in clinical service, education and research as we believe it should be (Cerniauskaite et al. 2011). Figure 1 shows the framework, on which the rest of this paper will be built.

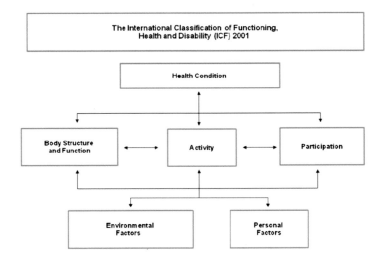

Figure 1. The International Classification of Functioning, Health and Disabilities framework

As can be seen, the ICF framework connects a number of ideas about health and health conditions to each other in an interesting way. Note that the concepts in the six boxes are all generic issues, and that none is specific to any disease or condition. Note as well that these ideas are interconnected without any hierarchy of implied importance. Having the health condition ('diagnosis') at the top traditionally directed our thinking towards the biomedical, whereas the ICF clearly presents the opportunity to consider all health issues within a broader social-ecological context that could be considered to turn the framework 'upside down'. This suggests that, within this 'dynamic system', changes in any area of the framework may potentially have influences elsewhere in the system. These ideas are elaborated below with an illustration of the connectedness of these concepts.

By taking a journey along the ICF 'trail', we can see how people are now beginning to think about disability. We hope to illustrate that by embedding the 'F-words' into relevant components of the framework, we open up possibilities for thought and action that should benefit children, parents, families and professionals.

THE FIRST 'F-WORD': FUNCTION

Function refers to what people do. Synonyms include 'role', 'job', 'occupation', 'task', etc.; for children, 'play' is their 'work'. In the ICF, we see functioning as belonging in both the ICF category 'Activity', which in WHO terms refers to 'execution of a task or action by an individual', and the ICF category 'Participation', defined in the WHO-ICF as 'involvement in life situations'. Most people who work in the field of childhood disability would of course argue that their efforts in counseling, treatment and management are all aimed at promoting and improving function. So one might ask: Is this different from before, and if so in what ways? We believe the answer is clearly yes: the emphasis we see in modern disability work represents an important advance on earlier thinking.

First, we used to believe that all our efforts needed to focus on 'impairments' in body function or structure, such as a significant deviation or loss at a biomedical level. The ICF refers to 'body functions (as) the physiological functions of body systems (including psychological functions)' and 'body structures (as) anatomical parts of the body, such as organs, limbs, and their components'. Thus, we have traditionally put much of our clinical effort into 'treatment' of impairments, and assumed that improvements in body structure and function would make a child better and thus would lead to functional gains. Unfortunately, this does not seem automatically to be the case (Wright et al. 2007), likely because any aspect of function is influenced by a myriad of factors (Chiarello et al. 2011), of which impairments are but one (even when they are 'treatable').

Second, we used to believe that from a very young age children's everyday activities – for example, walking or talking – had to be done 'normally', and we used typical ('normal') development as our standard. We agree that the idea of normality (what most people do) can be useful as a guide to function but it certainly need not be the only way that things are done. Consider, for example, how many well-functioning people are left-handed, or wear glasses, or only use a computer because their handwriting is slow or messy. We have likely inhibited children's development by stopping them doing things considered to be outside the normal – literally 'abnormally'. One need only think of preventing children with CP from pulling to stand and walking in a crouch gait, or expecting children to communicate only with spoken language. We have traditionally worried that such behavior would lead to the development of bad habits, and prevent 'normal' acquisition of skills and function. This approach may have sacrificed developmental progress in activities and participation on the altar of 'normality' (Gibson et al. 2011).

In considering other perspectives on function, two related concepts inherent in the ICF should be discussed. 'Capacity' is what we can do at our best, while 'performance' is what we ordinarily do. There is research indicating that capacity and performance are distinct constructs (Holsbeeke et al. 2009) and those data support the idea that a gap exists between the two. This is seen, for example, in mobility in school-aged children with CP, and can lead to a question, framed in ICF terms, about what to focus on in therapy: capacity or performance (Tieman et al. 2004; Smits et al. 2010).

Performance improves with practice, and hence our primary emphasis in counseling and intervention should be on promoting activity. This approach is consistent with developmental realities: children first learn to do things in their own way, and then (maybe) develop good skills in those activities. Picture a typical toddler learning to cruise and walk, first holding onto the furniture, and how that early 'developmental' gait progresses quickly over the second year of life. Children with unilateral spastic CP (hemiplegia) with a Gross Motor Function Classification System functional level of I or II, indicating they are independent on at least level surfaces without walking aids, are characterized by a wide spectrum of phenotypic variation in their gait patterns (Dobson et al. 2011). Note that how things are done is not initially considered important. Thinking in this way hopefully moves us towards 'achievement' of the activity and away from the tyranny of 'normal' as the only goal.

It is also important to recognize that children with disabilities can often be 'deprived' of experience. This may occur secondary to their functional challenges, and also because they have limited chances to practice skill development over and over unless the environment facilitates such possibilities (as might be done, e.g. through the provision of technical aids such as powered mobility; Butler 1986). To date, the perspectives and experiences of parents and children about their values and beliefs remain largely absent. We are excited to read a recent study in which children's and parents' beliefs about the value of walking were investigated, and to see how these beliefs inform rehabilitation choices and perceptions of 'success' (Gibson et al. 2011). Gibson and her colleagues found that the children under study are affected by normative ideas about walking as a moral good. This may contribute to parental feelings of angst and doubt, and negative self-identities for children; for this reason, we feel strongly that it is important to encourage the development and practice of function without regard to how 'nicely' it is achieved.

THE SECOND 'F-WORD': FAMILY

Family represents the essential 'environment' of all children. In ICF terms, parents are the central 'contextual factor' in their children's lives. One might well ask, 'Isn't this already obvious?' The answer, in many respects, is a mix of yes and no!

In child health, our 'patient' has always been the child, and at times parents have been tolerated but not engaged as well as they might be. Although things have changed in many ways, services have traditionally been very paternalistic, and professionals have often not explored families' issues and realities. This approach misses valuable opportunities to be helpful. For one thing, we know that parents' lives are 'complicated' with their extra concerns about their children with disabilities. There is evidence from both clinical and population-based research to show that parental physical and mental health is often challenged (Brehaut et al. 2004, 2009, 2011; Raina et al. 2005; Lach et al. 2009), and that having a child with CP in a family may lead to parents perceiving restrictions in family participation. These restrictions arise early in the life of a child with CP and may become more prominent as the child grows older (Rentinck et al. 2009). We also recognize that parents are frequently caught in a 'generational sandwich', being parents to their children, and (adult) children to their own parents! Grandparental voices, another contextual factor that is often in the background, can be powerful influences on the parents of children with whom we work, and these should be asked about and understood. Family -centred services provide the tools to address these concerns.

Research on family-centred services, undertaken with families as partners, has enabled us to see that engagement with parents, respect, continuity of care and informing people appropriately are key elements of service values by families (Rosenbaum 2004, 2011). We know that when services are more family-centred, parents report better satisfaction and mental health, and less stress in their dealings with providers. We have also learned that collaborating with parents to identify their goals can work to improve therapy outcomes effectively and efficiently (Ketelaar et al. 2001; Ostensjø et al.

2008; Øien et al. 2010; Darrah et al. 2011; Law et al. 2011). It has become apparent that it is not only the physical disability of children that contributes to parental stress. Maladaptive behaviour of children significantly contributes to parental stress scores and impacts attachment, the relationship with spouse, parental depression and, in particular, a sense of competence (Ketelaar et al. 2008). We therefore have to think of the various supports and resources for families as a whole, and help them to find the resources to make informed decisions.

THE THIRD 'F-WORD': FITNESS

The fitness of children with disabilities, a component of body structure and function in the ICF framework, has until recently been a neglected aspect of childhood disability. Research shows that children with disabilities and chronic illnesses are less 'fit' than other children, and less fit than they should be (van Brussel et al. 2011). This speaks to the need for an emphasis on a health promoting orientation to disabled children's lives and not one that simply focuses on remediation of their 'disabilities'. Although we know that exercise programs can be beneficial in children with disabilities, fitness training alone is not effective enough for them to stay physically active (Claassen et al. 2011). We need to understand what makes it easy or hard for children and adolescents with disabilities to become and to stay physically active. There is also a need for more and better recreational opportunities for all children, whether these are considered 'therapy' or not. Research by Colver and colleagues (Hammal et al. 2004; Fauconnier et al. 2009) shows the importance of environment, and of social and other policies that affect the lives of all children.

THE FOURTH 'F-WORD': FUN

Fun spans the ICF elements of 'personal factors' (What does/ might this particular child enjoy doing?) and 'participation', which in ICF terms refers to 'involvement in (meaningful) life situations'. More colloquially, life is about 'doin' stuff!' One might well ask: Isn't this what childhood should be about? Unfortunately, there is good evidence that people with disabilities have lower rates of participation than their able-bodied peers (Bult et al. 2010). This prompts the question: What can we do to increase and enhance the participation of young people with disabilities?

The answers are deceptively simple and straightforward. First, find out what they want to do! This can be accomplished informally by asking, and more formally with the Children's Assessment of Participation and Enjoyment (CAPE) measure, a tool developed and validated for this purpose (King et al. 2004). Note that activities may be formal (structured) or informal (free-range), and may be done on one's own or with others. Second, adapt those self-identified activities as needed, to allow children to pursue the things they want to do. Third, do not worry about expecting children to do things 'normally' (One need only think of the Paralympics to realize that disabled people can, with more or fewer adaptations, demonstrate remarkable feats of physical and psychological achievement. And indeed, there is now a 'disabled' young man from South Africa, missing the lower parts of both legs, who runs with the aid of prosthetic 'blades' against 'able-bodied' athletes at a world-class level!) Finally, use participatory activities to build children's confidence, competence, sense of achievement and capacity. It is the doing, rather than a superior level of accomplishment, that is most meaningful to most children.

THE FIFTH 'F-WORD': FRIENDS

Friends and friendships occupy the same ICF 'space' as 'fun' – namely 'personal factors' and 'participation'. Social development is an essential aspect of personhood, and we believe that considerable emphasis should be placed on facilitating this component of child development. It is the quality of relationships, rather than the number, that is important. Thus, as service providers we need to ask whether we include this dimension of children's development in discussing interventions – and if not, why not? We also need to consider what can be done to encourage, empower and enhance children's opportunities to develop and nurture meaningful peer connections. Being involved in peer group activities and opportunities for dating, rather than motor impairment or level of education, seems relevant for developing romantic relationships and sexual activity once children with CP reach adolescence and young adulthood (Wiegerink et al. 2010). Discussions with parents, right from the beginning of our relationship with them, should include counseling about this aspect of children's lives, and provide parents with ideas about how to address this.

SO, HOW DOES THE ICF HELP?

In Fig. 2, we have 'populated' the ICF framework with the first five 'F-words'. Consider the connections among these ideas. Imagine, for example, how an increase in a disabled child's self-identified meaningful participation might impact on the scope and intensity of their activities, and potentially lead to changes in body structure and function! In this scenario, engagement and participation (e.g. sport programs in the community) – in activities meaningful and fun to a child (and family) – might have an important impact on activity (e.g. improved physical and social functioning) and on body structure and function (e.g. fitness). The apparently 'backwards' direction of these connections certainly differs from traditional biomedical thinking – but it does work! This is how ICF thinking is making a difference!

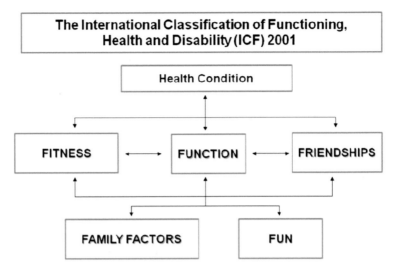

Figure 2. The International Classification of Functioning, Health and Disabilities framework: the interconnections among elements.

FINALLY, THE SIXTH 'F-WORD': FUTURE

This idea is included here to wrap the 'F-words' within the obvious but too often neglected idea that the future is what child 'development' is all about! All children, including disabled children, are in a constant state of 'becoming'. We believe that service providers need to think about the future – in a positive way – right from the start, and encourage parents to do so as well. This in no way implies that we should ignore the child's and family's present realities. Rather, we need to keep this horizon in view at all times. Addressing function, family, fitness, fun and friends will constantly remind us of what is important in the development of all children. We can ask parents and children with disabilities, at any time, about their expectations and dream for a future that is possible – and not decide for them what is impossible. These ideas present a challenge to professionals to acknowledge that 'modern' thinking provides many points of entry in our work with disabled children and their families.

> **Key messages**
>
> - The ICF provides a neutral framework for thinking about health as well as disability.
> - We believe that applying the 'F-word' ideas presented in this paper at the clinical level should allow service providers to 'populate' the ICF framework with each individual's special issues – including their strengths – in order to personalize interventions.
> - The authors encourage clinical and research colleagues to incorporate these concepts in all our work, and to evaluate whether good ideas actually make a difference!

ACKNOWLEDGEMENT

P. R. would like to acknowledge that it was J. W. G. who recognized the possibility to formulate our ideas about the ICF and childhood disability with 'F-words'. We have shared in the development of these ideas, but the credit for the title clearly goes to him. J. W. G., in turn, was first inspired by a presentation by colleague Johanna Darrah in Utrecht, the Netherlands, in May 2000; with her permission, the three research pillars family, function and fitness were created in the NetChild Network for Childhood Disability Research (http://www.netchild.nl).

KEYWORDS

childhood disability, chronic conditions ICF, family, fun, function

Correspondence: Peter Rosenbaum, MD, FRCP©, CanChild Centre for Childhood Disability Research, IAHS Building, Mc-

Master University, 1400 Main Street West, Hamilton, ON, Canada L8S 1C7 E-mail: rosenbau@mcmaster.ca

REFERENCES

1. Brehaut, J. C., Kohen, D. E., Raina, P., Walter, S. D., Russell, D. J., Swinton, M., O'Donnell, M. & Rosenbaum, P. (2004) The health of parents of children with cerebral palsy: how does it compare to other Canadian adults? Pediatrics, 114, e182–e191.

2. Brehaut, J. C., Kohen, D. E., Garner, R. E., Miller, A. R., Lach, L. M., Klassen, A. F. & Rosenbaum, P. L. (2009) Health among caregivers of children with health problems: findings from a Canadian population-based study. American Journal of Public Health, 99, 1254–1262. Epub 4 December 2008.

3. Brehaut, J. C., Garner, R. E., Miller, A. R., Lach, L. M., Klassen, A. F., Rosenbaum, P. L. & Kohen, D. E. (2011) Changes over time in the health of caregivers of children with health problems: growth curve findings from a 10-year Canadian population-based study. American Journal of Public Health (in press). van Brussel, M., van der Net, J., Hulzebos, E., Helders, P. J. & Takken, T. (2011) The Utrecht approach to exercise in chronic childhood conditions: the decade in review (Review). Pediatric Physical Therapy, 23, 2–14.

4. Bult, M. K., Verschuren, O., Gorter, J. W., Jongmans, M. J., Piskur, B. & Ketelaar, M. (2010) Cross-cultural validation and psychometric evaluation of the Dutch language version of the Children's Assessment of Participation and Enjoyment (CAPE) in children with and without physical disabilities. Clinical Rehabilitation, 24, 843–853. Epub 18 May 2010. PubMed PMID: 20483886.

5. Butler, C. (1986) Effects of powered mobility on self-initiated behaviours of very young children with locomotor

disability. Developmental Medicine and Child Neurology, 28, 325–332.

6. Cerniauskaite, M., Quintas, R., Boldt, C., Raggi, A., Cieza, A., Bickenbach, J. E. & Leonardi, M. (2011) Systematic literature review on ICF from 2001 to 2009: its use, implementation and operationalisation. Disability and Rehabilitation, 33, 281–309.

7. Chiarello, L. A., Palisano, R. J., Bartlett, D. J. & McCoy, S. W. (2011) A multivariate model of determinants of change in gross-motor abilities and engagement in self-care and play of young children with cerebral palsy. Physical & Occupational Therapy in Pediatrics, 31, 150–168.

8. Claassen, A. A., Gorter, J. W., Stewart, D., Verschuren, O., Galuppi, B. E. & Shimmell, L. J. (2011) Becoming and staying physically active in adolescents with cerebral palsy: protocol of a qualitative study of facilitators and barriers to physical activity. BMC Pediatrics, 11, 1.

9. Darrah, J., Law, M. C., Pollock, N., Wilson, B., Russell, D. J., Walter, S. D. & Rosenbaum, P. (2011) Context therapy – a new intervention approach for children with cerebral palsy. Developmental Medicine and Child Neurology 53, 615–620.

10. Dobson, F., Morris, M. E., Baker, R. & Graham, H. K. (2011) Unilateral cerebral palsy: a population-based study of gait and motor function. Developmental Medicine and Child Neurology, 53, 429–435. 6 P. Rosenbaum and J.W. Gorter © 2011 Blackwell Publishing Ltd, Child: care, health and development

11. Fauconnier, J., Dickinson, H. O., Beckung, E., Marcelli, M., McManus, V., Michelsen, S. I., Parkes, J., Parkinson, K. N., Thyen, U., Arnaud, C. & Colver, A. (2009) Participation in life situations of 8–12 year old children with cerebral pal-

sy: cross sectional European study. BMJ (Clinical Research Ed.), 338, b1458.

12. Gibson, B. E., Teachman, G., Wright, V., Fehlings, D., Young, N. L. & McKeever, P. (2011) Children's and parents' beliefs regarding the value of walking: rehabilitation implications for children with cerebral palsy. Child: Care, Health and Development, doi: 10.1111/ j.1365-2214.2011.01271.x.

13. Hammal, D., Jarvis, S. N. & Colver, A. F. (2004) Participation of children with cerebral palsy is influenced by where they live [see comment]. Developmental Medicine and Child Neurology, 46, 292–298.

14. Holsbeeke, L., Ketelaar, M., Schoemaker, M. M. & Gorter, J. W. (2009) Capacity, capability, and performance: different constructs or three of a kind? Archives of Physical Medicine and Rehabilitation, 90, 849–855.

15. Huber, M., Knottnerus, J. A., Green, L., van der Horst, H., Jadad, A. R., Kromhout, D., Leonard, B., Lorig, K., Loureiro, M. I., van der Meer, J. W., Schnabel, P., Smith, R., van Weel, C. & Smid, H. (2011) How should we define health? BMJ (Clinical Research Ed.), 343, d4163. doi: 10.1136/bmj.d4163.

16. Ketelaar, M., Vermeer, A., Hart, H., van Petegem-van Beek, E. & Helders, P. J. (2001) Effects of a functional therapy program on motor abilities of children with CP. Physical Therapy, 81, 1534–1545.

17. Ketelaar, M., Volman, M. J., Gorter, J. W. & Vermeer, A. (2008) Stress in parents of children with cerebral palsy: what sources of stress are we talking about? Child: Care, Health and Development, 34, 825–829.

18. King, G., Law, M., King, S., Hurley, P., Rosenbaum, P., Hanna, S., Kertoy, M. & Young, N. (2004) Children's Assessment of Participation and Enjoyment (CAPE) and Preferences for

Activities of Children (PAC). Harcourt Assessment, San Antonio, TX, USA.

19. Lach, L. M., Kohen, D. E., Garner, R. E., Brehaut, J. C., Miller, A. R., Klassen, A. F. & Rosenbaum, P. L. (2009) The health and psychosocial functioning of caregivers of children with neurodevelopmental disorders. Disability and Rehabilitation, 31, 741–752.

20. Law, M. C., Darrah, J., Pollock, N., Wilson, B., Russell, D. J., Walter, S. D., Rosenbaum, P. & Galuppi, B. (2011) Focus on Function: an RCT comparing child- versus context-focused intervention for young children with cerebral palsy. Developmental Medicine and Child Neurology, 53, 621–629.

21. Øien, I., Fallang, B. & Østensjø, S. (2010) Goal-setting in paediatric rehabilitation: perceptions of parents and professional. Child: Care, Health and Development, 36, 558–565. Epub 16 December 2009. PubMed PMID: 20030659.

22. Ostensjø, S., Oien, I. & Fallang, B. (2008) Goal-oriented rehabilitation of preschoolers with cerebral palsy – a multi-case study of combined use of the Canadian Occupational Performance Measure (COPM) and the Goal Attainment Scaling (GAS). Developmental Neurorehabilitation, 11, 252–259.

23. Raina, P., O'Donnell, M., Rosenbaum, P., Brehaut, J., Walter, S. D., Russell, D., Swinton, M., Zhu, B. & Wood, E. (2005) The health and well-being of caregivers of children with cerebral palsy. Pediatrics, 115, 626–636.

24. Rentinck, I. C., Gorter, J. W., Ketelaar, M., Lindeman, E. & Jongmans, M. J. (2009) Perceptions of family participation among parents of children with cerebral palsy followed from infancy to toddler hood. Disability and Rehabilitation, 31, 1828–1834. Rosenbaum, P. (2011) Family and quality of life: key elements in intervention in children

with cerebral palsy. Developmental Medicine and Child Neurology, 53 (Suppl. 4), 68–70. doi: 10.1111/ j.1469-8749.2011.04068.x.

25. Rosenbaum, P. L. (2004) Families and service providers: making the connection effectively. In: The Management of the Movement Disorders of Children with Cerebral Palsy, 2nd edn (eds. D. Scrutton, D. Damiano & M. Mayson), pp. 22–31. Mac Keith Press, London, UK.

26. Smits, D. W., Gorter, J. W., Ketelaar, M., Van Schie, P. E., Dallmeijer, A. J., Lindeman, E. & Jongmans, M. J. (2010) Relationship between gross motor capacity and daily-life mobility in children with cerebral palsy. Developmental Medicine and Child Neurology, 52, e60–e66. Epub 4 February 2010. Erratum in: Developmental Medicine and Child Neurology. 2010; 52, e60.

27. Tieman, B., Palisano, R. J., Gracely, E. J. & Rosenbaum, P. L. (2004) Gross motor capability and performance of mobility in children with cerebral palsy: a comparison across home, school, and outdoors/community settings. Physical Therapy, 84, 419–429.

28. Verschuren, O., Ada, L., Maltais, D. B., Gorter, J. W., Scianni, A. & Ketelaar, M. (2011) Muscle strengthening in children and adolescents with spastic cerebral palsy: considerations for future resistance training protocols. Physical Therapy, 91, 1130–1139.

29. Wiegerink, D. J., Roebroeck, M. E., van der Slot, W. M., Stam, H. J. & Cohen-Kettenis, P. T. (2010) South West Netherlands Transition Research Group. Importance of peers and dating in the development of romantic relationships and sexual activity of young adults with cerebral palsy. Developmental Medicine and Child Neurology, 52, 576–582.

30. World Health Organization (1980) International Classification of Impairment, Disability and Handicap (ICIDH). World Health Organization, Geneva, Switzerland.

31. World Health Organization (2001) International Classification of Functioning, Disability and Health (ICF). World Health Organization, Geneva, Switzerland.

32. Wright, F. V., Rosenbaum, P. L. & Fehlings, D. (2007) How do changes in Impairment, Activity, and Participation relate to each other? Study of children with cerebral palsy (CP) who have received lower extremity Botulinum Toxin Type-A (Bt-A) injections. Developmental Medicine and Child Neurology, 50, 283–289.

A BRIEF BACKGROUND TO THE TWO STORIES BELOW

Peter Rosenbaum, MD, FRCP(C), DSc (HC)
Professor of Paediatrics, McMaster University
Canada Research Chair in Childhood Disability 2001-14
Co-Founder, CanChild Centre for Childhood Disability Research

I am part of CanChild Centre for Childhood Disability Research at McMaster University. Among the many things we have done in our 30 years of research, writing and Knowledge Translation is to embrace the WHO's ICF framework for health and create a tongue-in-cheek operationalization of it in a 2012 paper called The F-words in Childhood Disability.

The impact of the ideas has been considerable: more 20,000 downloads of the paper, more than 200 citations and counting, and at least 25 translations of the poster co-created with Australian colleagues. We have done more 100 invited talks around the world about - or including - these ideas.

Two brief stories from colleagues about parents of children with impairments attest to the impact of these ideas:

1. From a senior colleague, sent October 2016 right after an F-words panel by young people at World CP Day:

Today in clinic I saw a child (who has CP and is functioning at a GMFCS V)– whose mother attended CP-NET Science and Family Day last Wednesday. She reported to me that her entire approach to raising her son has shifted from one of 'fixing' to embracing the F words and a wellness approach. She came to clinic with her goals related to the F words all worked out and felt very empowered! I couldn't be more pleased.

Thank-you to the entire CP-NET team for putting on such an excellent day and driving a wellness agenda (a goal of CP-NET)! Big kudos to Peter and Jan Willem for branding and promoting the F words!

2. From another colleague in our own community, sent July 2019:

Dear Peter and Jan Willem,

Today I saw a 6-year-old girl with CP GMFCS V, refugee from XXX via YYY, parents tried Stem cell therapy in ZZZ and came here (to Canada) with hopes to help her. We had a long consult with a whole team of therapists, social work, resident and myself, going way into our lunch hour trying to answer all the questions they had. I tried to explain what we understand by a functional approach and what the purpose of therapy is and that the exact etiology (nyd) probably won't change this approach. At the end, I showed them the F-words poster in Arabic, they read carefully, asked if these words are meant to be the child speaking and I confirmed. The mom commented under tears, "This is beautiful, that's what I wish for my daughter."

SCHIZOPHRENIA AND RELIGIOUS ENIGMA

Melissa Cowgill/ Melissa Hinostroza Saenz, M.D./M.B.B.S.
Ricardo Palma University, Lima-Peru

I was doing my internship in my home country of Peru. Working in the emergency room was very exciting because you can always get something you would never expect. One day I experienced an event that would impact my way of thinking about medicine and humanity.

An emaciated adolescent patient, too weak to walk and with apparent aphagia, was brought to the emergency room in the arms of his father. His appearance at such a young age stupefied me. I started making differential diagnoses in my head. I asked the patient how I could help him. He was very debilitated, and it was difficult for him to speak. I asked the parents and they could not articulate a sentence that could explain what happened to their son. They just said, "He does not want to eat."

Suddenly, the patient with weak hands grabbed my coat, pulled me towards him, and said, "Doctor, the only thing I want is to stop the voices in my head". I started formulating straightforward questions to his parents. They finally revealed that he was recently diagnosed with schizophrenia and that he stopped his medication because God would cure him on His own.

I consider myself to be a believer and a Christian, but I would have never imagined that another Christian could stop their medication for a religious reason. My heart broke to see my patient's state, and his parents' beliefs and actions could cost my precious patient his life. I stabilized my patient and he had to be transferred to a psychiatric facility where he was hospitalized and received the appropriate medication and care he needed.

Later, I had the fortunate opportunity to further educate my patient and his parents about schizophrenia and the importance of being consistent with medication. I reassured them that God could also work through medicine. They understood, and with regular visits, he adhered to his medication and improved.

Medicine is an art and also an opportunity to have the right platform to serve our patients, educate, and change the course of their lives. We have to be respectful and compassionate, assisting them in all stages of health and illness by promoting well-being, preventing diseases, diagnosing, and delivering proper treatment. Compassion and respect will remind us that each patient is unique, and our actions will have a direct impact on their lives and their loved ones.

HUMANISMS IN MEXICAN NEUROPEDIATRICS – REAL CASES OF A DEVELOPING LATIN AMERICAN COUNTRY

Daniel San-Juan, MD, MSc
Epilepsy Clinic at the National Institute of Neurology and Neurosurgery (NINN), Mexico City, Mexico

Rosana Huerta Albarrán, MD, MSc
Pediatric Service, Hospital General de México "Dr. Eduardo Liceaga," México City, Mexico

Efraín Olivas Peña, MD
Clinical Neurophysiology Laboratory, National Institute of Perinatology, Mexico City, Mexico

Tirso Zúñiga Santamaría, MD, PhD
Neuro-genetic Department at the National Institute of Neurology and Neurosurgery (NINN), Mexico City, Mexico

INTRODUCTION

The Mexican territory has an area of 1,964,375 km^2, making it the thirteenth largest country in the world and the third largest in Latin America. In 2015, according to the National Institute of Statistics and Geography (INEGI) of Mexico, there were was a population of 119, 938,473 and in 2018 there were 2,162,535 births registered; 17.5% of the mothers were under 20 years old (National Institute of Statistics and Geography (INEGI), 2020). In 2019, it was estimated by the National Population Council of Mexico that 31.4% of the population in Mexico was between 0 and 17 years old, a fertility rate of 2.08 children on average per woman and the mortality rate in children under 1 year was 13.1 deaths per 1000 live births (National Population Council Mexico, 2019.)

One of the fundamental challenges of the Mexican health system is that it provides health services in subsystems are disconnected. Each subsystem offers different levels of care, at different prices with different results. Individuals have the choice of choosing a private health plan or service provider, and their membership is determined by their employment. The Mexican Institute of Social Security is the main provider for patients or their families who have a formal job (serving 40% of Mexicans), if they lose their job they are treated through the Secretary of Health, which is dependent on the federal government (OECD Studies on Health Systems: Mexico 2016).

On the other hand, if they are federal government workers, other providers such as the Social Security and Services for State Employees or Petroleum of Mexico, etc., offer other health services (OECD Studies on Health Systems: Mexico 2016). In Mexico, out-of-pocket payment constitutes 45% of total health expenses (Caldera, 2014) and 4% of household expenses, being one of the highest in the OECD (OECD Studies on Health Systems: Mexico 2016). Mexico has one of the highest rates of disproportion between the OECD private and public health sector; 11.4 public hospitals vs 28.6 private hospitals per million inhabitants (OECD Studies on Health Systems: Mexico 2016). However, only 15% of the working population has life insurance for private medicine (AMIS, 2020).

In 2020, according to the Mexican Society of Pediatric Neurology, A.C. in Mexico, there are approximately 475 pediatric neurologists, and most are in large cities (SMNP, 2020). In this context, we propose to describe two real cases of children with neurological diseases who attended two public third-level health institutions that constituted medical and humanistic management challenges. For the second clinical case please read Always offer Greater well-being to the patient chapter.

DESCRIPTION OF THE CLINICAL CASES

Patient 1: Female neonate, first premature twin of 33.3 weeks of gestation, who was born on February 3, 2020, weighing 1745 gr, size 42 cm and an Apgar 8 - 9, who needed neonatal resuscitation with non-invasive mechanical ventilation of the airway and supplemental oxygen during the first 22 days of her life, she was discharged with gastroesophageal reflux with cisapride and esomeprazole, without data on neurological deficits and ultrasonography. The twins were the product of the first pregnancy of their 40-year-old mother, who was diagnosed with a bi-corial bi-amniotic pregnancy, and who developed polyhydramnios and pre-eclampsia with poor control with alpha methyldopa, steroids, and clopidogrel that caused decelerations of the fetal heart rate, so it was decided to perform an urgent cesarean section, which passed without complications. She was the first twin. Her twin was diagnosed with Down syndrome, duodenal agenesis, pulmonary hypoplasia and intraventricular hemorrhage grade II; because of this, she underwent a gastrojejunal anastomosis and she was left with a gastrostomy; however, she developed septic shock and respiratory complications for which she died 28 days after birth.

On March 14, 2020 (18 days after being discharged), twin 1 (39.1 weeks of gestation) was admitted for clinical data of urosepsis, so she received treatment with cefotaxime and amikacin, however, that same night of her readmission she had a bronchoaspiration with milk that induced cardiorespiratory arrest so it required advanced cardiopulmonary resuscitation maneuvers for 20 minutes, so she was transferred to intensive pediatric therapy, where bronchial aspiration pneumonia was diagnosed and she was managed with vasoactive amines, mechanical ventilation, fluticasone, meropenem and vancomycin for 2 weeks, in addition to being diagnosed with hypoxic-ischemic encephalopathy after cardio-respiratory arrest (Figure 1), EEG monitoring was started in which a non-convulsive electrical epileptic state was diagnosed, due to which started treatment with Levetiracetam IV (80 mg / kg / day), midazolam IV (300 µg / kg / h), phenytoin IV (9 mg / kg / d) and phenobarbital IV (5 mg / kg /day); and due to his refractoriness, she underwent therapeutic hypothermia with monitoring of integrated amplitude EEG (aEEG) for 72h until the epileptic state was aborted. Simple skull tomography showed grade III intraventricular hemorrhage in the left hemisphere involving the ipsilateral thalamus, so she underwent drainage of intraventricular hemorrhage (Figure 2) and developed periventricular leukomalacia in the right hemisphere and multicystic encephalomalacia in the left hemisphere, so she was discharged from the hospital (Figure 3).

In her follow-up by telemedicine at 86 days (2 months, 3 weeks, 3 days of age; 45.5 weeks of age) she was alert and reactive with weak crying, axial hypotonia, and spastic diplegia in lower limbs, asymmetric tonic reflex, and incomplete weak moron. She continued breastfeeding on levetiracetam, phenobarbital, cisapride, spironolactone, esomeprazole, supplemental oxygen, and in physical rehabilitation. She received pneumococcal and tetravalent vaccines. At 46.5 weeks of gestation, the evoked potentials showed moderate right sensorineural hearing loss and demyelination of the bilateral cortical retinal visual pathway, and she was diagnosed with severe bronchopulmonary dysplasia and West syndrome.

Figure 1. Scalp EEG (chronological age 45 days of life, 39.6 corrected weeks, shows disorganized background activity: severe asynchrony, inter-outbreak with intervals of 26 seconds, brief bi-temporal rhythmic abnormal acute waves. Filters 1-70Hz, Notch: 60Hz

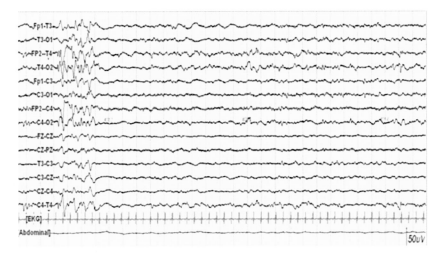

Figure 2. Simple skull tomography. At 40.5 weeks of gestation, showing grade III intraventricular hemorrhage in the left hemisphere involving the ipsilateral thalamus.

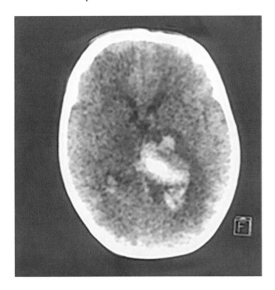

Figure 3. Simple MRI of the brain at 42 weeks of gestation, showing in T2 FLAIR (A: Transversal, B and C: Coronal), periventricular leukomalacia in the right hemisphere, multicystic encephalomalacia in the left hemisphere and intraventricular hematic remains.

519

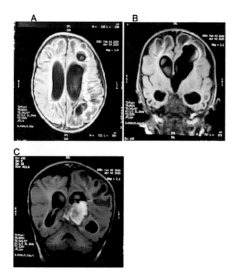

Figure 4. Awakened scalp EEG (chronological age: 3 months of life, 46.4 corrected weeks of gestation), shows disorganized background activity with severe asynchrony and left front-center-temporal epileptiform activity. Filters 1-70Hz, Notch: 60Hz.

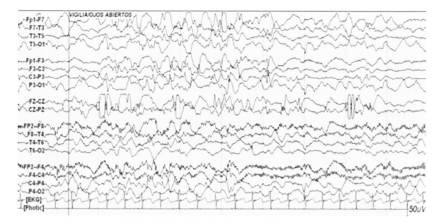

DISCUSSION

In this case, a mother who has factors that classify her as a high-risk pregnancy (age over 35 and multiple gestations) that predisposed her to maternal and pediatric complications

(Holness, 2018), such as preeclampsia and acute fetal distress (Adank et al., 2020) is illustrated. A French study that included 1102 twins (551 pregnancies) found that 9.8% of these infants had a poor outcome; 40.7% of the times one of the twins dies (Chitrit et al., 1999), as happened in this unfortunate situation that derived from multiple organic anomalies, being the pulmonary anomalies and intraventricular hemorrhage, the critics to define their survival, and have associated premature births in multiple pregnancies (Wong et al., 2015). In the surviving neonate, bronchoaspiration was key to the development of pneumonia that led to the cardio-respiratory arrest that required intensive medical management with mechanical ventilation and management with amines and antibiotics, however, the brain developed hypoxic-ischemic encephalopathy.

So continuous electroencephalographic monitoring was started, which in this context is considered a crucial part of a critically ill child since it allows up to 14% of critically ill patients to be diagnosed with a non-convulsive epileptic state (DeLorenzo et al., 1998) and subsequently guide treatment in particular when therapeutic hypothermia was indicated, which has been successful in cases of refractory epileptic states (Casey et al., 2011; Guilliams et al., 2013). Derived from all these multifactorial etiologies is that intracranial hemorrhages developed that directly impacted the neurological development of twin 1, regardless of the gestational age at birth (Ment et al., 2015) and with a normal initial transfontanelar ultrasound. Many of these critical events and their follow-up occurred in the context of the SARS-CoV2 pandemic, given that in Mexico the first case was reported on February 28, 2020 (Ornelas-Aguirre, 2020), which made its intra attention very complex. In-hospital and out-of-hospital care, so that all the measures and guidelines currently followed in the world were being developed in parallel and not much information was available (Griffin et al., 2020).

Looking at it from a humanistic point of view, the patients (mother and daughters) received "excellent in-hospital and out-of-hospital care," especially during the global health emergency for SARS-CoV-2 (COVID-19). Unfortunately, the mother suffered from pre-eclampsia and the pregnancy had to be terminated due to fetal distress, twin 2 died at 28 days from severe congenital complications. Fortunately, the mother and twin 1 were discharged without becoming infected with SARS-CoV-2 during their 22-day hospital stay.

This reflection leads us to delve into the peculiarities of the clinical relationship. The term "excellence," from its origins in classical Greek culture, translates a basic term of ethics, that of "areté." Today we can translate it into "virtue" and understand it as a positive moral quality (the ability to do something well). Therefore, a good health professional is one who has the proper name of his activity (medical activity). This undoubtedly means that said professional is virtuous in search of the best well-being of their patient (Gracia, 2004).

This situation is reflected in the medical care received by the patients (mother and daughters) and the framework in which the clinical relationship developed; A quick tour of specific aspects are presented, such as personalized care, the organization of care within the teamwork and the doctor's decision to send the mother and daughter home and continue with the medical care and the therapy of early stimulation by means of telecare, given the conditions of the health crisis and the risk of contagion by SARS-CoV-2. These actions guaranteed equal and effective access to health benefits on an equal basis for all Mexicans.

The clinical relationship is, therefore, a complex relationship between two or more human beings in which, in a situation of great uncertainty such as the situation of disease and vulnerability, technical and informative elements of medical science are brought into play together with elements of values in order to make decisions, as in this specific case in a situation of great uncertainty to offer the greatest possible well-being to both patients. Many authors have studied and characterized these different models of clinical relationships (Veatch 1981, Gracia, 2004; Quill, 2001). However, there is an important fact to mention in this clinical case. The fact that this is a single mother who aged with the desire to have a pregnancy, which is complicated by the presence of pre-eclampsia, which contributes significantly to twin 1 having severe and irreversible neurological damage despite the therapeutic efforts made to offer the greatest possible well-being.

Uncertainty plays a very important role in medicine, especially when making decisions. It is precisely this uncertainty, which threatens to render ethical knowledge ineffective in future responsibility in daily medical practice, such as this specific case that we present and, of course, that this ethical theory of responsibility has to be incorporated into said clinical practice as a new principle that can be effective as a practical precept (Jonas, 1995).

From the ethical analysis, there is a consensus in affirming that not everything technically possible is necessarily ethically admissible, and hence we have reasons to limit the therapeutic effort, reasons that, obviously, were very well justified, as in the case of twin 2. The team of physicians from the beginning, with non-maleficence, made the decision not to put procedures that are clearly contraindicated to firstly avoid causing harm, this is clearly observed in both cases (twin 1 and twin 2). Prudence calls for a shared framework in decision-making based on the recognition that individualized it which requires both contributions (the precautionary principle and the non-maleficence principle) because what is at stake is life, health, and the dignity of both twins. These ethical principles or values converge in promoting the well-being of both patients (Buchanan and Brock, 1989).

REFERENCES

1. Adank, M.C., Broere-Brown, Z.A., Gonçalves, R., Ikram, M.K., Jaddoe, V.W.V., Steegers, E.A.P., Schalekamp-Timmermans, S., 2020. Maternal cardiovascular adaptation to twin pregnancy: a population-based prospective cohort study. BMC Pregnancy Childbirth 20, 327. https://doi.org/10.1186/s12884-020-02994-wAMIS [WWW Document], n.d. URL https://sitio.amis.com.mx/ (accessed 6.15.20).

2. Bagley, C.A., Pindrik, J.A., Bookland, M.J., Camara-Quintana, J.Q., Carson, B.S., 2006. Cervicomedullary decompression for foramen magnum stenosis in achondroplasia. J. Neurosurg. 104, 166–172. https://doi.org/10.3171/ped.2006.104.3.166

3. Buchanan, A.E., Brock, D.W., 1989. Deciding for Others: The Ethics of Surrogate Decision Making [WWW Document]. BRL:KIE/32047. http://dx.doi.org/10.1017/CBO9781139171946

4. Caldera, A., 2014. Working Papers No . 873 Towards a Better Understanding of the Informal Economy Dan Andrews , Aida Caldera Sánchez ,. https://doi.org/10.1787/5kgb1m-f88x28-en

5. Casey, D.M., Tella, N., Turesky, R., Labrecque, M., 2011. Therapeutic hypothermia: treatment for hypoxic-ischemic encephalopathy in the NICU. Neonatal Netw. NN 30, 370–380. https://doi.org/10.1891/0730-0832.30.6.370

6. Chitrit, Y., Filidori, M., Pons, J.C., Duyme, M., Papiernik, E., 1999. Perinatal mortality in twin pregnancies: a 3-year analysis in Seine Saint-Denis (France). Eur. J. Obstet. Gynecol. Reprod. Biol. 86, 23–28. https://doi.org/10.1016/s0301-2115(99)00037-8

7. Consejo Nacional de Población | Gobierno | gob.mx [WWW Document], n.d. URL https://www.gob.mx/conapo (accessed 6.15.20).

8. DeLorenzo, R.J., Waterhouse, E.J., Towne, A.R., Boggs, J.G., Ko, D., DeLorenzo, G.A., Brown, A., Garnett, L., 1998. Persistent nonconvulsive status epilepticus after the control of convulsive status epilepticus. Epilepsia 39, 833–840. https://doi.org/10.1111/j.1528-1157.1998.tb01177.x

9. Estudios de la OCDE sobre los Sistemas de Salud: México 2016, 2016. , Estudios de la OCDE sobre los Sistemas de Salud: México 2016. https://doi.org/10.1787/9789264265523-es

10. Gracia, D., 2004. ÉTICA EN LA PRÁCTICA CLÍNICA. TRIACASTELA, Madrid.

11. Griffin, I., Benarba, F., Peters, C., Oyelese, Y., Murphy, T., Contreras, D., Gagliardo, C., Nwaobasi-Iwuh, E., DiPentima, M.C., Schenkman, A., 2020. The Impact of COVID-19 Infection on Labor and Delivery, Newborn Nursery, and Neonatal Intensive Care Unit: Prospective Observational Data from a Single Hospital System. Am. J. Perinatol. https://doi.org/10.1055/s-0040-1713416

12. Guilliams, K., Rosen, M., Buttram, S., Zempel, J., Pineda, J., Miller, B., Shoykhet, M., 2013. Hypothermia for pediatric refractory status epilepticus. Epilepsia 54, 1586–1594. https://doi.org/10.1111/epi.12331

13. Holness, N., 2018. High-Risk Pregnancy. Nurs. Clin. North Am. 53, 241–251. https://doi.org/10.1016/j.cnur.2018.01.010

14. Hoover-Fong, J., McGready, J., Schulze, K., Alade, A.Y., Scott, C.I., 2017. A height-for-age growth reference for children with achondroplasia: Expanded applications and com-

parison with original reference data. Am. J. Med. Genet. A. 173, 1226–1230. https://doi.org/10.1002/ajmg.a.38150

15. Instituto Nacional de Estadística y Geografía (INEGI) [WWW Document], n.d. URL https://inegi.org.mx/default.html (accessed 6.2.20).

16. Jonas, H., 1995. El principio de responsabilidad: ensayo de una ética para la civilización tecnológica. Barcelona, España: Herder.

17. Kubota, T., Adachi, M., Kitaoka, T., Hasegawa, K., Ohata, Y., Fujiwara, M., Michigami, T., Mochizuki, H., Ozono, K., 2020. Clinical practice guidelines for achondroplasia. Clin. Pediatr. Endocrinol. 29, 25–42. https://doi.org/10.1297/cpe.29.25

18. Ment, L.R., Ådén, U., Bauer, C.R., Bada, H.S., Carlo, W.A., Kaiser, J.R., Lin, A., Cotten, C.M., Murray, J., Page, G., Hallman, M., Lifton, R.P., Zhang, H., 2015. Genes and Environment in Neonatal Intraventricular Hemorrhage. Semin. Perinatol. 39, 592–603. https://doi.org/10.1053/j.semperi.2015.09.006

19. Ornelas-Aguirre, J.M., 2020. The new coronavirus that came from the East: analysis of the initial epidemic in Mexico. Gac. Med. Mex. 156.

20. Quill, D.T.E., 2001. A Midwife through the Dying Process: Stories of Healing and Hard Choices at the End of Life, 1 edition. ed. The Johns Hopkins University Press.

21. Ronen, G.M., Rosenbaum, P.L., 2017. Reflections on Ethics and Humanity in Pediatric Neurology: the Value of Recognizing Ethical Issues in Common Clinical Practice. Curr. Neurol. Neurosci. Rep. 17, 39. https://doi.org/10.1007/s11910-017-0749-7

22. Simón, P., Barrio, I.M., 2004. ¿Quién puede decidir por mí? Una revisión de la legislación española vigente sobre las

decisiones de representación y las instrucciones previas. Rev. Calid. Asist. 19, 460–472. https://doi.org/10.1016/S1134-282X(04)77743-X

23. Sisk, B.A., Canavera, K., Sharma, A., Baker, J.N., Johnson, L.-M., 2019. Ethical issues in the care of adolescent and young adult oncology patients. Pediatr. Blood Cancer 66, e27608. https://doi.org/10.1002/pbc.27608

24. SMNP - Sociedad Mexicana de Neuro Pediatría [WWW Document], n.d. URL https://neuropediatria.org.mx/#/nosotros/red (accessed 6.15.20).

25. Trotter, T.L., Hall, J.G., 2005. Health supervision for children with achondroplasia. Pediatrics 116, 771–783. https://doi.org/10.1542/peds.2005-1440

26. Veatch RM A Theory of Medical Ethics by Robert M. Veatch New York, Basic Books, 1981. 387 pp. Theol. Today 39, 216–216. https://doi.org/10.1177/004057368203900219

27. White, K.K., Bompadre, V., Goldberg, M.J., Bober, M.B., Campbell, J.W., Cho, T.J., Hoover-Fong, J., Mackenzie, W., Parnell, S.E., Raggio, C., Rapoport, D.M., Spencer, S.A., Savarirayan, R., 2015. Best practices in the evaluation and treatment of foramen magnum stenosis in achondroplasia during infancy. Am. J. Med. Genet. A. 170, 42–51. https://doi.org/10.1002/ajmg.a.37394

28. Wong, L.F., Holmgren, C.M., Silver, R.M., Varner, M.W., Manuck, T.A., 2015. Outcomes of expectantly managed pregnancies with multiple gestations and preterm premature rupture of membranes prior to 26 weeks. Am. J. Obstet. Gynecol. 212, 215.e1–9. https://doi.org/10.1016/j.ajog.2014.09.005

HUMANISM IN NEONATAL NEUROLOGY – PERSPECTIVE FROM A NOT YET DEVELOPED REGION

Varnit Shanker, MBBS, DCH (UK), MRCPCH
ALM Biology degree candidate, HES, Harvard University
Consultant, Department of Neonatal Neurocritical Care,
DACH, Jaipur, India

Children born with metabolic errors, severe hypoxic brain injuries or other neurological insults are living longer in the twenty first century. Several generations of clinicians and researchers have provided insights regarding these complex pathologies. Parents are now able to see hope in contrast to their counterparts a few decades earlier. However, without advanced medical interventions, were these severely disabled and genetically erred neonates destined to survive? As much as we want it, the answer is probably not. This raises the question if intensivists and neurologists are attempting to alter the natural course decided by the mighty evolution? The answer is again, probably not. As an example, certain bacteria have rapidly incorporated antimicrobial genes, helping them survive the antibiotics when they were ought to die. This highlights that seldom utilizing, seldom overcoming the genetic and environmental obstacles has been the hallmark of evolutionary progress. Humans are inevitably acting out to protect their kind in accordance with natural instincts and an advanced neocortex.

But that very sophisticated brain also holds us responsible for the consequences following our interventions. Emotions and logical reasoning are as much critical components of human existence as the very instinct of survival. Clinicians are uniquely placed to make a judgment call based on parental wish and their own experience, whether to proceed with a life-saving intervention or not. For example, if a child with severe chronic neurodisability lands up in the ICU after aspiration, clinician's opinions carry a huge impact on the final parental decision regarding the DNR consent.

General consensus is that medical fraternity is hard wired to "save" life. In any acute illness or emergency situation it is out of reflex to think about preserving life. Extreme preterms born as low as 500 grams, Hypoxic Ischemic Encephalopathy Grade III neonates with no spontaneous respiration, neonatal septicemia cases with intraventricular hemorrhage or mechanically ventilated neonate without clinical improvement in the last forty eight hours – in all these situations, the clinician always attempts to reverse the damage compelled by duty, skills and medical optimism. In many cases, unfortunately, horizon of optimism is reached and there remains no other alternative to accept the reality that the child cannot be cured.

In our neurocritical care practice, we have realized that there is a huge space between absolute optimism that the child will be cured and realization that nothing more can be done. Few critical cases carry favorable prognosis right from the beginning. A case of neonatal seizures with hypocalcemia, hypoglycemia, hypothermia and septicemia is critical, but we have rarely lost a newborn with such diagnosis. On the other end of the critical spectrum, a non-responsive intubated neonate on inotropes, with twelve days of illness, hypotension, anasarca, refractory seizures, bilateral severe pneumonitis and·

anuria will most likely succumb. However, there are numerous instances, when situation is not clear enough to predict the outcome. This is typically relevant for primary neurological insults. After each assessment, the confusion only deepens if the child will come out healthy or not. Further, it remains uncertain about the long-term neurological outcome of the child even if he / she survives. At this juncture, principles of Humanism in clinical decision-making start getting blurred.

Humanism is a state of democracy with medical ethics as its constitution. The constitutional rule book (medical ethics) remains objective but its (humanism) interpretation in democratic setting is subjective. This makes humanism a perspective based philosophy. Despite agreeable code of medical ethics, a singular patient scenario can have multiple versions of humanism. Additionally, these versions of humanism in medicine can evolve temporally.

For instance, evaluation and role of parental emotions in the long-term management of pediatric neurological conditions is an understudied area. Modern medicine is largely evidence based with established flowcharts. The patient management is considered successful following a completed checklist. By default, it is an understood position that such approach will incorporate principles of medical ethics. Ethics not only protect the patient but also help treating physicians justify their actions taken in the patient's "best interest." In complex ethical dilemmas, an objective consensus can be reached with discussions between stakeholders. But in this process, especially in the developing world where universal health coverage is unavailable, socio-economic constraints, cultural factors, level of parental education, availability of medical resources, social support and impact of saving a disabled life on the family and siblings is ignored. Humanism in neonatal neurology cannot be limited to holistic care of the patient, but has to also account for a holistic care of the family.

In the last year (2019), our unit (DACH Neonatal Neurocritical Care) catered to 880 neonatal neurology cases. The vast majority of them (549) had delayed cry after birth. 53 of these neonates were born roadside, non-home non-hospital deliveries, of whom 18 developed fulminant septicaemia. Of these 53 neonates, 47 were born in below poverty line families. 218 neonates out of 549, required mechanical ventilation for more than 3 days. 64 of these neonates were labelled as Grade III HIE. 32 of them belonged to lower socio economic strata and 12 neonates belonged to families below the poverty line. 87 out of 880 neonates were diagnosed as bacterial meningitis and 8 neonates developed some form of complication. 4 of these 8 neonates were born in families living below the poverty line. Of 880, only 330 families could understand nature of the disease, prognosis and possible complications. The rest of all the families were dependent on family friends, neighbours or others for getting an idea of the situation. Based on our estimates, close to 250 neonates will be lost on follow up because of economic constraints. Most of these families belong to rural India, with primary care facilities within a few miles reach at best. We suspect, of these 880 cases, at least 65 neonates will have some form of neurological deficit and close to 24 neonates will likely have severe neurological sequalae. Strikingly, 18 out of 24 families belong to lower economic strata or below the poverty line.

I clearly remember 4 neonates from economically backward families, who were extremely critical and carried little chances of survival. However in these neonates, neurological deficits were clearly apparent. In all 4 independent scenarios, the parents communicated their wish to not continue the treatment anymore. It went against my instinct to agree to their wish but eventually our team did respect their opinion to withdraw the care in view of possible severe neurological sequalae. Retrospectively, I feel it was a painful decision to make. At the same time it was a correct one.

Parents coming from rural India tell frightening stories. To afford a quality clinical care for child, means loss of lifelong savings for many families. When a family doesn't have guaranteed meals twice a day, when the children have no footwear, no schooling and the nearest primary healthcare facility is at a distance of 40 miles; how can anyone expect the family to take care of child with cerebral palsy? Despite this reality, there are instances when clinicians, with no fault of their own, are adamant on continuing care of the newborn with evident signs of brain damage. And unfortunately, I have been one of those clinicians in the very early stages of my career.

Like all residents, as a young paediatrician all I wanted was to diagnose and treat the child at all costs. Patient counselling is fluidic in nature – the reality may be critical but words of physicians can give or take away hope. Even after an objective explanation of the child's condition, most of times I saw parents joining their hands asking me to do whatever "I" feel is right. As a resident, discharging a child meant successful patient management. But on several occasions I have wondered if saving the child's life was wise or mere stubbornness. It is a difficult conversation to have and to face the realities in developing countries with humongous resource constraints. The healthcare models of developed countries can't be copied in an absolutely different and dismal scenario. There has to be a consensus on continuing the care in light of evidence of severe brain injury. Keeping patient's dignity and families' limitation in mind, while avoiding single minded approach to save lives at all costs might be the humanism that we need.

Yes, every effort must be made to ensure universal health coverage and social support systems. But for many populations in the world this is a tough and long journey. While these populations make their journey to reach at a point where healthcare becomes a natural right, attention must be paid to the thought process of all stakeholders. Their wish at times might sound cruel and even unethical, but it must be remembered that unlike medical ethics, humanism can encompass both the former and the latter.

Jade Vine flower or Strongylodon macrobotrys is a unique species with a turquoise flower color, varying from blue-green to mint green. It seems to be endemic to the Philippines and is usually found in dense forests. But because of difficult propagation due to limited number of its natural pollinators – this species has become endangered. Despite a stunning visual treat, it cannot survive in the absence of a medium to thrive. To summarize, I propose The Jade Vine Conjecture of Humanism – despite purest of intentions to preserve life, a deficient healthcare and social support can make lives of the resource-limited family as difficult as a loss of life.

A STORY OF RESURRECTION

Ornella Ciccone, (SFMA) MD
Consultant Paediatric Neurologist
Istituto Serafico, Assisi, Italy
University Teaching Hospitals - Children's Hospital
Lusaka, Zambia

It was a quiet rainy day when I saw a shining car entering our gate and stopping in the parking area of the Convent. A gentleman dressed in "a suit and tie" came out of the car, accompanied by a simply dressed young woman. She was carrying something that could be a baby, wrapped in a typical Zambian cloth. It was a day of the week in which I used to remain home from the hospital to offer free neurological assessments for children with disabilities looking for possible school placement and rehabilitation in our facility. Most of the children referred to our Centre by other missionaries were from distant villages or from shanty compounds in the periphery of Lusaka. The gentleman stopped in front of the door and greeted me in a polite and shy manner.

I asked them to come in and let me see the baby. When they uncovered him, I was caught by both surprise and sorrow to see a very small, wasted child with the facial expression of a much older child. He had multiple limbs contractions, several black dental caries, and long nails on his hands and feet. His clothes were very old and his skin was so dry, but what struck me the most was the fear in his eyes and the expression of pain on his face. I tried to call him by name "Gift" and talk to him, but he was just crying, arching his back in a spastic-dystonic posture.

I did not know how to start asking questions. I asked the young lady if she was the child's mother, but she told me that she was just the "maid," and pointed at the gentleman. The man started narrating that he was the child's father and he explained to me, in clear and correct English, the complications that occurred during his son's birth, and how they later tried to take him to some doctors, hoping that he could get well. He was working in a large company and his wife was a teacher. Mum was very busy with school and the child was at home, with the maid, most of the time. This man was looking down, and speaking in a very low tone, as he narrated the story. I could feel all the pain and embarrassment passing through his heart... and I could not put together the severe state of child neglect I was witnessing with the educational and social background of the man.

I looked again at the child and I noticed a cluster of focal seizures. Dad told me that they occurred several times a day. The child was not on anti-seizure medications (ASM) as they tried one drug, without effect, and they thought that it was not possible to control them; they tried prayers but "they did not work" as well. I decided to start from the matter of the seizures; after explaining the possibility of controlling them with proper medications, Dad agreed to put him on treatment, which also meant that he would take Gift regularly to my clinic for follow-up. I was happy to see them back in a few days' time reporting an initial reduction of seizures. I could then start to adjust doses of ASM, introduce some more treatment to reduce spasticity and pain, and orient the maid on how to feed Gift and care for him, including talking, playing music, and trying to play with him.

Some weeks later, I was surprised when the maid brought Gift for review at the clinic, accompanied by Gift's mother. Mum was looking very tense; she sat down and kept quiet. I asked her how her child was doing in the last weeks, and she said "much less seizures", and followed with these words: "I did not believe that it was possible to control them." I waited for her to continue; her eyes became red and filled with tears. After some seconds of silence, she started narrating what happened at birth: the baby did not cry, he was resuscitated and put in oxygen and later discharged during the day. In the following month, she noticed that the baby had abnormal movements, he could not look and smile at her, he was unable to hold his head early on and to sit and stand later. She went to a clinic where she was told that the child's brain got spoiled at birth and there was nothing that could be done; the child was not going to talk or to walk, even if he were to receive physiotherapy. Mum said that she fell into great disappointment and depression. She felt that whatever effort she was putting into helping the child improve was just a waste; "from that time on, I stopped caring for him," she said among her tears; Gift was now 8 years old. I let her cry, then I slowly started to tell her how many things we could do, with them and the clinic's staff, to make Gift feel better and happy. We then started a journey together, which lasted from months to years.

I will never forget one sunny morning when Mum and Dad came for the medical review of the son at the clinic; Mum was holding her child. Gift was smiling and he looked relaxed; his skin was shining and clean; he had beautiful clothes and new shoes. Mum and Dad were looking at him with loving smiles. He was the same child with spastic quadriplegia, unable to talk and walk, but a new gaze, radiant of joy and peace was now shining in Gift's and his parents' eyes.

ALWAYS OFFER GREATER WELL-BEING TO THE PATIENT

Daniel San-Juan, MD, Msc
Epilepsy Clinic at the National Institute of Neurology and
Neurosurgery (NINN), Mexico City, Mexico

Rosana Huerta Albarran, MD, Msc
Pediatric Service, Hospital General de México "Dr. Eduardo
Liceaga," México City, Mexico

Efrain Olivas Pena, MD
Clinical Neurophysiology Laboratory, National Institute of
Perinatology, Mexico City, Mexico

Tirso Zuniga Santamaria, MD, PhD
Neuro-genetic Department at the National Institute of Neurology and Neurosurgery (NINN), Mexico City, Mexico

Patient 2. 2-year, 9-month-old female with achondroplasia,
without any history of the disease in the family or history of
repeated respiratory disease, only with chronic constipation.
It was the product of the third gestation of a 41-year-old mother, with prenatal control at the expense of 8 consultations
with three obstetric ultrasounds, the mother studied during
pregnancy with urinary tract infection and cervicovaginitis
in the first trimester, receiving unspecified treatment and remission, achondroplasia was diagnosed in the product at the
eighth month of gestation, the breast did not consume folic
acid or received immunizations during pregnancy, and the
rest of the pregnancy was normal. She was born by cesarean
section for achondroplasia at 38 weeks gestation, weighing
2450 grams, height 43 cm, discharged after 72 hours without
complications. Her neurological development was appropri-

ate for her age. Her CT scan of 1 year and 3 months after admission showed data on the narrow medullary canal.

She went to the emergency room due to falling from the ladder, getting hit in the back of the neck, the mother did not see the fall, and found her unable to move, with loss of alertness for two minutes, with the subsequent presence of pallor and perioral cyanosis. Upon admission, she was alert, without verbal response, hypoactive, with integumentary pallor, with the cranial-face relationship altered by macrocephaly, a prominent frontal region, a depressed nasal bridge, with 80% saturation that improved with the placement of a mask with supplemental oxygen; she presented neurological deterioration with quadriparesis and bradypnea, a new tomography of the skull was performed with cortico-subcortical atrophy predominantly frontoparietal with more marked ventricular dilation in the lateral ventricles and discrete in the third ventricle, with no data on the joint bone lesion or physiological evaluation, the reason why a rigid Philadelphia type collar was placed. The neurological examination with an incomplete medullary syndrome, muscular strength 1/5 in the upper extremities and 0/5 in the lower extremities, reactive to sensory stimulation and its magnetic resonance imaging of the brain showed a stenosis of the foramen magnum associated with achondroplasia, which conditioned compressive myelopathy and Cystic myelomalacia from C1 to C7 with the medulla oblongata. During her hospitalization, she presented sudden and severe arterial hypotension that did not improve with fluid replacement, which required mechanical ventilation and management of spinal cord shock with amines and methylprednisolone for one month. Medullary decompression was proposed by means of suboccipital craniectomy and posterior C1 arch resection, but the adequately informed parents did not initially accept the surgical procedure, they were given enough time to reconsider, and the intervention was reconsidered, explaining the complications of it not happening.

In its evolution 30 days after hospitalization, she was neurologically established with adequate interaction with the environment, respiratory automatism, persistent quadriplegia, and response to painful stimuli. However, in-hospital pneumonia was diagnosed with segmental atelectasis in the left upper lobe and later left pulmonary total atelectasis, which resolved, persisting with poor functional prognosis, due to immobility, a tracheostomy was performed to manage the airway. Severe chronic malnutrition related to low intake was documented despite orogastric tube feeding and parenteral nutrition. In addition, she developed urinary tract infections with Enterococcus faecium managed with ceftriaxone and a sacral ulcer infected with Escherichia coli and Acinetobacter baumani. taking that into account, an early physical rehabilitation program was started to manage immobility and contractures.

At 3 years, 4 months, she presented respiratory distress, requiring hospitalization with mechanical ventilation. She developed community-acquired pneumonia managed with ceftazidime and clindamycin, but manifested clinical deterioration due to fever, with increased transtracheal secretions, severe hypoxemia, and increased ventilation parameters, she received multiple antimicrobial regimens: imipenem - amikacin, vancomycin, colistin, piperacillin. - tazobactam, fluconazole, tigecycline; polyculture at each isolated scheme change during their stay Candida albicans and Pseudomonas aeruginosa. She developed a urinary tract infection with Escherichia coli, Klebsiella pneumoniae, and Enterococcus faecalis. Unfortunately, this led her to present two cardiorespiratory arrests with a duration of 6 minutes and a difference of 15 days each, with subsequent neurological sequelae at the expense of loss of interaction with the environment, with no ocular response to light in the right eye, only the left one with a response, sudden saccadic movements in the horizontal axis, normal intraocular pressure, normal fundus, with spontaneous ocular opening and closing associated with a circadian cycle, no follow-up or fixation of objects, persistent quadriplegia, with manifest pyramidal data from exhaustible clonus in both feet, she continued with rehabilitation and received management with gabapentin. In her evolution, she presented a clonic focal seizure in the right hemibody of onset in the leg after ipsilateral upper limb with evolution to bilateral, lasting 30 seconds, she was administered an IV of phenytoin and then orally. Her simple skull tomography with cortico-subcortical atrophy with increased volume of the ventricular system, visual evoked potentials without a response at the level of the optic nerves. Pressure ulcers in the sacral region (3 cm in diameter, with scant serous secretion and a fundus that reaches deep dermis with fibrin cream) were documented with patches since the previous hospitalization; another ulcer in the occipital region of 1 cm in diameter, with little serous secretion, in management with bepanthen, toilet, mobilization, and an air mattress. The parents on this occasion were anxious to offer her a surgical possibility that improves conditions and requested a multidisciplinary session, but it was explained that the current conditions are not favorable for a surgical procedure and the prognosis of the procedure given the evolution and spinal damage is not good for the function. She remained hospitalized accompanied at all times by her parents until she died three months after her re-entry.

DISCUSSION

Achondroplasia is a skeletal dysplasia that presents limb shortening characterized by rhizomelia and short stature, an incidence of 1 per 10,000 to 30,000 births is estimated. It is caused by abnormal endochondral ossification of the skeleton, affecting the extension of the long bones and most of the bones of the vertebral bodies, as well as the base of the skull, manifesting with stenosis of the foramen magnum, ventriculomegaly and hydrocephalus due to poor circulation of cerebrospinal fluid and spinal canal stenosis, as well as compression myelopathy of the medullary canal. This is due to a gain-of-function mutation in the fibroblast growth factor receptor 3 gene (FGFR3), in ≥ 97% of patients in which glycine is replaced by arginine (Gly380Arg) located on chromosome 4p26.3, with an autosomal dominant inheritance; although in 80% of cases it is due to spontaneous mutations in healthy parents (Kubota et al., 2020; White et al., 2015) as is our patient.

Clinically, features such as an elongated skull, prominent forehead, flattened nasal bridge, medial facial hypoplasia, relative protrusion of the jaw, and a trident hand configuration are also observed. The clinical characteristics and radiological findings are observed from the neonatal period, although 20% of patients are not diagnosed at this time. As development progresses, spinal kyphosis and joint hyper-extensibility become more noticeable, obstructive sleep apnea may occur due to upper airway stenosis or even central apnea due to spinal cord compression or vertebral arteries due to stenosis of the foramen magnum with cervical myelopathy, with reports of sudden death in 2 to 10% of cases (Kubota et al., 2020; Trotter and Hall, 2005; White et al., 2015).

That is why monitoring and early intervention are recommended through multidisciplinary management that includes a clinical history with neurological exploration and polysomnography (Kubota et al., 2020; Trotter and Hall, 2005; White et al., 2015); If these alterations are suspected, magnetic resonance imaging should be requested. Monitoring is essential, every two months up to one year (White et al., 2015), then every 3 months up to two years, and then every year, evaluating the neurological clinical history with an emphasis on searching for respiratory sleep disorders (White et al., 2015), hypotonia, weakness, asymmetry in movement and reflexes, sustained clonus, weak sucking at feeding, presence of seizures and developmental delay; that is why growth monitoring (weight, height, and head circumference) (Hoover-Fong et al., 2017; Trotter and Hall, 2005) and neurodevelopment, with standards in achondroplasia (Trotter and Hall, 2005). Requesting a neuroimaging study for all children with achondroplasia is controversial. In 2005 the American Academy of Pediatrics suggested even from the neonatal period for the opportunity to avoid sudden death through a bone window skull tomography, because it has measurement standards in people with achondroplasia of the length of the foramen magnum, with the opportunity to avoid sedation or by means of magnetic resonance imaging that would allow the brain structures to be seen with better quality (Trotter and Hall, 2005). However, the last consensus in 2015 through a Delphi process, carried out by 11 multidisciplinary experts from the United States, South Korea, and Australia, does not suggest neuroimaging for all patients; this due to radiation exposure in the case of tomography and sedation in the case of magnetic resonance imaging, leaving the request for the study in cases where there is an alteration in the medical history, neurological physical examination or in polysomnography with data from sleep apnea, primarily of the central type (White et al., 2015). The most recent clinical practice guidelines for achondroplasia published in Japan in January 2020, citing the 2015 consensus and comment that there is still no consensus to evaluate the complications of foramen magnum stenosis and the optimal time for its intervention; but they suggest magnetic resonance imaging of the brain to identify the lesion and handle the cervical cranial junction in childhood with care, with special care in baby carriers (Kubota et al., 2020). Although medullary compression due to foramen magnum stenosis is common, the frequency of symptomatic medullary compression is low. Decompression of the foramen magnum is recommended suboccipital (White et al., 2015) in case of image-detected abnormalities (signal changes in the spinal cord, myelomalacia, indentation of the spinal cord) associated with neurological symptoms or signs including disorders of the respiratory center(Kubota et al., 2020; White et al., 2015), this intervention has been necessary in 6.7 to 13.3% of patients at the age of 2 years (Kubota et al., 2020); and in case of communicating hydrocephalus, bypass valve placement is suggested. In the case of only having abnormal findings on MRI, surveillance is indicated every three months (White et al., 2015).

Regarding the risks of the intervention, in an 11-year review (1993-2003), 43 cases of pediatric patients with achondroplasia and stenosis of the foramen magnum were reviewed (one of them asymptomatic, but with evidence of severe cervical-medullary compression by resonance). The patients received decompression of the foramen magnum and superior cervical laminectomy with or without duralplasty, as well as placement of a bypass valve prior to or during decompression in whoever required it; the average age at the intervention was 70 months (2-199 months) and the average duration of symptoms was 7 months (1 to 12 months), no patient died, and most had clinical benefits that persisted at an average follow-up of 62.5 months (1-123 months, two patients lost follow-up), with no regression of symptoms. Postoperative hospitalization was on average 14 days (3-48 days), the most frequent complication was a cerebrospinal fluid leak in 7 patients and 4 of them with infection (9%) who responded to a systemic antibiotic, no patient had clinical deterioration. Immediately, but the symptoms returned in 5 of the patients due to recurrence of stenosis of the foramen magnum, so a new intervention was made with complete resolution of the symptoms, with transient involvement of the cranial nerves V and VII (Bagley et al., 2006). In summary, spinal decompression is useful for managing the spinal canal associated with neurological symptoms (Kubota et al., 2020).

In our patient, the severe limitation of movement predisposed to malnutrition and very difficult to manage nosocomial pneumonia that led to cardiorespiratory arrest with severe hypoxic-ischemic neurological damage, seizures and systemic complications with a frank deterioration of her health status until her death without being a candidate for surgical intervention in the latter scenario, but she was initially when she presented to the emergency room.

From the ethical point of view, the main criteria that should guide the tutors when deciding should be the search for the "direct benefit" of their client. This search authorizes to reject or withdraw any medical treatment or intervention (Simón and Barrio, 2004). Given the parents' refusal of an initial proposal for surgical treatment, health professionals are faced with a conflict of values. On the one hand, the life value, which in case of not applying the proposed surgical treatment will be seriously threatened. On the other hand, the will expressed by the parents (guardians), who are the legal representatives to express their decisions and exercise their right to refuse treatment, since the criteria of best interest must prevail, so the medical group must support in the guideline expressed by the tutors.

The therapeutic effort is limited in the intensive care units in different ways: not accepting the admission of certain patients, not initiating life support measures (including cardiopulmonary resuscitation),or withdrawing these measures once they have been established. One of the fundamental and most important aspects when withdrawing or not starting life support treatment is determining how the decision is made. In this case, the parents have to make the decision to continue with life support measures or to start palliative care, so that the tutors take on a fundamental role, being responsible for the decision. When it comes to chronic patients it is best to make a collegial decision by the group of treating doctors. The case is presented in a clinical session and after discussing it, the course of action is followed, which has received the support of the professionals involved in assisting the case and subsequently communicates the decision to the tutors (Ronen and Rosenbaum, 2017).

Prudence plays a very important role in decision-making based on promoting the best possible well-being for the patient, but ultimately what is at stake is health, quality of life and why not say it, the life of the patient. In this sense, preserving or maintaining life is not always or necessarily a benefit for the patient, it will depend on the type of life that is going to be maintained, as is clearly seen in this specific case when the tutors at a second time, request the surgical treatment, however, the health conditions, functional reserve and the presentation of the complications of the immobility syndrome are adverse to the quality of life for the patient (Gracia, 2004).

In the context of urgency, the so-called "duty of non-abandonment to the patient" acquires the particular characterization of "duty of relief," a natural duty of solidarity existing in a human collective. No one can avoid this feeling of collective solidarity, which is why support is given to the person in need, even if their well-being is compromised (Sisk et al., 2019). Artificial hydration and nutrition are medical treatments and can be uninitiated or withdrawn under the same conditions as any other form of medical treatment. This analysis of the girl's quality of life should be based primarily on clinical criteria such as the degree of suffering, pain, and recurrent complications of the immobility syndrome (pressure ulcers, pneumonia, and urinary tract infection, muscle pain, among others) and not in other social criteria. The three basic criteria for decision-making in minor patients are the subjective criterion, the substitute judgment criterion, and the best interest criterion.

In this case, we present a conflict of values between health personnel, who consider it necessary to carry out the surgical treatment in the first place to offer greater well-being to the patient and improve their quality of life based on available medical evidence. However, parents object to this. The professionals' conflict occurs between two values: on the one hand, the search for the best patient care, suggesting medullary decompression and avoiding their suffering; on the other hand, the respect of the will of her parents, who, in addition, and given the age of the girl, are under her tutelage. In this scenario, the treating medical group enables communication with the tutors to help them make the best decision both in the first time that they offer the surgical treatment that is indicated to improve their quality of life, and in the second time that the tutors request the surgical treatment and that the risk is greater than the benefit, and also would not improve their quality of life. Unfortunately, in the end, the girl passed away.

My Apology to Myself

Sarah Hisham Hassan Wagdy, BA
Faculty of Al-Alsun Ain Shams University,
Cairo, Egypt.

Dear self, this year is full of surprises and we have seen so many till now. You know I always knew that one day I must apologize to you and make amends with you, it had started with a doubt then this doubt had increased to a strong thought each day, but I never thought that that day may be so soon.

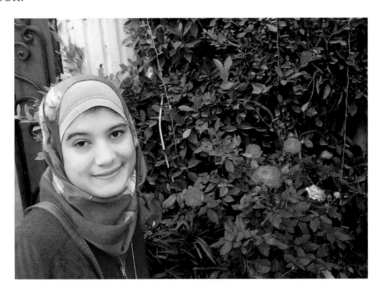

I am really sorry for the different forms of emotional abuse that you faced: sorry for suffering from the idiocies of the others, sorry for the bad things that you had started to believe that to be in you although they are not, sorry for paying less attention to you and blaming you, sorry for every time you believed you are cheesy, detested, opportunist, inconsiderate and a jerk. Sorry for every tear you had shed specially at night, sorry for every time you had to suffer in silence, sorry for every time you cried and the suffer is shown, sorry for every time you tried to hold on at any gathering and when you couldn't, tears appeared so you felt ashamed and to make things ok you forced yourself to smile and the same for the photos like this one.

Sorry for every time you suffered and cried when your favorite people are not around and being not able to tell them what you really wanted them to know and instead you are checking on them or changing the subject so that they won't be sad. Sorry for every time you wouldn't be able to sleep peacefully at night and sorry for every time you were upset that you almost forgot your goal.

But let me tell you this, I am really proud of you, yup, I really am: I am proud of you, of who you have become, I mean the fighter you have become. I am really proud of how you handled these previous situations, I am proud of every time you insisted and were persistent to find the exit and how you planned to find it, I am proud of every time you insisted to help others and soothe them with the same calmness of the natural views or may be less I am proud of how you show them the way calmly. Finally, thank you: for showing me that growing up could be easier than I thought and thank you for not only reminding me but also proving to me something my grandfather once told me " Suffering may cause hurt and pain but among of its benefits is helping others to grow and learn safely in this life by preventing its effect and the feeling of pain from reaching them."

TO THE SICK CHILD

Gladys Guerrero de Torres
Past President of the Committee of Pediatrics Ladies
Quito, Ecuador

I saw you on the bed of pain suffering
Angelic God Creature
And seeing your little body destroyed
I asked to save your soul from evil

The generosity of the human heart
Turn over today in your sorrows to relieve
That is why there is an illusion and there is hope
That tomorrow your orphan hood improves

You have taught me so many things, child ...
Your sad face helped me think
That the only ones who live are the ones who at all times
Knows how to suffer, love, fight and give

I would like to tell you so many things ...
I would like to transform the world
So that you grow up smiling and healthy
And may enjoy the tomorrow

I do not want to say goodbye because I cannot
Forget your heartaches and pain
I will continue working every day
For changing the sourness in love.

UNFORGETTABLE

David L. Coulter, MD
Associate Professor of Neurology at Harvard Medical School
Senior Associate at Boston Children's Hospital
Boston Children's Hospital
Boston, Massachusetts

I was young when I met Larry. Well, not that young: I was thirty-one. My medical training–thirteen years in all–was finally over, and I was working as an instructor in the child-neurology clinic at the University of Michigan, Ann Arbor, and caring for kids with epilepsy.

My patient Larry was seventeen. A stocky, dark-haired, non-athletic boy with borderline intellectual disability, he suffered from depression, and my notes mentioned his "pugnacious personality."

From age eight, Larry had had epileptic seizures. Typically, he would lose consciousness and fall down, sometimes with grand mal convulsions. Despite taking several medications, he had seizures at least once a week.

Larry was unhappy and unloved. "His father was extremely angry and verbally abusive," my notes read. "He had canceled the most recent clinic appointment as punishment because Larry had not done some things he was supposed to do." Another note described how his father "would throw Larry into a cold shower or force him to eat cigarettes because of misbehavior."

At school, Larry's classmates taunted him, saying, "So Larry, are you going to flip out on us now?" He had few, if any, real friends. In the eleventh grade, he dropped out. His father put him into foster care for a while, but he drifted back home. Later that year, though, he returned to school and reported getting along better with his father.

I was young enough to look past Larry's clinical labels–borderline intellectual disability and temporal-lobe epilepsy–and see a teenage boy who was hurting. We connected, although I didn't quite understand why. I was just starting out as a doctor, figuring out how to relate to patients; I tried to see the world through Larry's eyes.

In fact, I had just recently recovered from my own suicidal depression. I knew what it is to feel worthless and unloved, and I was trying to understand Larry's life the way I understood my own–to see him as I saw myself. At any rate, I am sure Larry knew that I liked him and cared about him.

One day, I was seeing patients in the clinic when the secretary told me that I had a phone call. It was Larry.

I could tell he was upset. His voice was shaky; he may have been crying. I asked him about his meds, which he recited correctly, and I checked his chart and saw that his medication levels were fine.

He was upset about school. "My teacher isn't treating me right. She doesn't give me any attention. She doesn't help me. No one helps me. No one likes me. I don't have any friends. My father hates me."

I had zero experience with talking to a teenage boy in distress, especially in the midst of a busy epilepsy clinic, but I did the best I could.

"Tell David to take as much time as he needs," my training director, Dr. Allen, told the secretary. "We'll talk later. Don't worry about the clinic."

Larry and I talked for over an hour. "I've been thinking about calling you for a week," he said. "My teacher and my counselor aren't helping me, and the other kids call me 'spaz' and make fun of me."

"How can I help?" I asked. "Do you want me to talk to your teacher and counselor and ask them to be more helpful?"

"No, that's okay," he said.

As we talked, he seemed to grow calmer. "I want to finish high school and then go to a vocational rehab program, get a job and move on with my life," he confided. By the hour's end, he sounded like the kid I'd known, with none of his earlier shakiness.

Again I said, "Larry, please let me know if there's anything I can do for you."

"No," he answered. "But thanks, doc, for talking to me."

As we said goodbye, I said, "I'm looking forward to seeing you again."

He didn't answer.

Later that day, the clinic secretary came to me again. "Dr. Coulter, I think you need to take this call."

Larry's mother was on the line, sobbing.

"When I came home from work, I went into the basement and found Larry hanging from the pipe....Larry is dead. I called the police. They checked the phone and said that you were the last person he ever talked to. That's why I called you."

She put the officer on the phone, and I told him what Larry and I had talked about and offered to help in any way I could. Afterwards, I told Dr. Allen.

"David, go home," he said. "I'll take care of the clinic. Talk to Joanna." (She was our social worker.) "Let's talk tomorrow."

At home, I wrote four pages of notes describing my conversation with Larry, in case the police would find it helpful

I felt stunned. None of my experience or training had prepared me for this. My patient–the boy I'd loved and cared for–was dead. What more could I have done to save his life?

Like all doctors, I blamed myself. But Joanna offered a different perspective.

"David, the reason Larry called you was to say goodbye," she told me. "He knew what he was going to do. Larry could have called a lot of other people, but he called you, because he knew you cared about him. I think he'd been planning it for a while, but he didn't want to die until he'd talked to you one last time. You did the best you could, and you obviously meant a lot to him. So be grateful for that."

I found Joanna's counsel very comforting. For the first time, I realized what a unique relationship Larry and I had had.

The day after Larry's death, I wrote to his parents.

"I am terribly shaken by what happened because I could not help him enough," I wrote. "Through his memory, though, I will do all I can to prevent such a tragedy from happening to other children with epilepsy."

Larry was buried in a small rural cemetery. The coroner certified the cause of death as an epileptic seizure so that he could receive a Christian burial. His family asked that contributions in his memory be made to our clinic.

Despite Joanna's comforting words, Larry's death was devastating for me. I felt personally responsible, and medically incompetent: I couldn't save him from the demons that tormented him, I couldn't control his seizures, and I felt that I'd failed him in our last phone call.

In the days that followed, Dr. Allen gave me space to grieve, and Joanna helped me to deal with my feelings of guilt. But I will always regret my inability to help Larry deal with his depression.

Looking back, I've wondered, How could I have missed seeing that he was suicidal? Why didn't I call a teenage-suicide hotline? But I know that nothing in my medical training had prepared me for this, and back in 1979 there were no such hotlines.

I'm no longer young. In the forty years since Larry died, I've had the great privilege of caring for more than 10,000 children with epilepsy and intellectual disability. We have better medications now, but the stigma of epilepsy remains, and thousands of these young patients still need our love and support.

Larry's memory has stayed with me throughout my career. I have never forgotten the teenage boy who first showed me how to care deeply for the patients who need our love the most.

FROM DARKNESS TO LIGHT

Dr. Kshitij Mankad MRCP, FRCR, PG Dip Hospital & Healthcare Mgmt., Lean 6 Sigma (Black Belt)
Clinical Lead for Paediatric Neuroradiology & Associate Professor
Great Ormond Street Hospital, University College London Hospital

I was already regretting putting myself forward to meet the parents of this fifteen-month-old boy in the Neurodisability clinic on Monday morning to show and tell the scan findings. There was this uneasy queasiness all through the weekend. 'I am a radiologist, what the hell will I do in clinic seeing these parents and breaking the diagnosis? Why did I volunteer to do this? ....And now, I don't even know what to wear, ...and yes I have to remember to shave!' It felt like a performance waiting to happen. A very restless weekend, indeed. I had not taken up Radiology as a specialty to go and have difficult conversations with parents, surely?

At the time I revealed the findings to the Neurodisability physician during one of the multi-disciplinary team meetings, I had felt all-powerful, like superman, even silently patting my back for my amazing diagnostic skills: the satisfaction of search, the precise genotype-phenotype correlation, and the sheer élan with which I had done it! The boy himself was a globally delayed child with the diagnostic tag of severe autism, the scans having been previously reported at two other centres as 'unremarkable' and 'non-specific'. Having detected the subtle perisylvian polymicrogyria, the thickened and horizontally disposed superior cerebellar peduncles, and the even more subtle superior cerebellar vermian dysfoliation, I exclaimed: "This is a ciliopathy, within the spectrum of Joubert's", even perhaps ridiculing the other two centres. Only to further subconsciously boost my own ego, I had gone ahead and added "I am very happy to come to your clinic and show these findings to the family". I had also gone on and suggested a few genes, because paediatric neuroradiologists these days memorise well a few of these alphabet soups and release them like bullets to impress – mostly these ideations are born out of aggressive Googling on the side. In this case, however, one of the bullets had hit its target and a PIBF1 mutation was confirmed.

The clinic had, therefore, been organised to discuss the 'new' findings with the parents. And there I was, uncomfortably overdressed in a suit trying to appear 'consultoid' while within I was broken into a thousand nervous fragments – completely out of my comfort zone and yearning for the solace of the dimly lit radiology reporting room.

"This is Dr Mankad, one of our Neuroradiologists, and he has kindly given up his time to come and help us understand the imaging findings that he showed at our meeting", said the Neurologist in a soft, calm tone.

I just cannot forget the look on the mother's face at that very moment in time – she was trying to squeeze a smile towards me, acknowledge my presence, and perhaps saying thank you, but all I saw were a million furrows of anxiety suddenly contour all over her face. A face that had aged rapidly, I thought, given the burdensome yolk of caring for a disabled child with an unknown diagnosis.

I could see that she was clenching her husband's hands tightly, the veins of her neck engorging as her face flushed, and her eyes began floating... The little boy, however, cherubic and struggling to hold his rather large head steady as he crawled on the play mat in the clinic, was in a different world – breaking out the broadest smile ever as he shrieked in delight when the clinic assistant handed him an inflated blue glove that probably reminded him of a peacock.

I sat there frozen, my sweaty toes digging into my shoes. The child looked up at me and made a calling gesture. Was this even real – the face behind the scan, the actual life behind a fixed screen. This real world was so alien to me. My emotions were getting the better of me. I sat there, pursing my lips desperate to burst into tears or burst out of the room.

I had to stop myself. I could not show it. This was the real endpoint of all that confident, boastful diagnosis and the satisfaction of search that I was trained for. But I just wasn't prepared for it.

"Hello, you can call me Kish, and I will take you through this scan on the screen here." I knew I was barely audible. "Please feel free to interrupt me and ask any questions that you may have... this is an MRI scan and what you see here are the different sequences we can acquire..." I was fumbling with words. I was used to describing everything so technically as T1 shortening, and T2 prolongation, and jumping to big words like leukodystrophy, dysgyria, dysfoliation and polymicrogyria – overtly confident that my audience would understand everything verbatim. This was, however, a different place, a different audience, and it was not my comfort zone – I was, in fact, miles from it!

"And here, as you can see, there is a difference in the way the brain is formed... let me show you what normal should look like... and this can explain why your boy has the odd eye movements and inability to coordinate activities... and because the cortex of the brain is folded as such here, it can explain the seizures..."

I was just beginning to speak the language they understood when the boy's father spoke: "Are you a doctor?" Words that fell on my ears like a hammer.

It's the perception that we have built in others of ourselves, I could not blame him for asking. We relegate ourselves to the dark spaces we have dwelled in for eons and it has become our impervious fortress.

"Sorry, I mean why did it take fifteen months for anyone to tell us these things were on my baby's scan?" he went on, as his wife dug her face into his sleeve and fought against her tears. "We were told the scan is normal, from both hospitals. Are you sure of these new findings? We didn't know what to expect."' His face was flushed. We were all looking at the baby as we spoke, hardly making any eye contact with each other. "Are you confident and sure?"

"I am a Radiologist", I said – softly. "We are doctors who report on scans and discuss them with the clinicians... I am really sorry these findings were not detected earlier on, but I hope that they help us understand why your child is not developing as expected. I can understand your frustration..." I was learning to empathise and take responsibility – not just compete with others around to prove my superiority in the dissociated, disconnected, sterile environment of the dimly lit reading room.

Moments passed in silence. It felt like an eternity. I sat there, probably looking at the screen, scrolling through the images- just to avoid further eye contact. Their anguish was palpable throughout the room.

Suddenly, the mother touched my wrist and said, "thank you so much, doctor... we were actually living in darkness, we knew something was wrong, but no one knew what... for the first time in all these fifteen harrowing months, I am actually relieved that we have an answer." There was a strange calmness on her face as she spoke. "All this time we were blaming ourselves and our parenting... fighting the system... waiting for a miracle, when what we really needed was closure, acceptance, and something to jolt us back towards life". And, with that, she picked up her baby boy and kissed him on his forehead, smiled at me through her streaming tears, and gave me some reassuring nods.

I left the clinic a few moments later, to return to my world. On the way, I stopped by the restroom, locked myself in, and sobbed uncontrollably.

I will never forget those echoing nods: "closure, acceptance, moving on".

Since that day, every time I open a scan to report I am reminded of her face and her baby's broad oblivious grin. I am reminded of her anxious facial furrows, her husband's anxiety, and of the strange calmness I had left them in.

It's not just scans anymore for me, but each scan a face speaking to me, asking for help, seeking answers, and hoping that I come out of my dimly lit reporting room and meet them in the real world to share with them their problems and help them understand that elusive diagnosis better.

DISCUSSION AND CONCLUSIONS

The goal of the Namaste Project was to realize a global vision of humanism in child neurology and neurodevelopmental disabilities and to share that vision with our colleagues in every country in the world. The results presented in this volume illustrate that vision with clarity and insights that exceeded our expectations. The authors who contributed to this effort deserve all of the credit for sharing their knowledge and experience with the world. Our intention as co-editors was to be as inclusive as possible and to respect the diversity of the authors. Each chapter is a gem that illuminates our global vision of humanism in child neurology.

These results provide an opportunity to discuss several conclusions. First, the authors demonstrate that humanism in child neurology is universal. It is not limited to one culture or tradition. Humanistic care of children and youth with neurological disorders and their families is a unifying element of the practice of child neurology worldwide. Humanistic care is the reason most of us became child neurologists in the first place and is the reason why we continue to practice our profession in spite of all of the other challenges we face. Those challenges are daunting in different ways in many different countries all over the world, but the authors who contributed to this volume demonstrate that a stubborn reliance on humanism still makes the clinical practice of child neurology meaningful and rewarding.

Second, the authors demonstrate that humanism in child neurology is particular. It is truly specific to each individual context. Similarly, the definition and meaning of humanism vary from one place to another. The chapters in this book offer a number of approaches to understand humanism, each of which is relevant in that particular context. Nonetheless they also share a common ground. To paraphrase US Supreme Court Justice Potter Stewart's famous line, "We may not be able to define humanism, but we can recognize it when we see it." The authors demonstrate that humanism in the practice of child neurology can be seen in every continent, country and culture across the globe. One of the objectives of the Namaste Project was to present and respect the particularity of every author through the inclusiveness and diversity of their contributions to this volume.

Third, this volume recognizes that humanism can be religious or not. Some definitions of humanism specifically exclude any religious meaning and insist that it must be a purely secular process. Those who advocate for secular humanism reject any role for religion or spirituality. But the authors of the chapters in Part Two of this volume clearly demonstrate that humanism can indeed spring forth from religious and spiritual traditions, teaching and experience. Indeed, the chapters illustrate how humanism is an integral part of all of the major religions. Humanism can be considered as a representation of the Golden (or Universal) Rule, which asks us to "Treat others as you would wish them to treat you." The Golden Rule can be found in some form in most of the world's religions as well as in many non-religious ethical guides. For that reason, there should be no conflict between secular and religious humanism.

Fourth, the authors demonstrate that humanism is practiced and sustained through personal relationships between caregivers, patients and families. The chapters in Part Three provide a systematic illustration of how humanism affects the clinical practice of child neurology. The chapters in Part Four provide personal stories describing the humanistic care of children with neurological disorders and their families in many different settings all over the world. Sharing these stories is a powerful way to help us to support one another and to work together to improve our ability to provide humanistic care. Accessing the free website of Pulse: Voices From the Heart of Medicine https://pulsevoices.org/ is another way to listen to other caregivers' stories and to share our own experiences.

We understand that in compiling this volume as co-editors, we have almost certainly left out some important voices. We hope that those voices will be heard in subsequent publications on humanism in child neurology. We have much to learn from one another and hope that this volume will be useful in advancing that conversation.

Now is the time to practice humanism in child neurology, to study and to learn global perspectives on humanism in child neurology as we have presented it here, to teach humanism to our child neurology students, residents, fellows, and colleagues, and to promote humanism globally to a world that may not always be receptive. In the end, our most fervent wish as co-editors is that this volume will help all of us to create a more humanistic world for children with neurological disorders and their families who are living in every country all over the world.

David L. Coulter, MD
Associate Professor of Neurology at Harvard Medical School
Senior Associate at Boston Children's Hospital
Boston Children's Hospital
Boston, Massachusetts

Alcy R. Torres, MD, FAAP
Associate Professor of Pediatrics and Neurology
Assistant Dean of Diversity and Inclusion
Director of the Pediatric Traumatic Injury, International and
Bilingual Programs
Boston University School of Medicine
Boston Medical Center
Boston, MA, USA